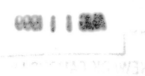

Hippocrates

MEDICINE & CULTURE

Sander L. Gilman
SERIES EDITOR

Robert Michaels, M.D., Linda Hutcheon, Ph.D., and
Michael Hutcheon, M.D.
EDITORIAL BOARD

Georges Minois, *History of Suicide: Voluntary Death in Western Culture,*
translated by Lydia G. Cochrane

Jacques Jouanna, *Hippocrates,* translated by M. B. DeBevoise

Laura Otis, *Membranes: Metaphors of Invasion in Nineteenth-Century
Literature, Science, and Politics*

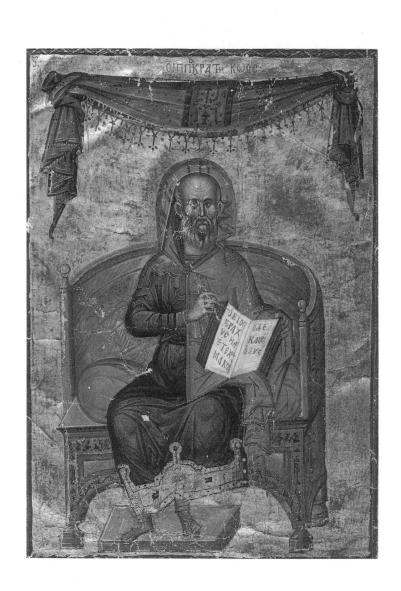

Hippocrates

JACQUES JOUANNA

TRANSLATED BY
M. B. DeBevoise

The Johns Hopkins University Press
BALTIMORE AND LONDON

The translation was prepared with the generous assistance of the
Association des Études Grecques and the French Ministry of Culture.

Originally published as *Hippocrate*, © Librairie Arthème Fayard, 1992
© 1999 The Johns Hopkins University Press
All rights reserved. Published 1999
Printed in the United States of America on acid-free paper
2 4 6 8 9 7 5 3 1

The Johns Hopkins University Press
2715 North Charles Street
Baltimore, Maryland 21218-4363
The Johns Hopkins Press Ltd., London
www.press.jhu.edu

Frontispiece: Portrait of Hippocrates of Cos. Bibliothèque
Nationale, Paris. Greek manuscript Z144, folio 10v (14th c.).
Photo B.N.

Library of Congress Cataloging-in-Publication Data

Jouanna, Jacques.
    [Hippocrate. English]
    Hippocrates / Jacques Jouanna ; translated by M. B. DeBevoise.
        p.   cm — (Medicine and culture)
    Includes selections from Hippocrates' works.
    Includes bibliographical references and index.
    ISBN 0-8018-5907-7 (alk. paper)
        1. Hippocrates. 2. Medicine, Ancient. 3. Physicians—Biography.
    I. Hippocrates. Selections. English and Greek. 1998. II. Title. III. Series.
    R126.H8J6813 1999
    610'.92—dc21
    [B]
                                                                        98–6999
                                                                        CIP

CONTENTS

viii   *Contents*

Citation to the treatises of the Hippocratic Collection is made on the whole with reference to the chapter and section numbering found in Littré's Greek-French edition. Because the numbering of these texts occasionally differs in the Greek-English edition prepared over the last eight decades as part of the Loeb Classical Library series by W. H. S. Jones and others, I have indicated this numbering in those cases—and only those cases—where a passage from the Loeb edition is reproduced in the present work; in all other cases, the reader may assume that it is the Littré edition to which reference is made in the notes, as in the relevant entries of the index of passages cited.

For ancient authors other than Hippocrates, I have tended to rely on Loeb translations for the sake of convenience and, illusorily perhaps, consistency. In the case of certain writers, however, for instance Aristophanes, I have translated directly from the Greek, following the author's interpretation of the text in preference to alternative renderings in English. In the case of Plato, I have cited to the new Hackett edition of the complete works. For Homer, Hesiod, and Pindar, as for historians and dramatists of the classical period, I have drawn upon a variety of other sources.

On the vexed question of transliteration and whether to anglicize titles of treatises in Greek and Latin, I join with my predecessors—in view of the highly variable practice that has arisen from the fact that no rule is universally obeyed—and cheerfully admit to embracing inconsistency, almost as a policy. In the main I have romanized Greek personal and place-names in the conventional manner, with various exceptions sanctioned to one degree or another by tradition: among Hippocrates' relatives, for example, Epione, Nebros, and Chrysos (though Phaenerete is used); also assorted Persians and, of course, Greek persons and places customarily referred to by their given names. With regard to titles, I have tried to give English versions in the case of major authors, while deferring from time to time to the authority of the *Oxford Classical Dictionary*, which not infrequently shows a preference for Latin versions. Thus Aristotle is cited for the most part in Latin, which I trust will not inconvenience many readers; Galen, on the other hand, whose works, like those of other medical authors of the period, are almost invariably referred to by scholars by their Latin names, I have occasionally Englished. With respect to the titles of the Hippocratic treatises themselves, I have mostly followed the practice of Jones and his successors, while taking certain small liberties here and there. And with regard to the transliteration of Greek terms in the text, I have followed the author in using a grave accent to indicate the letter eta (as opposed to epsilon) rather than the macron that is customarily placed over this vowel by authors writing in English.

Finally, a good amount of bibliographical material has been added to the English edition, reflecting recent literature in the field that has appeared since the book's first publication in 1992, together with an *index locorum* to enable the reader conveniently to locate passages cited in the work. This index has the incidental virtue of serving to cross-reference discrepant citations to the Hippocratic Collection in the Littré and Loeb editions. Because the Loeb translations of Hippocrates are in many instances flawed, or have otherwise been superseded by later scholarship, minor corrections have been made as necessary and indicated in the corresponding notes. Regrettably, it has not been possible to quote from the new English translation of the collection now being prepared by Professor Heinrich von Staden of Yale University.

I am indebted to Larry Kim, a doctoral candidate in classics at Princeton University, for research assistance and guidance on questions of technical detail; and, most especially, to Jacques Jouanna himself for his careful review of the final draft as well as his patient cooperation in answering a range of queries on matters of substance and interpretation. Whatever errors remain are my responsibility alone.

"Hippocrates," Sganarelle declares to Géronte in Molière's *The Physician in Spite of Himself*, "says that we should both keep our hats on."

"Pray tell," asks Géronte with surprise, "in what chapter?"

"In his chapter on hats," replies Sganarelle learnedly.

Hippocrates obviously never wrote a chapter on hats. But Molière's joke, which probably stems from the peculiar discussion recorded by biographers about the reasons Hippocrates was pictured with his head covered (see page 39), is symbolic of the mythic aura that still surrounded Hippocrates and his work in the seventeenth century, and even later.

Hippocrates, a Greek physician of the fifth century before Jesus Christ, has long been considered the Father of Medicine. Over time he came to be credited with a semilegendary life and an enormous body of work, the contours of which are poorly defined yet whose authority, to judge from Molière, was comparable only to that of the gospel: no one challenged the word of Hippocrates any more than the word of God. "Since Hippocrates says so, it must be done," concedes Géronte, bowing, and putting his hat back upon his head.

Various biographies, more or less late, including a purely fictive cycle of Byzantine accounts of the life of Hippocrates, had the effect of blurring the image of the physician, making him into an ideal and mythic figure not altogether unlike Homer. Just as one finds the stone said to mark the place where Homer taught on the island of Chios, at Dascalopetra, so on Cos one looks with wonder upon the "tree of Hippocrates." And just as the Homeric poems were long taken to mark the absolute beginning of poetry, so, too, the Hippocratic writings were long regarded as the cornerstone of medicine. The study of these texts, known directly or indirectly through commentaries, guided medical theory and practice through the middle of the nineteenth century—to say nothing of the famous Hippocratic oath, which still today is taken by students in many schools of medicine throughout the Western world upon completion of their studies.

One might suppose that an excess of credulous respect should have been succeeded by deep skepticism, attaching as much to the person of Hippocrates as to the extensive body of work that antiquity has bequeathed to us under his name. One might further suppose that from the moment when scientific advances in the nineteenth century led medicine to follow paths different than those indicated by the physician of Cos, Hippocrates, having once been praised to the skies, should have survived only as a half-forgotten figure, a mere footnote of medical history. But not at all! Owing to the volume of this work, and the various readings of it that have been proposed over the course of twenty-five centuries, Hippocrates emerges once more as a vital figure in the history of science, having profited from the renewed interest in this discipline in our own century. Thanks to the combined efforts of philologists, historians, philosophers, and other specialists in antiquity, he is now at last coming to find his true place in the history of classical Greece. The life and works of Hippocrates provide invaluable evidence about the life, literature, and thought of the Age of Pericles. This evidence is, in certain respects, no less fascinating than that supplied by Thucydides, Euripides, and Plato— Hippocrates' most eminent contemporaries in the fields of history, drama, and philosophy—all three of whom drew upon his work, each transposing and adapting what he borrowed to suit his own purposes.

The some sixty treatises that have come down to us under the name of Hippocrates surely could not all have been written by the great physician himself, nor even by his disciples of the school of Cos; some of these treatises plainly come from other sources, or are to be dated to later periods. But the main part of this work is prior to that of Aristotle, and it forms, despite certain undeniable discrepancies, an ancient and globally coherent core that can be seen as constituting a distinctly Hippocratic style of thought. Even if we must renounce the impossible dream of definitively identifying the authors of so rich and varied a body of work, we may therefore legitimately refer to them as *Hippocratic physicians*, in the broad sense of the term. What is more, even if some measure of doubt inevitably remains, the personality of Hippocrates himself no longer remains blurred as it once was. As philological analysis and epigraphical investigations continue to provide fresh insight into the life and works of Hippocrates, the Father of Medicine now gradually begins to free himself from the limbo of hagiography and to reenter the living world of human history.

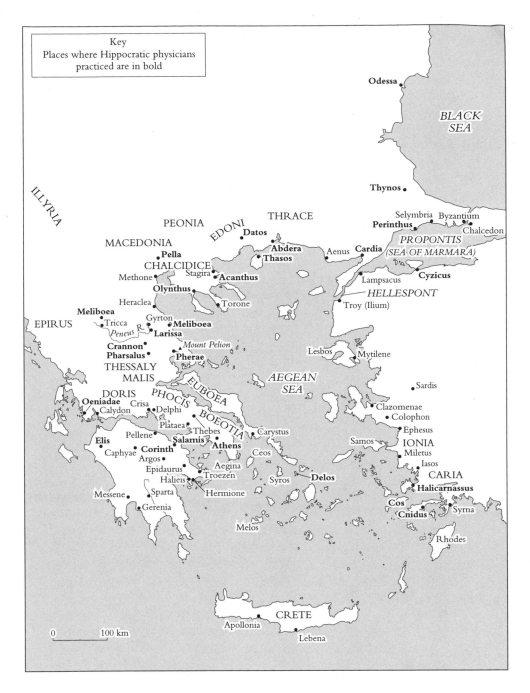

ILLYRIA

BLACK
SEA

Odessa

Thynos

THRACE

PEONIA

EDONI

Selymbria   Byzantium

Perinthus

Chalcedon

MACEDONIA

Datos

PROPONTIS
(SEA OF MARMARA)

Pella

Abdera

Aenus   Cardia

CHALCIDICE

Thasos

Cyzicus

Methone   Stagira   Acanthus

Lampsacus

HELLESPONT

Olynthus

Heraclea   Torone

Troy (Ilium)

Meliboea

Gyrton   Meliboea

Lesbos   Mytilene

Tricca

Peneus R.   Larissa

EPIRUS

Crannon   Mount Pelion

AEGEAN
SEA

Pharsalus   Pherae

THESSALY

Sardis

MALIS

DORIS   PHOCIS   EUBOEA

Clazomenae

Oeniadae   Crisa

Colophon

Calydon   Delphi   BOEOTIA

Carystus

Ephesus

Pellene   Plataea   Thebes

Samos   IONIA

Elis   Salamis   Athens

Miletus

Caphyae   Corinth   Ceos

Iasos

Argos   Aegina

CARIA

Epidaurus   Troezen   Syros   Delos

Halieis

Halicarnassus

Messene   Hermione

Sparta

Cos

Gerenia

Cnidus   Syrna

Melos

Rhodes

0   100 km

CRETE

Apollonia

Lebena

Greece in the Time of Hippocrates

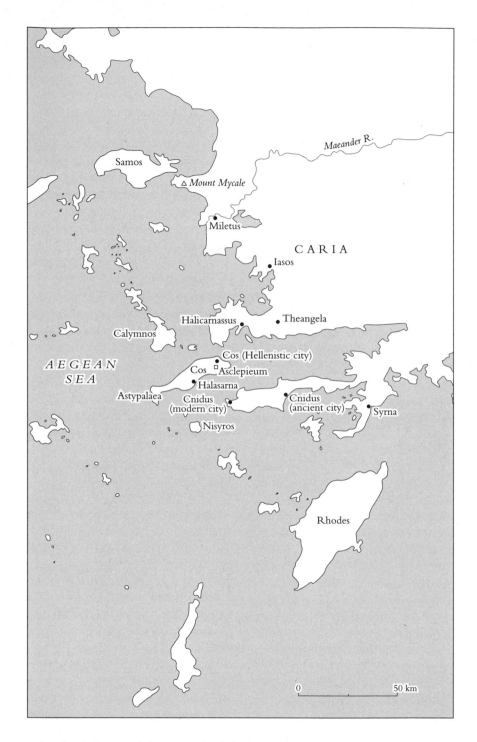

The Island of Cos and the Peninsula of Cnidus

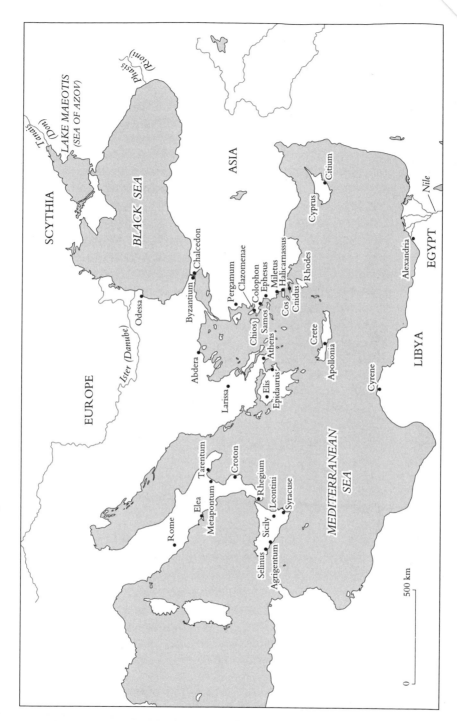

The Mediterranean and Black Seas: Centers of Medicine and Learning

PART I

Hippocrates the Asclepiad

ONE

Hippocrates of Cos

"Hippocrates of Cos, the Asclepiad." Thus the celebrated physician was designated during his lifetime to distinguish him from others called Hippocrates, for this was a common name. The epithet contains two fundamental pieces of information, one of which—having to do with his native land—is well known, while the other one—having to do with his family, which took its name from Asclepius—is little known. In fact he passed only a part of his life on Cos, the island of his birth, moving later to continental Greece, more specifically to Thessaly, the mythic cradle of the family of the Asclepiads, where he died. But it is with Cos, his birthplace, where his family had been settled for many generations, that his name is permanently linked.

The Trail of Hippocrates on the Island of Cos

The tourist who goes to the island of Cos to follow in the footsteps of Hippocrates will return home with deceiving memories. On disembarking and proceeding to the handsome Plateia Platanou, not far from the imposing castle of the knights of Rhodes, one sees the enormous platan, or planar tree, in the shadow of which Hippocrates is conventionally said to have gathered with his disciples. Even granting that this venerable tree might be as much as five centuries old, as the *Blue Guide* to Greece suggests, it is still far younger than Hippocrates—younger by about twenty centuries. This considerable gap does not prevent the myth from surviving, however, even among physicians, who have planted offshoots with more or less success in the lands of the New World at places where congresses of history of medicine have been held, and placed commemorative plaques next to them, notably in Venezuela.

Moving on next to the museum at Cos, the tourist will see a statue of Hippocrates standing prominently in a rotunda to the left of the entrance.

Confirmation can be found in the *Blue Guide*, though somewhat less confidently: "Statue from the end of the Hellenistic period, but modeled on a classical original, which might represent Hippocrates." In fact, the attribution is certainly false, for the long-haired head of the statue does not match that of the physician, who according to biographical testimony was bald and who was so pictured on coins of Cos from the Roman period, where the identity of the head is authenticated by the two Greek letters ΙΠ, the standard abbreviation for Hippocrates.[1] The tourist then proceeds to within several kilometers of the present-day city, to the imposing sanctuary of Asclepius, from which a vast panorama opens upon the plain below, stretching as far as the sea. Looking down to one of the middle terraces, one sees the remains of pools and fountains that were used for the treatment of the sick who came from all over Greece in search of a cure for their ills, and naturally imagines Hippocrates caring for these patients—all the more easily as the artfully designed tickets sold at the entrance to the shrine bear the image of the false statue of Hippocrates seen earlier in the museum. But until now excavations have revealed nothing at this site prior to the fourth century before Christ. It is therefore not certain that Hippocrates knew this Asclepieum, and there is no evidence that he was a priest of Asclepius.

Still, returning to the current town of Cos and strolling along the street named after Hippocrates, where merchants hawk busts of the Father of Medicine, one supposes that one is at least walking on the same ground where Hippocrates walked. But, again, not at all! The present-day town of Cos, located at the eastern end of the island, was not built on the site of the classical city. The vast groups of ruins in the very heart of the modern town, along with the many blocks of ancient marble used again later to build the walls of the castle of the knights of Rhodes, come from the Hellenistic and Roman city founded in 366/365 B.C. It was at this time, as the result of a dispute, that the inhabitants of Cos relocated their home. The ancient city that they left was called Astypalaea (Old Town) and was situated in another part of the island, equally close to the sea.[2] This was the city that Hippocrates knew. Archaeologists are agreed in locating it at the other end of the island, in the southwest part called Palatia, not far from the present-day town of Kephalos, surrounding an acropolis that overlooks the harbor of Kamari. This magnificent and well-protected harbor is the site today of—Club Méditerranée! From the top of the acropolis above, one can still see vestiges of ramparts and blocks of marble from an ancient temple that were reused in the chapel, now abandoned, of Panaghia Palatiane, and, not far from there, the modest remains of temples and of a theater of the fourth century B.C. While it is true that we do not have an inscription proving it was here that the family of Hippocrates lived and that the ancient Hippocratic school met, systematic excavations have not yet been conducted at this site.

By an irony of fate, it is not the tourist desiring to retrace the steps of Hippocrates who sees the scenes of the physician's childhood on the island, but the tourist who has come in search of surf and sun at Club Med. The one will go away thinking he has seen them; the other will leave having seen them, but without knowing it. The only souvenir that the historically minded tourist will bring back home is a photograph of the mosaic in the museum representing the elderly Hippocrates, together with an anonymous inhabitant of Cos, welcoming the young god Asclepius as he disembarks on the island.[3] But this mosaic, from the Roman era (second or third century A.D.), tells us nothing about the historical Hippocrates. Literary accounts alone permit a corner of the veil to be raised, and the real Hippocrates to be revealed.

Hippocrates as Judged by His Contemporaries

Unlike Homer, who remains for us a figure of legend, Hippocrates is a historical figure about whom we possess an ancient literary record of inestimable value due to a younger contemporary—Plato.

In Plato's youthful dialogue *Protagoras*, named for the celebrated Sophist who had come to teach in Athens, one of the characters is a young Athenian, himself called Hippocrates, who is wild with excitement at the Sophist's presence in the city. Socrates questions this Hippocrates, using his maieutic method, trying to get him to say exactly what he expects to gain from instruction by Protagoras. For this purpose, Socrates asks him to reflect upon other, clearer examples:

"I mean, suppose you had your mind set on going to your namesake, Hippocrates of Cos, the famous physician, to pay him a fee for his services to you, and if someone asked you what this Hippocrates is that you were going to pay him, what would you say?"

"I would say a physician," he said.

"And what would you expect to become?"

"A physician."

"And if you had a mind to go to Polyclitus of Argos or Phideas of Athens to pay them a fee, and if somebody were to ask you what kind of professionals you had in mind paying, what would you say?"

"I would say sculptors."

"And what would you expect to become?"

"A sculptor, obviously."[4]

This early dialogue, written by Plato at the beginning of the fourth century B.C., is supposed to have taken place much earlier, sometime around 430. The reference to the physician Hippocrates therefore attests that by the end of the fifth century he was known for his teaching and that he was already regarded by his contemporaries as the paradigmatic representative of the art of medicine, in the same way that Polyclitus of Argos and Phidias of Athens were taken to represent the art of sculpture. Hippocrates was therefore the most celebrated physician of the Periclean Age.

Plato alludes to Hippocrates again in one of his mature dialogues, the *Phaedrus*. There Socrates is seeking to define the true art of rhetoric. This art, he holds, presumes a knowledge not only of public speaking but also of the psychology of the public needing to be persuaded. Socrates then questions Phaedrus about the method to be followed in order to understand this psychology, or "science of the soul":

> *Socrates*: Do you think it possible, then, satisfactorily to comprehend the nature of soul apart from the nature of the universe?
>
> *Phaedrus*: Nay, if we are to believe Hippocrates, of the Asclepiad family, we cannot learn even about the body unless we follow this method of procedure.
>
> *Socrates*: Yes, my friend, and he is right. Yet besides the doctrine of Hippocrates, we must examine our argument and see if it harmonizes with it.
>
> *Phaedrus*: Yes.
>
> *Socrates*: Observe, then, what it is that both Hippocrates and correct argument mean by an examination of nature.[5]

This passage confirms the previous one while making it more precise.[6] The physician of Cos was known in Athens not only by reputation; his teaching was also known in detail, though he had never lived nor taught there. This account therefore reveals the importance of Hippocratic thought and, at the same time, the influence of medical thinking in the intellectual history of Greece during the classical period. Here was a philosopher making reference to the thought of a physician; and medicine, the science of the body, serving as a model for philosophy, the science of the soul.

It is therefore not surprising that another philosopher, Aristotle, should have alluded some forty years later to Hippocrates. Aristotle had all the more reason to be familiar with Hippocrates and his work since he was himself the son of a doctor, and recommended that philosophers learn medicine. In the *Politics*, he cites Hippocrates, in passing, as an example of a man who was great by reason of his science rather than of his size: "One would pronounce

Hippocrates to be greater, not as a human being but as a physician, than someone who surpassed him in bodily size."[7] In this brief passage, the name of Hippocrates is no longer accompanied by the details about his place of origin and family that were still necessary to identify him during Plato's time. This is proof of an unchallenged celebrity.

For the average Athenian of the fifth century, by contrast, the name Hippocrates was not yet enough by itself to uniquely pick out the physician of Cos. The plays of Aristophanes testify to this. It was believed for a time that the Athenian comic playwright was referring to the Hippocratic oath in this passage from the *Thesmophoriazusae*:

> *Euripides*: I swear by Ether, the dwelling place of Zeus.
> *Mnesilochus*: No, that won't do. Might as well swear by the [household of Hippocrates].
> *Euripides*: Then I'll swear it by the gods, the whole lot of them.[8]

In the nineteenth century it was believed that the "household of Hippocrates" referred to the "brotherhood" of the physician of Cos and that Aristophanes was thus alluding, in advance of Plato, to his work and, in particular, to the Hippocratic oath. In fact, the reference is both more prosaic and more specific. It involves the sons of an Athenian general named Hippocrates, a nephew of Pericles, known throughout the city for their foolishness and objects of ridicule in Aristophanes' earlier play *Clouds*.

Almost a century divides the *Thesmophoriazusae* of Aristophanes and the *Politics* of Aristotle.[9] Hippocrates' renown, apparent already during his lifetime, had grown after his death to the point that it eclipsed that of all others named Hippocrates, not only the various political figures of antiquity known by that name, but even that other distinguished man of learning of his own time who shared it, Hippocrates of Chios, the mathematician.

The ancient accounts due to Plato and Aristotle attest therefore to the historical existence of Hippocrates the physician, his ties to place and to family, the fame of his teaching during his lifetime, and the magnitude of his reputation in the years after his death.

Other Accounts of the Life of Hippocrates

Other accounts are less sparing with details about the life of Hippocrates. But they appeared later, and are of uneven value.

In the works collected under his name, several passages provide biographical information. For the most part, especially in the case of the *Letters* addressed to or from Hippocrates, they are to be used with the greatest caution. This epistolary literature dates from the Roman era, between the first century B.C. and the first century A.D. For this very reason, the events of the life of Hippocrates to which it alludes and the opinions that it attributes to him are highly suspect. For example, in one of the letters concerning the hypothetical acquaintance of Hippocrates and the philosopher Democritus of Abdera, who was suspected of madness by his countrymen, the physician of Cos, summoned by the Abderites to treat the philosopher, recounts to his friend Philopoemen the premonitory dream that had been sent by Asclepius to him prior to his departure, and concludes: "I do not deny dreams, especially when they retain coherence. Medicine and prophesy are very closely related, since of the two arts Apollo is the single father. He, who is my ancestor, declares the diseases that are and that will be and he heals those on whom disease is coming and has come."[10] This profession of faith in the close connection between medicine and soothsaying does not accord with the spirit of the ancient Hippocratic treatises, where medical prognosis, based solely on the resources of observation and reason, is silent on the subject of Apollinian divination.

Even so, it is not necessary to reject this epistolary literature altogether. Certain passages may rely upon an ancient tradition, accounts of which have been lost. An example can be found in the same collection of letters concerning the relations between Hippocrates and Democritus. The Abderites have just officially called upon the physician to come treat the philosopher. Hippocrates' reply begins thus:

Hippocrates to the Senate and People of Abdera. Greetings.
Your fellow citizen Amelesagoras came to Cos. It chanced to be the day of the Assumption of the Staff, which you know is an annual festival and elaborate procession to the cypress grove customarily led by people related to the god.[11]

The details given about the religious festival at the shrine of Asclepius on Cos in this passage are so specific that they did not fail to catch the attention of historians. Each year, the staff of the votive statue was replaced. An elaborate procession made its way up to the sacred cypress grove, led by the relatives of the god—that is, by the very family of the Asclepiads to which Hippocrates belonged. It is of course true nothing is known that proves this ritual existed during Hippocrates' time. But neither does anything tell against it.

Ever since Émile Littré's positivist and indiscriminate rejection of the documentary aspects of the legend, an undue skepticism has surrounded everything in the work attributed to Hippocrates that supplies information about his life or about the history of his family. While the *Letters* manifestly contain elements that are recent and romanticized, other works belonging to the corpus are more reliable. This is the case above all with the *Presbeutikos*, or the *Speech of the Envoy*.[12] This speech is supposed to have been delivered by Hippocrates' son Thessalus before the Athenian assembly on the occasion of a dispute between the island of Cos and Athens at the end of the fifth century. It contains a good many specific details, some of which have been confirmed fairly recently by new epigraphic discoveries.

Aside from the Hippocratic writings themselves, the best-known biographical account is the *Life of Hippocrates* attributed to Soranus. This short biography stands as the canonical source, for it figures at the head of the manuscripts and earliest editions of Hippocrates' works. Traditionally attributed to Soranus of Ephesus, a physician of the first and second centuries A.D., this account draws upon more ancient sources, the most outstanding of which is the director of the library of Alexandria during the Hellenistic era, Eratosthenes of Cyrene.

A second biography of Hippocrates is conventionally called the *Vie de Bruxelles* since it is preserved in a manuscript held by the Belgian royal library in Brussels. This document is far less well known than the Soranus, having been rediscovered only at the beginning of the century.[13] Though anonymous and incomplete, and written in a barbarous Latin, it is not without interest to the extent that it provides certain new details not found in Soranos.

Otherwise, additional information about Hippocrates can be found in the encyclopedic articles of the Byzantine era, notably the article "Cos" by Stephanus of Byzantium and "Hippocrates," from the *Suda* (tenth century). Finally, there is the verse account of Hippocrates by Johannes Tzetzes, a scholar of the Comnenus period, in his *Chiliades* (twelfth century).

To all of this must be added the many allusions to Hippocrates with which the physician Galen, a great admirer and commentator on Hippocrates, sprinkled the immense body of work that he composed during the second century of the present era. One of his treatises in particular, *Quod optimus medicus sit quoque philosophus* (The best physician is also a philosopher), includes a substantial number of allusions to Hippocrates' life.

Critical examination of these various sources yields information about the family background and life of Hippocrates that is either certain or probable. What matters above all here, in any case, is retracing the way in which the ancients themselves saw and experienced their past. The boundary between legend and history was not the same for them as it is for us.

Hippocrates' Birth and Background:
The Family of the Asclepiads

Hippocrates was born on Cos, an island of Doric dialect, in the first year of the Eighty-Fourth Olympiad, which is to say in 460 B.C. The exact day of his birth is in fact known thanks to a local scholar, a certain Soranus of Cos, who consulted the archives of the island. Hippocrates was born on the twenty-seventh day of the Dorian month of Agrianos—the eighth month of the local calendar—under the "monarchy" of Abriadas.[14]

Hippocrates belonged to the Coan branch of the Asclepiad family "by male descent," to use the formula that was customary both in the Hippocratic corpus and in the epigraphy of Cos itself.[15]

It is necessary at this point to clarify what is meant by *Asclepiad.* This term was often used in a broad sense to denote physicians in general, to the extent that their art falls under the patronage of Asclepius, the god of medicine in the classical period. It was thus that in Plato's *Symposium* the Athenian physician Eryximachus, representing his fellow doctors, speaks of "our ancestor Asclepius [who] first established medicine as a profession."[16] The term originally possessed a more restricted and precise sense. It designated the two sons of Asclepius, Podalirius and Machaon, as well as their descendants; that is, a noble family that claimed to descend directly from Asclepius. This fundamental distinction, sometimes neglected by modern historians and philologists but better known to epigraphists,[17] is clearly made by the Byzantine Johannes Tzetzes: "Those whose line descends from this origin [that is, from Asclepius] are called Asclepiads in the proper sense of the term, whether they are physicians or whether they practice another activity, as Hippocrates and many others. But all physicians are called, by an improper extension [of the term], Asclepiads from the fact of such an art."[18]

Like all great aristocratic families, the Asclepiads (in the narrow sense of the term) carefully preserved the tradition of their illustrious genealogy, transmitted orally from generation to generation. According to this tradition, the family of Hippocrates belonged to the Asclepiads descended from Podalirius. The founding ancestor of the family as a whole, Asclepius, was not yet a god in Homer's time, but an earthly prince, from Tricca in Thessaly. He was renowned for his medical knowledge, which he had learned from the centaur Chiron. He sent his two sons Podalirius and Machaon, also physicians, to fight in the Trojan War. Already, then, medical knowledge was handed down within families.[19] Worthy sons of their father, during the course of their expedition they rendered important service as warriors, but above all as doctors in the camp of the Achaeans:

As for Machaon and Podaleirios, who are healers, I think Machaon has got a wound, and is in the shelters lying there, and himself is in need of a blameless healer, while the other in the plain is standing the bitter attack of the Trojans.[20]

It was with reference to one of them, Machaon, that Homer put in the mouth of one of his heroes this formula, which was to become proverbial: "A healer is a man worth many men in his knowledge."[21]

The fate of these two sons of Asclepius, the first two Asclepiads, was well known to the Greeks through the epic literature called the cyclic poems (or the Epic Cycle), which completed the *Iliad* and the *Odyssey.*

Machaon belonged to the elite band of warriors hidden in the famous horse that by trickery was smuggled into Troy. He died during the taking of the city from wounds sustained in combat with the son of Telephus,[22] and his remains were brought back by Nestor to Gerenia in Messenia. There is found his grave, along with a shrine to which men came to seek treatment for their illnesses.[23]

Podalirius, the more fortunate of the two for having survived the war, nonetheless encountered a host of difficulties in trying to make his way home, like so many other Achaean heroes. Unlike Ulysses, however, whose navigation of the seas landed him on shores where lived the likes of Calypso and Circe, Podalirius ended up on the coast of Asia Minor, at the city of Syrna, in Caria, where he decided to settle. A detailed version of his arrival there has come down to us from Stephanus of Byzantium:

Podalirius, having strayed from his route [during his return from the Trojan War], was saved by a goatherd and led by him to Damaethus, the king of Caria, whose daughter Syrna, who had fallen from the roof, was treated by him. As Damaethus was completely desperate, Podalirius, it is said, saved his daughter by bleeding her in each arm; and the king, full of admiration, gave him his daughter in marriage and granted him the Chersonesus [of Caria]. There Podalirius founded two cities, one [called] Syrna, from the name of his wife, the other from the name of the goatherd who had saved him.[24]

The physician who saves is saved by his own art. Though this version is no doubt romanticized, it is not necessarily as recent as its source.[25]

It was from Syrna, the cradle of the family of Asclepiads in Asia, that the descendants of Podalirius departed, splitting into two great branches. The one established itself on the small island of Cos, just off the Asian coast: this is the branch of the family to which Hippocrates belonged. The second did not leave the Asian continent, settling instead at Cnidus, on a peninsula directly across from Cos. This fact is attested by a quite ancient source, the historian Theopompus of Chios, who was born at about the time that Hippocrates died.[26]

Given that medical science was handed down from father to son, it is not surprising that this dual resettlement resulted in the creation of two famous medical centers, though it is true that Hippocrates' importance was to cause the reputation of Cos to eclipse that of Cnidus. There was even an incipient third branch, which settled on the isle of Rhodes, not far from Cos and Cnidus, but it rapidly disappeared. Galen mentions the history of this branch in a celebrated passage: "[F]or there were still two schools of Asclepiads in Asia, even when the school of Rhodes had fallen into decline."[27]

Galen's contemporary Aelius Aristides refers to a tradition of Cos in analogous terms, saying that the sons of Asclepius and their descendants settled on Cos, Rhodes, and on the Carian coast at Cnidus. The only great descendant whose name he mentions on this occasion is Hippocrates, the supreme heir of the art.[28]

According to certain biographies, Hippocrates was said to be the nineteenth male descended from Asclepius; according to others, to be the seventeenth or the eighteenth.[29] Several of these even propose genealogical trees, which in the main agree while differing with respect to details. The most complete is that of Johannes Tzetzes:

The great Hippocrates is the seventeenth descendant from Asclepius. After the Trojan War, on the mainland across from Rhodes, Podalirius, the son of Asclepius, had for a first son Hippolochus of whom Sostratus was born. This latter had for a first son Dardanus. Of Dardanus was born Crisamis, who had for a son Cleomyttades. He had a son Theodorus. Of this son was born another Sostratus. Of this Sostratus was born Crisamis the second. Of this Crisamis was born in his turn a second Theodorus and of this Theodorus a third Sostratus, who had for a son Nebros. Of this latter was born Gnosidicus, who had for a son Hippocrates. Of this first Hippocrates, son of Gnosidicus, the son was Heraclides. Of him and Phaenerete was born the great Hippocrates, who is the second.[30]

But even if the historical details of such a descent are open to question, it is clear from this account that Hippocrates was not the first to have distinguished the family of the Asclepiads.

Hippocrates' Illustrious Ancestors

When Hippocrates was born on Cos, the family was already doubly celebrated by reason both of its medical knowledge and of the services that several of its members had rendered either to Greece or to their homeland. Two members in particular had added to the luster of the family's reputation since its arrival on Cos, one in the sixth century, the other in the fifth.

The more famous of the two is the sixth-century ancestor, Nebros, who probably played a role in the First Sacred War. It is known that Greece experienced several "sacred wars," so called because they were fought over control of the shrine to Apollo at Delphi. The first took place at the beginning of the sixth century b.c. and grew out of an expedition led by the league of tribes charged with responsibility for protecting the shrine, the Amphictionies, against the neighboring city of Crisa in order to punish its citizens for their sacrilege.[31] According to the *Speech of the Envoy*, a pestilential disease broke out in the confederate camp during their siege of Crisa. Here is how Thessalus, the son of Hippocrates, describes what happened next:

But finally, rankling at their suffering and disagreeing among themselves, they turned to the god and asked what they ought to do. He bade them fight, and promised that they would win if they went to Cos and brought back for assistance a deer's child with gold, hurrying so the Criseans did not loot the tripod in the inner sanctum beforehand. If they did not do it, the city would not be captured. When they heard that, they went to Cos and made an announcement of what the oracle had said. The Coans were at a loss and did not understand the oracle, but a man stood up, an Asclepiad by family and an ancestor of mine, by common agreement the best physician of the Greeks of that time, whose name was Fawn (Nebros). He said that he believed that the oracle was directed to him. "If in fact the god so advised you to come to Cos and fetch a deer's child for assistance, this is Cos, the offspring of deer are called fawns, and Fawn is my name. What better assistance to a sick army could there be than a physician? And as for what was joined with that, indeed, I do not believe that the god directed those who excel the Greeks so much in wealth to come to Cos to ask for gold currency. Rather this oracle comes on my house. Gold (Chrysos) is the name of my youngest male child. He is in all respects, in form and in excellence of mind, if a father may say so, outstanding among citizens. I, therefore, unless you decide otherwise, will come myself and bring my son, with a fifty-oared ship equipped at my expense with medical and military assistance so that we can give aid in both."[32]

Father and son therefore set off to take part in the siege, where they both distinguished themselves. The father introduced a drug into the water supply of the besieged city that gave its inhabitants diarrhea.[33] The son, for his part, met a heroic death upon scaling the town's ramparts in the front rank. The importance of this ancestor Nebros was such that his descendants were sometimes styled as "Nebrides": "Hippocrates belonged to those who are called the Nebrides. Nebros was the most brilliant of the Asclepiads, the one in favor of whom the Pythia testified. Of him was born Gnosidicus, of Gnosidicus Hippocrates [the grandfather], Aenius, and Podalirius. Of Hippocrates was born Heraclides, of whom was born Hippocrates, the most illustrious of the name, who left admirable works."[34]

The exploits of Nebros and his son did not remain alive only in memory; there is tangible evidence of their influence as well. The son was buried in the hippodrome at Delphi and was entitled to a public cult. This also marked the beginning of privileged relations between the Asclepiads and the Delphic shrine. In recognition of their help, the Asclepiads were accorded the privilege of consulting the oracle, enjoying access on the same terms with the hieromnemones, or sacred recorders, of the sanctuary.[35]

Such in any case is the service that Nebros is supposed to have rendered to Greece in the course of the First Sacred War. Hippocrates could also boast of another ancestor who, a century later, served his country during the First Persian War: Hippolochus, fourth in line of descent from Nebros. Hippocrates' son Thessalus could take pride in counting not one but two forebears who distinguished themselves in this conflict. A relative on his mother's side, named Cadmus, also played a decisive political role—proof, moreover, that Hippocrates, himself born to a great aristocratic family of Cos, had married a wife whose ancestors were likewise figures of consequence.[36]

One of the darkest moments in the history of the island of Cos occurred during the First Persian War. The entire coastline of Asia Minor, including the islands near the coast, was populated by Greek colonists. The colonists had been until this time on fairly good terms with Persia, to which they paid tribute. At the beginning of the fifth century, however, these cities, with Miletus at their head, tried to throw off the Persian yoke. Their revolt, rapidly put down by Darius, who destroyed Miletus in reprisal, was the occasion of the First Persian War. Darius launched a punitive expedition against Greece for having encouraged the rebellion. It was aimed, in particular, against Athens and Eretria as the most active supporters of the Ionian revolt. Before setting off, the Persian king demanded that the Greek cities of Asia supply him with warships. These cities thus found themselves confronted with a cruel dilemma: either to accede to the demand, and so cooperate in a war against their fellow Greeks, or to refuse to obey the Persians, with all the risks that this entailed. According to the *Speech of the Envoy*, Cos chose the second course of action. Thessalus, the son of Hippocrates, describes the decision in this way:

When the Great King with the Persians and other barbarians made war on those Greeks who did not give him earth and water, our country chose rather to perish all altogether so as not to take up arms and set out in a naval expedition against you and those that agreed with you. In this refusal the Coans exhibited a greatness of mind worthy of our forefathers, who are said to be earth born and Heraclids. They decided, though there were four fortified towns on the island, to abandon them all, and to take flight to the mountains and there to cling to their salvation. And from this what evil did not come to pass? Their land was devastated, their free persons were enslaved and killed by the law of enemies, the city and all other defenses, and the sacred places were burned, and finally they were given over to Artemisia, daughter of Lygdamis, in accordance with an ancestral quarrel, to catch with a dragnet everything that was left. Still, it seems, we were not neglected by the gods. There were extraordinary storms and the ships of Artemisia were all in danger of destruction. Many were destroyed and many thunderbolts fell on her army, but the island was hardly touched by lightning. And it is said that visions of heroes were seen by the woman. And terrified at all this she departed with her work undone, having made a bitter agreement, too bitter to describe, so let it go. But I will here give to my ancestors the dignity, no false one, that the Coans never took up willing arms against you, nor against the Lacedemonians nor any other Greeks, though many of the surrounding people who lived on the islands and mainland of Asia joined with the barbarians in the war when they were not forced. Cadmus and Hippolochus were at that time in charge of the city. And it is in the realm of truth that Cadmus and Hippolochus are my forebears. Cadmus who formed the plan itself is in the line of my mother, and Hippolochus is an Asclepiad, fourth in line from Fawn, who destroyed the Criseans. And we are Asclepiads by male descent. Therefore, it was some of our ancestors who undertook this excellent work also.[37]

If the *Speech of the Envoy* is to be credited, then, Hippocrates' ancestor Hippolochus and his wife's ancestor Cadmus both occupied a preeminent place in the political life of Cos at the beginning of the fifth century,[38] and played a decisive role in the island's resistance when the Persians demanded that a contingent of ships take part in the expedition.

The revolt against Persia must have occurred in 490, when the Asiatic fleet, departing from Cilicia en route to Samos, sailed along the coast of Cos. It may seem surprising that Herodotus, the historian of the Persian Wars, and a man who knew the region well, having been born in the neighboring city of Halicarnassus, does not mention this crisis in the island's history. His silence can be explained, however, by local rivalries between Cos and Halicarnassus. Queen Artemesia of Halicarnassus, for instance, is referred to unfavorably in the *Speech of the Envoy* by a source from Cos. Herodotus, by contrast, does not hide his admiration for the energetic woman who ruled over the city of his childhood, and he praises (not unhumorously) her bravery in fighting at sea ten years later among the ranks of the barbarians in the battle of Salamis.[39] Despite the historian's silence in the matter of the Cos revolt, indirect confirmation of it may be found in his work. Herodotus, having described the defeat of the barbarians at Plataea in 480, mentions the case of a rich woman, the concubine of a Persian, who came, covered in gold from head to toe, to beseech the protection of the Spartan chief Pausanias, exclaiming: "King of Sparta, I am your suppliant. Save me from the slavery of being a prisoner of war. Till now you have been my benefactor in that you have destroyed these people, who regarded not the wrath of god or hero. I am a Coan by race, the daughter of Hegetorides, son of Antagoras. The Persian took me prisoner in Cos and has kept me ever since."[40]

This anecdote is symbolic of the Asian Greeks' taste for liberty, which barbarian gold did not succeed in corrupting. But the poignant words of this woman, the daughter of a leading Coan family, acquire special meaning if one considers them in the context of what the *Speech of the Envoy* tells us about the Persian repression after the revolt of Cos, the burning of the island's shrines and the enslavement of free persons. It was probably in the aftermath of this revolt, in 490, that the daughter of Hegetorides was taken far away from her country to become the concubine of the Persian Pharandates, son of Teaspis.

Despite the desperate resistance of the natives of Cos, before long the island fell again under foreign domination. Herodotus indicates that during the Second Persian War, in 480, Artemesia's rule extended not only over Halicarnassus but also over the three neighboring islands, Cos, Nisyros, and Calymnos.[41] What became of the leaders of the revolt? Cadmus, leaving wife and children behind on Cos, preferred to quit his native island in the company of a group of citizens who shared his views. He went to Sicily, where he continued to play an important role, first at Zancle, then at the court of Gelon, at Syracuse, where he was the tyrant's confidant during the Second Persian War.[42] By contrast, nothing is known about the fate of Hippocrates' ancestor, Hippolochus, who seems to have remained on Cos.

When Hippocrates was born on Cos, twenty years after the Second Persian War, the memories of the heroic conduct of this ancestor must have still been quite vivid. Cos finally freed itself from the Persian yoke after the naval victory over the Persians at Cape Mycale in 479.[43] Henceforth the city belonged to the Athenian confederation, founded for the purpose of preventing the return of Persian domination, and paid an annual tribute to Athens.

Hippocrates' Descent from Heracles

Hippocrates was descended not only from Asclepius but also from Heracles. He was therefore both Asclepiad and Heraclid. Biographers explain this relationship with Heracles in various ways. An isolated source says that the Asclepiads were also Heraclids on the ground that Asclepius's two sons, Podalirius and Machaon, were borne by Epione, a daughter of Heracles.[44]

This view allows us to make sense of the name of Hippocrates' father, Heraclides, which etymologically signifies "descendant of Heracles." But the most widespread version is that Hippocrates is Asclepiad through his father and Heraclid through his mother Phaenerete (sometimes identified as Praxithea, daughter of Phaenerete).[45]

One often tends to suspect biographers of taking liberties, even when they cite their sources.[46] Sometimes it happens, though, that inscriptions confirm what would otherwise seem extraordinary. The claim of dual descent from both Asclepius and Heracles is asserted by two residents of Cos in two inscriptions from the Roman period on the island: the one mentions a "descendant of the Asclepiads and of the Heraclidae," the other "a descendant of Asclepius on one side and of Heracles on the other side."[47] The latter formulation makes it clear that being an Asclepiad did not mean that one was automatically descended from Heracles.

It is tempting, too, to smile on reading in the *Life* of Hippocrates according to Soranus that he "was the twentieth in descent from Heracles and the nineteenth from Asclepius." But the second inscription likewise states that the Coan in question is "a descendant of Asclepius of the thirty-fifth generation." Such calculations are therefore not the invention of biographers. They are part of the history of the race, avowed by the aristocratic families of the island themselves. That this history may seem legendary to us is another matter. Aristocratic families, for their part, believed in the factual basis of their genealogies sufficiently to go to the trouble of engraving them in stone inscriptions that were meant to be read by everyone.

Hippocrates' Training

Born of a doubly illustrious line, and bearing the name of his grandfather, Hippocrates received the education thought suited to all children of the aristocracy.

But unlike the majority of other noble children, his future was strongly determined by his family background, since medical knowledge was transmitted from father to son.

Asclepius, the founder of the family, had first communicated the art of medicine to his sons Podalirius and Machaon. Since then the transmission of medical knowledge had been passed down without interruption among the Asclepiads, both before and after the split of the family into two branches. In the Cos branch we have seen that Nebros was, according to the *Speech of the Envoy*, the most celebrated physician of his time. Hippocrates, as the son and grandson of doctors, received his medical education within the family, in keeping with tradition. In this family, at this time, teaching was in all likelihood essentially oral and practical in nature. "[Children] practiced dissection from childhood under parental instruction, as they did reading and writing," writes Galen in his influential treatise *Anatomical Procedures*.[48] Medicine, it is true, is better suited to oral teaching combined with practical instruction than to written teaching. "[I]t is not easy," declares the author of the Hippocratic treatise *On Joints*, "to give exact and complete details of an operation in writing; but the reader should form an outline of it from the description."[49] Nonetheless Hippocrates was also able to profit during his apprenticeship from a written tradition issuing from his own family: his grandfather had written works on medicine, perhaps ones dealing with surgery.[50]

Did Hippocrates receive instruction outside his family? Certain accounts maintain that he was also a disciple of the physician Herodicus,[51] the Sophist Gorgias of Leontini,[52] and the philosopher Democritus of Abdera.[53] All this is very unlikely. But such claims have the merit of reminding us that the training of a good physician in antiquity was not thought to be restricted to a knowledge of things human. It indubitably encompassed rhetoric, and very probably philosophy as well, insofar as these disciplines gave knowledge of the universe.

With regard to Hippocrates' training, a relatively ancient tradition maintains that he learned medicine with the aid of accounts of healing inscribed on steles in the shrine of Asclepius on Cos. In the first century B.C., the Greek geographer Strabo declared: "And it is said that the dietetics practised by Hippocrates were derived mostly from the cures recorded on the votive tablets there."[54]

This tradition was known also in the Latin world: Pliny the Elder, writing in the first century A.D., repeats a slanderous version that he found in Varro. Retracing the history of medicine at the beginning of book 29 of his *Natural History*, he says:

[M]edicine [was already] famous in Trojan times, in which its renown was more assured, but only for the treatment of wounds.

The subsequent story of medicine, strange to say, lay hidden in the darkest night down to the Peloponnesian War, when it was restored to the light by Hippocrates, who was born in the very famous and powerful island of Cos, sacred to Aesculapius. It had been the custom for patients recovered from illness to inscribe in the temple of that god an account of the help that they had received, so that afterwards similar remedies might be enjoyed. Accordingly Hippocrates, it is said, wrote out these inscriptions, and, as our countryman Varro believes, after the temple had been burnt, founded that branch of medicine called "clinical." Afterwards there was no limit to the profit from medical practice.[55]

The mention of the legend of the burning of the temple is explained by the Latins' mistrust of Greek medicine. But what are we to think of this tradition, attested by both Greeks and Latins, according to which Hippocrates learned medicine in the temple of Asclepius at Cos? It seems to have derived from the development of priestly medicine at the Asclepieum of the Hellenistic city of Cos after the time of Hippocrates. Although archaeologists have not uncovered steles of this kind in the shrine there, it is certain that medical inscriptions existed during the Hellenistic era. Pliny the Elder indicates that a very famous preparation against venomous animals, written in verse, had been engraved on a stone in the shrine of Aesculapius at Cos.[56] But what is true of the Hellenistic period does not necessarily hold for the classical period. No archaeological trace prior to the fourth century has been uncovered in the great shrine to the east of the island. In any case, since Hippocrates lived at a time when the city was still in the west, if a sanctuary of Asclepius is supposed to have existed where he could have read medical inscriptions, it would have had to have been that of Astypalaea. The cult of Asclepius is attested epigraphically there. But no medical stele has been discovered at the site. The only medical steles that are known are those of the Asclepieum at Epidaurus, and the miraculous healings that they describe have nothing to do with Hippocratic medicine.[57] The rational medicine of the Asclepiads did not emerge from the temples of Asclepius. If such a legend exists regarding Hippocrates' medical training, it is probably because it was put into circulation by the Asclepiad clergy in order to appropriate the glory of the great physician of Cos for its own purposes.[58]

Hippocrates' Wife and Children

Having completed his education within the family circle, Hippocrates first practiced medicine on his native island, and married. Biographers have not recorded the name of his wife, but it is clear she belonged to a great family. As we have seen, one of her ancestors, Cadmus of Cos, was the tyrant of the island at the time of the First Persian War. Three children were born of this marriage: two sons, Thessalus and Dracon, whom Hippocrates trained in medicine in accordance with family tradition, and a daughter. About this daughter, the imagination of poets and storytellers has made up for a lack of information. She inspired the Byzantine legend that figures in a medieval account by Jean de Mandeville, having been carried back to France by the Crusades.[59] Turned into a dragon by a magic spell, Hippocrates' daughter lies stooped in the basement of an old castle ("gist es voutes au bout d'un ancien chastel") on the "ille de Cohos," of which Hippocrates is "prince et sire." There she awaits a knight whose kiss will restore her to human form. In reality, Hippocrates' daughter lived a quiet life at Astypalaea, where she married Polybus, one of her father's medical students.

Hippocrates of Cos and Democritus of Abdera

Hippocrates seems to have achieved fame during the first part of his career at Cos. According to biographers, he was summoned by the city of Abdera, situated on the Thracian coast across from the isle of Thasos, to treat the philosopher Democritus, whom the Abderites believed to have become mad.[60] This anecdote has been popularized by a group of the Letters.[61] These letters are presented in the form of a short romance that La Fontaine later recalled in his fable "Democritus and the Abderites" and that in the eighteenth century delighted Stendhal's grandfather as well as, in the nineteenth, Stendhal himself.[62] After having received the petition of the Abderites, who were plunged into despair by the apparent illness of the philosopher who laughed at everything, Hippocrates made his preparations. He asked his friend Dionysius of Halicarnassus to come in his absence to watch over his house (and his wife), begged his friend Damagetus on the neighboring island of Rhodes to lend him a ship in which to sail to Abdera, and applied to yet another friend, Crateuas, a slicer of roots, to obtain the necessary medicinal plants for treatment. At Abdera he was to be met by his host, Philopoemen. These preparatory arrangements having been made, Hippocrates arrived after an uneventful trip in the city of Abdera, where a subdued crowd, overcome by sadness, awaited him. He went immediately to see Democritus, whom he found seated under a tree, next to a stream, surrounded by his books and the corpses of animals that he had dissected. The philosopher was in the process of composing a work on—madness! Thus the physician discovered that Democritus's laugh, far from being a symptom of illness, was a sign of wisdom: Democritus was laughing, as it turned out, at the folly of human beings. Prior to this meeting, the physician and the philosopher knew each other only by reputation; afterwards, they held each other in high regard as personal friends.

Does this legend have a basis in truth? It is impossible to say. All that can be said is that Hippocrates and Democritus were contemporaries, and that Hippocrates (or his disciples) did actually treat patients at Abdera.[63]

The Invitation of the King of Persia

The reputation of the physician of Cos was not only widespread in Greece; it had penetrated the barbarian world as well.

The king of the Persians, Artaxerxes I (464–424 B.C.), son of Xerxes, wished to engage Hippocrates' services in order to put an end to the pestilence that had fallen upon his army, which he had been unable to check.[64] Through one of his governors, the Great King made enticing offers. Here is the letter that Hystanes, governor of the Hellespont, is supposed to have sent to Hippocrates of the Asclepiad family: "The Great King Artaxerxes, desiring you, sent subordinates to me and bade me give you silver and gold and abundantly all else you want and need and bade me send you to him quickly. You will be honored equally with the foremost of Persians. Please come immediately."[65]

There is nothing implausible, in and of itself, about the Great King Artaxerxes I appealing for help to a Greek physician. His grandfather Darius had reason to value the services of one before him. Traditionally, the physicians of the Persian court were Egyptian.[66] From earliest antiquity, in fact, Egyptian physicians had been regarded as the most expert in the world.[67] Accordingly, it was upon them that Darius called when he dislocated his ankle in dismounting from a horse. But these doctors, as Herodotus reports,[68] twisted the foot too sharply and worsened his suffering: for seven successive nights the king could not sleep. It was thus upon learning of the presence of a Greek physician among his prisoners—Democedes of Croton—that Darius summoned him and obliged him to treat his injury: "Democedes, using Greek remedies and gentle rather than forcible means, after the latter had been tried by others, succeeded in getting Darius his share of sleep and, in a while, healed him completely, though the King had never expected to have the proper use of his foot again."[69] Some time later, Democedes demonstrated the full extent of his talents in successfully treating Darius's queen, Atossa, for an abcess in her breast.[70]

It is true that Democedes did not serve as a physician in the court of the Persian king of his own free will, and that he managed by a ruse to return to his homeland of Croton in southern Italy, where he married the daughter of the celebrated wrestler Milo of Croton. But he unquestionably helped draw the attention of the Persian sovereigns to the skill of Greek doctors. Several subsequently became physicians to the court.

It was during the reign of Artaxerxes I, in fact, that a doctor named Apollonides, originally from Cos but older than Hippocrates, was appointed court physician. Apollonides' fate is a good example of both the glory and the agony these doctors were liable to experience. He lived at court for many years, and no doubt was held in the same high esteem as the leading nobles of the land, just as Artaxerxes promised Hippocrates he would be regarded. The king was grateful to him for having saved Megabyzus, who had been grievously wounded in the struggle to suppress a conspiracy against Artaxerxes at the beginning of his reign. But some thirty years later he met a dreadful end, for after the death of Megabyzes he dared seduce his widow Amytis, who was also the sister of the Great King. Apollonides did, it is true, abuse his position as physician: having fallen in love with Amytis, he took advantage of her illness (a uteral ailment) to advise that she would recover her health if she had sexual intercourse with men: thus he became her lover. But Amytis continued to waste away. She therefore broke off relations with her doctor and, as she was going to die, told the whole story to her mother, Amestris. Amestris, with Artaxerxes' consent, had Apollonides tortured on the rack for two months, then buried alive when her daughter died. Apollonides had broken one of the rules that later were to constitute the basis of Hippocratic ethics: "Into whatsoever houses I enter," says *The Oath*, "I will enter to help the sick, and I will abstain from all intentional wrong-doing and harm, especially from abusing the bodies of man or woman, bond or free."[71] In defense of the doctor, it must be said that the woman he seduced, as well as her mother, were well known for their dissolute ways. The profession of court physician evidently was not without its dangers.

The story of Apollonides is recounted by an author who knew whereof he spoke, a Greek physician who was to serve some years later as physician to the Persian Court, during the reign of Artaxerxes II (405–359). This man, named Ctesias, was a younger relation of Hippocrates who belonged to the Cnidus branch of the Asclepiads. He had, among other achievements, successfully treated the wound that the Persian king had received from his brother Cyrus II at the battle of Cunaxa in 401.[72] But the fate of Ctesias cannot be compared with that of Apollonides. Ctesias managed to return to his native land, where he composed a history of Persia in twenty-three volumes, the *Persica*. It is in this work that the story of his predecessor as court physician, Apollonides, is told.[73]

Recalling the examples of Apollonides of Cos and Ctesias of Cnidus, it seems entirely plausible to suppose that Artaxerxes I did in fact invite Hippocrates to his court. To this invitation, conveyed by Hystanes, Hippocrates is said to have replied with a haughty refusal:

Hippocrates the physician to Hystanes, governor of the Hellespont. Greetings.
In response to the letter you sent which you said came from the King, write to the King and send him as quickly as possible what I say: I have enough food, clothing, shelter and all substance sufficient for life. It is not proper that I should enjoy Persian opulence or save Persians from disease, since they are enemies of the Greeks. Be well![74]

By the second century A.D. this refusal had become a very well known theme among historical writers. Galen mentions it in his portrait of the ideal physician, inspired by the life of Hippocrates: "The excellent physician will disdain Artaxerxes and not be able to show himself to his view, even for a single moment."[75]

Hippocrates' attitude in this regard has usually been interpreted as an example of patriotism and disinterestedness. In the Roman context, however, it was used to justify mistrust of Greek doctors of medicine, who were considered xenophobic. Plutarch, in fact, referring to Cato's hatred for the Greeks, says this:

However, Cato's dislike of the Greeks was not confined to philosophers: he was also deeply suspicious of the Greek physicians who practiced in Rome. He had heard of Hippocrates' celebrated reply, when he was called upon to attend the king of Persia for a fee amounting to many talents, and declared that he would never give his services to barbarians who were enemies of Greece. Cato maintained that all Greek physicians had taken an oath of this kind, and urged his son not to trust any of them.[76]

There is no real reason to doubt the Persian king's invitation and Hippocrates' refusal, even if the terms of the response given in the *Letters* are not authentic, and even if the event did come to acquire a legendary character during the Roman era. His refusal accords rather well with the attitude of his forebear Hippolochus, who, according to the *Speech of the Envoy*, incited the revolt of Cos against the Persians; and it occurred in a period when the island of Cos, now delivered from Persian domination, belonged to the Athenian confederation.[77]

In the late eighteenth and early nineteenth century, this episode from the life of Hippocrates was still famous. It was painted in 1792 by Girodet, whose "brush always dipped into the most literary sources." His canvas was noticed by Baudelaire at an exhibition in 1846: "Girodet's *Hippocrates Refusing the Presents of Artaxerxes* has come back from the School of Medicine to make us admire its superb organization, its excellent finish and its spiritual details."[78]

The whole first part of Hippocrates' life unfolded therefore on Cos, where, if the Artaxerxes episode is to be believed, his fame was already great. However, his career surely would not have won him exceptional renown during his lifetime had he not left his native island. At some unknown date, but in any case at a time when he had reached full maturity and had already attained the mastery of his art, this man, who was not yet the ideal physician that he was later to become in Plato's eyes, but who was yet heir to the mantle of a long line of celebrated doctors, left Cos, not for the East and the Persian Empire, but for the West and Greece—more particularly for Thessaly, the birthplace of his ancestors.

TWO

Hippocrates the Thessalian

It was not unusual for medical doctors during the classical period to leave their birthplace, or the place where they received their training, to make their career in another or several other cities, either as a private or a public physician.[1]

A Traveling Physician Prior to Hippocrates

The best-known example, prior to Hippocrates, was Democedes, son of Calliphon, originally of Croton in southern Italy. He was regarded as the foremost physician of his time. We have already noted that he had successfully treated King Darius and Queen Atossa.[2] But it was only after a brilliant medical career that he found himself the prisoner and slave of the Persian king. This career is recounted in considerable detail by Herodotus:

In Croton he had to deal with his father, who was very harsh-tempered, and Democedes, being unable to put up with him, left and went to Aegina. Having set up there, within the first year he surpassed all the other doctors, although he was quite unfurnished and lacking all the things that are, for a doctor, working equipment. In his second year the people of Aegina took him for public physician at a fee of one talent [= 60 minas or 6,000 drachmas]; in his third year the Athenians, for the same work, gave him a hundred minas; and in the fourth year Polycrates hired him for two talents. So he came to Samos, and it was because of this man not least that the Crotoniates gained their reputation as doctors. For this was the time when the Crotoniates first became spoken of as doctors throughout Greece; the second place was held by the Cyrenaeans.[3]

The product of the Pythagorean milieu of Croton (like another celebrated physician, Alcmaeon, who left there as well), Democedes is the very model of the itinerant medical doctor who occupied a variety of positions. He began in private practice, and then went on to become a public physician in municipal service before taking up residence in the court of a Greek prince. His career in Greece was an immediate success: within two years his initial salary had doubled, with Polycrates of Samos offering twice what the city of Aegina was paying him.

The rest of his career proceeded less smoothly. Being the personal physician of a tyrant was not free of disadvantages, as he was to learn. When Polycrates was traitorously assassinated by Oroetes, the Persian governor of Sardes, Democedes, like all foreigners in Polycrates' entourage, found himself enslaved. He must have shown evidence of his talents as a doctor at once, for his name was soon mentioned in conversation at Sardes. But Oroetes was himself assassinated, on the orders of Darius, and Democedes was transferred to Susa along with the members of Oroetes' court. He then fell back into anonymity for a time, until the failure of the Egyptian doctors gave him the opportunity, as we have seen, to successfully treat Darius's foot. Thus it was that he suddenly found himself, most reluctantly, the new court physician. A large house was placed at his disposal, and he became the king's dining companion. He took advantage of his new position to secure the freedom of a former fellow slave, a soothsayer from Elea who, like him, had been attracted by the luxury of the court of Polycrates. His generosity extended even to his unlucky medical colleagues: he obtained pardons for the Egyptian physicians, whom Darius had intended to impale in punishment for their failure. In short, Democedes became a very important figure in the king's circle. His art saved him from slavery.

One would like to have equally detailed information about the career of Hippocrates. Unfortunately, what we have is far less complete. His career seems to have been rather more peaceful, and less romantic, than that of the physician of Croton.

Hippocrates' Departure for Thessaly

When Hippocrates departed Cos, it was in any event not because, as in the case of Democedes, he did not get along with his father. He went away only after the death of his parents.[4] Regarding the causes for his leaving, biographers give differing accounts.

One traditional version, a malicious one, scarcely deserves attention, though we have it from a relatively ancient source. According to Andreas,[5] in his work on the *Genealogy of Physicians*, Hippocrates left Cos because he had burned down the library at Cnidus. Stories of arson are very frequently encountered in biographies of Hippocrates. We have already noted that he was accused of burning down the temple of Asclepius at Cos after having consulted the medical inscriptions there.[6] These two accounts share the same malevolent purpose: to accuse Hippocrates of plagiarism, to suggest that the great physician's knowledge was the result of theft, which he sought to hide by destroying his sources. In the one instance, he was supposed to have destroyed the medical archives of the temple of Asclepius at Cos, and in the other, the archives of the medical library at Cnidus. A third tale of arson, recorded by the Byzantine Tzetzes,[7] seems to blend the two preceding versions. In this account, Hippocrates was the curator of the archives of the medical library at Cos, and was exiled after having burned the ancient works contained in this collection. Thus Hippocratic science was erected on the ashes of the very learning of the school of Cos.

None of this can be taken seriously. But such accounts, at least one of which comes down to us from the Hellenistic period, testify to the existence of an anti-Hippocratic movement antedating the Roman mistrust of Greek doctors. A certain hostility with regard to Hippocrates already existed in Egypt during the Hellenistic period, among the pupils of the great physician Herophilus. This, at any rate, is what our most ancient source, Andreas, a disciple of Herophilus and physician to Ptolemy IV, suggests.

Another version, relying upon a better source, since it goes back to a local scholar, Soranus of Cos, maintains that Hippocrates left as a result of a dream enjoining him to settle in Thessaly.[8]

The most probable explanation is that he wished to enrich his experience through examination of the practices of other lands. One of the most important ideas of Hippocratic medicine, in fact, is that the natural environment of a place has an influence upon health and disease. This explanation is given by Galen in his portrait of the ideal physician, inspired by the example of Hippocrates: "He will leave to his fellow citizens of Cos Polybus and his other disciples, while he himself will go away, travelling throughout all of Greece. For it is necessary for him also to write about the nature of places. In order therefore to judge by experience what he has learned through discourse, it is necessary that he see different cities himself."[9]

When did this departure occur? No specific indication is given directly in the biographical writings. The fact that he left after the death of his parents provides only very limited information. He did not leave his native island before having raised his sons, who followed him, and before having married his daughter to his disciple Polybus, who remained at Astypalaea and took over responsibility for medical instruction from his teacher.[10] Hippocrates' maturity coincides with the Peloponnesian War (431–404). His departure must have taken place sometime during the decade after 430, if one can trust the chronology based on information found in the *Speech of the Envoy*. Hippocrates was already settled in Thessaly when a pestilence broke out that may be dated to the years 419–416.

Hippocrates in Thessaly

This voyage undertaken by Hippocrates, which took him far away from Cos, is not to be thought of as the rite of initiation of a provincial student, but as the voluntary relocation of a physician who was already celebrated for his expertise, and whose retinue attests to his fame and importance. Some idea of how great this was can be had by considering the way in which those other "stars" of the period moved from place to place—the great Sophists such as Gorgias or Protagoras, whose arrival, so vividly evoked by Plato in the *Protagoras*, did not fail to produce a great sensation wherever they went. Hippocrates, however, must have avoided overly theatrical effects.

Just as Democedes of Croton, once he had settled in Aegina, rapidly surpassed his colleagues in reputation, so the reputation of Hippocrates must have spread through Thessaly and passed beyond its borders. "My name has gone further than I have," Hippocrates is made to say in the *Address from the Altar*. One would like to know if Hippocrates was a private or a public physician, like Democedes, or whether he was in the service of the great aristocratic families of Thessaly. All surviving accounts are silent on this point. He did not restrict himself, in any case, to treating the poor, as Galen tried to make it appear in his praise of an idealized Hippocrates.[11] One would also like to know if Hippocrates settled at Larissa upon his arrival in Thessaly, using it as a base from which he could travel about the region, or if he was an itinerant physician for a time; that is, if he stayed for more or less extended periods in various cities. When the biographical writings speak of Hippocrates' time in Thessaly, they do so in general terms. The *Speech of the Envoy*, for example, indicates simply that Hippocrates made his home in Thessaly. However, as it is said in the *Address from the Altar* that Hippocrates was known in many cities in Thessaly, it may be thought that he practiced in several or more of them. This was Galen's opinion. In support of it he relied upon the names of the places mentioned in the Hippocratic corpus.

The information found in biographical accounts is in fact supported by indirect evidence contained in the corpus, notably in the *Epidemics*. These treatises supply notes on individual patients and recapitulate, sometimes on a day-to-day basis, the evolution of their illnesses. The place of origin of these patients is often mentioned, which makes it possible to follow on the map the different places where Hippocratic medicine was practiced. Reference is made, unsurprisingly, to patients living in Larissa,[12] but also to ones living in various other Thessalian cities: Meliboea, Crannon, Pharsalus, and Pherae.[13] There is no chance whatever that the whole of the *Epidemics*, the three major parts of which were successively produced between the end of the fifth century and the middle of the fourth century, might have been the work of Hippocrates alone.[14] But it is remarkable that all three parts refer to these Thessalian cities. Such allusions confirm the presence of Hippocrates and his disciples in Thessaly, and mark off fairly precisely the territory within which the better part of their practice took place over the course of a half century.

Hippocrates and Northern Greece

Did Hippocrates also practice outside of Thessaly? While the *Speech of the Envoy* speaks only of this country, other sources cite, along with Thessaly, the part of Thrace occupied by the Edoni, and continental Greece.[15] These accounts, which have the physician of Cos residing in Macedonia, because he was a friend of the king, Perdiccas,[16] point mainly to the north of Greece.

The place-names outside of Thessaly found in the *Epidemics* mostly refer to northern Greece as well: Thrace and the Propontis are mentioned, but also Macedonia.

Epidemics I and *III* were composed by an itinerant physician who lived not only in Thessaly but who spent at least four years on the island of Thasos, who treated patients in Abdera, the city on the Thracian coast across from Thasos where Democritus lived, and who traveled as far away as Cyzicus on the Asiatic side of the Propontis (the modern Sea of Marmara).[17] And as this author was not content simply to give the name of the city where he treated his patients, but sometimes adds a more specific address with reference to a known landmark of the city, one has the impression of following the route of the doctor extremely closely as he visits patients confined to their beds, all the more when these places have been identified by archaeologists working in the field. In Abdera, only two places are mentioned, the Sacred Way and the Thracian Gate. On Thasos, by contrast, a whole crowd of places comes back to life. Here one finds reference to ramparts old and new: ramparts that today still stand in the western part of the city with their towers and gates. There one finds shrines and temples: first the Heracleion and the Artemision, both identified by archaeologists from the École française d'Athènes, next the

Heraion and the temple of Earth, which have not yet been identified by field archaeologists. Elsewhere there is the evocatively named Liars' Market; here there is a freshwater fountain; there again, finally, places that take their names from the configuration of the land, such as the Platform and Herdsman's Gully.[18]

In the second group of the *Epidemics* (*II*, *IV*, and *VI*), the regions named outside of Thessaly are the same, Thrace and Propontis. Alongside the names of cities already known through *Epidemics I* and *III*, however, new localities appear, particularly Acanthus, in the Chalcidice, and Perinthus, in the Propontis.[19]

In the final group of the *Epidemics* (*V* and *VII*), the situation with regard to Thrace and Thasos appears largely unchanged. But a new region now makes its appearance, Macedonia, with its capital, Pella, while the Propontis seems no longer to be represented.[20]

The list of the place-names of the sick contained in the Hippocratic Collection surely gives a rather faithful picture of the sphere in which Hippocrates' school exercised its influence. If so, this was essentially in Thessaly and the north of Greece (Thrace, Propontis, and Macedonia). The fact that Thasos and Abdera are the only two cities outside Thessaly that figure in all three groups of the *Epidemics* attests that outside of Thessaly, which was the center of the Hippocratic school following his departure from Cos, the ties between Hippocratic physicians and this part of Thrace were strong.

Doctors of the Hippocratic school must have traveled as a group. Indeed, one finds the first person plural used in the *Epidemics*, in phrases such as "when we arrived at Perinthus."[21]

The Frontiers of Hippocratic Activity

Outside of Thessaly and northern Greece, local references in the Hippocratic corpus are rare. The most distant city to the north where a Hippocratic physician is mentioned practicing was Odessus, on the western shore of the Euxine (or Black) Sea, the present-day Varna in Bulgaria.[22] South of Thessaly, there was Athens and the island of Salamis, and, in the Peloponnesus, Elis and Corinth; in the Aegean Sea, the islands of Syros and Delos.[23] What is remarkable is that the island of Cos is very rarely mentioned in the medical works attributed to Hippocrates. The only writing that makes reference to a patient from Cos is *Prorrhetic I*.[24] One may conclude from this that the clinical work of the Hippocratic school as a whole dates from the time after Hippocrates left Cos, and that its height is to be associated with the career of Hippocrates and his disciples during the Thessalian period.

Hippocrates and Perdiccas, King of Macedonia

Two facts stand out in biographical accounts of Hippocrates' career during this period. The first concerns his relations with a prince, Perdiccas II, king of Macedonia.

Officially summoned to tend to Perdiccas, who was believed to have been stricken with consumption following the death of his father, Alexander I, Hippocrates is said to have diagnosed lovesickness and in this way cured the king, who was enamored of Philè, the courtesan of his late father.[25] This is a nice story. But is it true? A similar anecdote is related in connection with the great physician of the Hellenistic era, Erasistratus, who diagnosed King Antiochus as being sick with love for Stratonice, the wife of his father, Seleucus I.[26] In both cases, a great doctor discovers that a young prince suffers from a hidden love for the lover or the wife of his father. The sameness of the two narratives tends to cast doubt upon the authenticity of the underlying story. However there is nothing absurd about supposing that Hippocrates came into contact with Perdiccas. The *Speech of the Envoy*, while not alluding to this particular story, confirms ancestral bonds of hospitality between the family of the Asclepiads and the kings of Macedonia.[27] These ties continued after the time of Hippocrates, since his son Thessalus became physician to Archelaus, Perdiccas's bastard son and successor.

Whether real or invented, this episode from the life of Hippocrates has remained famous. The story was still being told in the fifth century A.D., in a poem entitled *Aegritudo Perdicae* ("The Illness of Perdiccas") and attributed to Dracontius, a Christian poet of North Africa, although many new elements were introduced, as even a brief description of the tale indicates: the young prince, whom Venus caused to fall in love with his own mother, Castalia, for having neglected to honor her, falls ill and wastes away while refusing to reveal to anyone the cause of his disease. Only Hippocrates, feeling the young man's pulse when Castalia comes into his bedroom, succeeds in diagnosing the sickness. Unfortunately, he is not able to save Perdiccas for all of this, for the young man hangs himself rather than succumb to his incestuous passion.[28]

Hippocrates and the Plague in Greece

The second outstanding fact of the Thessalian period was to have far greater consequences for Hippocrates' reputation. It was not a question in this case of service rendered to an individual of great eminence but of assistance, during a plague, refused to the barbarians and granted instead to Greece. Here is the beginning of the account given in the *Speech of the Envoy*:

In the time in which the plague was running through the barbarian land north of the Illyrians and Paeonians, when the evil reached that area, the kings of those peoples sent to Thessaly after my father because of his reputation as a physician, which, being a true one, had managed to go everywhere. He had lived in Thessaly previously and had a dwelling there then. They summoned him to help, saying that they were not going to send gold and silver and other possessions for him to have, but that he could carry away all that he wanted when he had come to help. And he made inquiry what kind of disturbances there were, area by area, in heat and winds and mist and other things that produce unusual conditions. When he had gotten everyone's information he told them to go back, pretending that he was unable to go to their country. But as quickly as he could he arranged to announce to the Thessalians by what means they could contrive protection against the evil that was coming.[29]

Let us first of all observe that this plague is not to be confused, either in its origin or its date, with the great attack of the "plague" of Athens, described by Thucydides. Whereas the "plague" of Athens developed far to the south, in Ethiopia, and was propagated in Egypt, Libya, and thence the majority of the territories of the Great King before finally penetrating Athens through the port of Piraeus,[30] the plague that figures in the Hippocratic tradition came from the north, from the barbarian territories located beyond Illyria and Paeonia. And while the "plague" of Athens occurred in 430–429, the plague of Hippocratic tradition was rife only after the year 421, if the chronology found in the *Speech of the Envoy* is to be credited, and most probably during the years 419–416.[31] Hippocrates' attitude is consistent with the one that is traditionally attributed to him in connection with the offer of the Persian king Artaxerxes. Once again, not allowing himself to be seduced by the promises of the barbarians, he refused to care for them. But his devotion to the Greek cause was more positively demonstrated in this case. Hiding his real motives, he questioned the barbarian envoys about climatic conditions and wind patterns in their countries, and took advantage of their replies to predict the spread of the disease in Greece and to prescribe a treatment for those infected. His zeal in this matter was not limited to Thessaly. He dispatched his son and disciples to various countries, Thessalus to Macedonia, for example, and Dracon to the Hellespont. He himself, after having ministered to the Thessalonians, traveled to bring relief to populations as far away as Athens and in the Peloponnesus, passing along the way through Doris, Phocis, with its city of Delphi, and Boeotia. In return, he was rewarded with honors by the Greek cities, notably Athens, where he was presented with a gold crown and initiated into the mysteries of Eleusis.[32] Hippocrates' cordial relations with the Athenians, at least until the end of the Sicilian expedition (415–413), no doubt explain his offering to send his son Thessalus at his own expense to accompany the expeditionary force, in which Thessalus was to serve without salary for the length of the campaign. Thessalus adds that in his turn he, too, received a gold crown from the Athenians.

The facts mentioned in the *Speech of the Envoy* are specific. But are they accurate? It is striking that no accounts other than those of the Hippocratic tradition allude to a plague in Greece in the years 419–416. Thucydides, in particular, does not speak of one.[33] The lack of confirming evidence calls the authenticity of the tradition into question. It should be noted that this anecdote, like the one about the treatment of Perdiccas, did not cease to evolve over time. As the centuries passed, though less was known about it, more details were made up. The plague of Hippocratic tradition that originated in the north came to be confused with the great Athenian plague, which arrived from the south[34] (we moderns, it must be admitted, are no less liable to confusion on this point) and Hippocrates was credited with having put an end to the illness it brought by lighting great fires that purified the air.[35] In the Byzantine period, legend went so far as to attribute to Hippocrates the discovery of an antidote to the plague, for which the Athenians bestowed upon him the crown already mentioned.[36]

Hippocrates and Delphi

Not all of the details contained in the ancient version given in the *Speech of the Envoy* can have been invented, however. What is said there in connection with Hippocrates' visit to Delphi merits special attention.

On arriving at Delphi, Hippocrates addressed a plea to the god for the safety of the Greeks and made a sacrifice. He also took advantage of the occasion to reaffirm the privileges that his family, the Asclepiads, had obtained as a result of the services rendered by Nebros during the First Sacred War. Here is what Thessalus says: "And to the Asclepiads from Cos was given, for [Nebros]'s sake, the right of priority in consulting the oracle, the same as the Hieromnemones. . . . Because what I am saying is true, when my father and I went there the Amphictyons renewed those things and granted them to us, and they inscribed it on a column which they set up at Delphi."[37]

The proof Thessalus gives is specific, and the epigraphy at Delphi indirectly confirms it. To be sure, the stele referred to in the *Speech of the Envoy* has not been recovered. But several inscriptions attest that Hippocrates did indeed go to Delphi and that the Asclepiads did in fact enjoy privileges in the sanctuary of Apollo.

The coming of Hippocrates to Delphi is confirmed by a dedicatory in-scription bearing his name.[38] Despite the highly incomplete character of this inscription, for which no translation could be proposed without vigorous interpolation, it unquestionably concerns Hippocrates. Indeed, apart from the fact that his name is perfectly legible, the inscription speaks of diseases. Moreover Hippocrates' name is preceded by the term "[Thess]alus," which allows of three possible interpretations. It may be taken to refer either to the "Thessalian Hippocrates," as in the funereal epigram of the *Anthologia Graeca*, or to "Thessalus son of Hippocrates," or to "Thessalus and Hippocrates."[39] According to this last interpretation there were two dedicators, Hippocrates and his son, which matches the account of the *Speech of the Envoy*, where Thessalus makes it clear that he accompanied his father on the trip to Delphi. In that case, what we would have are the remains of an inscription recording a dedication by both Hippocrates and Thessalus during their stay in Delphi in the 420s. In any case, the inscription attests at a minimum to Hippocrates' association with the Delphic shrine.

This association may also be deduced from the existence of a statue of a patient suffering from consumption that stood in the sanctuary at Delphi and was taken to be an offering of Hippocrates. The statue still existed when Pausanias visited Delphi in the second century B.C. Here is what he said of it: "Among the votive offerings to Apollo was a representation in bronze of a man's body in an advanced stage of decay, with the flesh already fallen off, and nothing left but the bones. The Delphians said that it was an offering of Hippocrates the physician."[40]

As for the privileges enjoyed by the Asclepiads of Cos at Delphi as de-scribed in the *Speech of the Envoy*, they have been confirmed by an important inscription at Delphi whose relatively recent discovery throws new light on the trustworthiness of the information contained in the Hippocratic corpus. The discovery involved a decree issued by the association (*koinon*, in Greek) of the Asclepiads of Cos and Cnidus toward the end of Hippocrates' life.[41] Since the inscription has fewer lacunae than the dedication by Hippocrates, a trans-lation can be suggested: "Decree of the *koinon* of the Asclepiads of Cos and of Cnidus: the Asclepiad arriving at Delphi, if he desires to consult the oracle or to sacrifice, must swear, before consulting the oracle or sacrificing, that he is Asclepiad by male descent [gap]. He who breaks these rules will not have access to the oracle as an Asclepiad, and any other privilege granted by the Delphians will not be accorded to him if it is not in conformity with the preceding prescriptions."

The inscription does not specify the nature of the privileges enjoyed by the

Asclepiads at Delphi in detail, but it leaves no doubt about the existence of these privileges, among which precedence may reasonably be assumed to have been one; that is, the privilege of consulting the oracle first indicated by the *Speech of the Envoy*.[42] There is a slight difference, however, between the literary text and the inscription: where the *Speech of the Envoy* talks of the privileges belonging to the Asclepiads of Cos, which is to say, the line descended from Nebros, the inscription refers to privileges shared by both branches of the family, on Cos and Cnidus.[43] On the other hand, the inscription confirms the importance of descent through the male line of the aristocratic family of the Asclepiads. "We are Asclepiads by male descent," says Thessalus in the *Speech of the Envoy*, speaking of himself and his father. "It is necessary to swear that one is Asclepiad by male descent," reads the inscription. Encountering the same characteristic but rare expression (*kat'androgeneian*)[44] in each case is a strong reason for believing that the information found in the *Speech of the Envoy* is taken from a good source. Even if it is not authentic, the speech of Hippocrates' son to the Athenians contains valuable material that goes back, in the final analysis, to the Asclepiad family archives on Cos.

Hippocrates' Continuing Ties with His Native Land

Following his departure from Cos, Hippocrates' ties to his native land must have remained close. Some time after the episode of the plague, shortly following the Athenian expedition to Sicily, he interceded in a dispute between Athens and Cos.[45] It was precisely this dispute that gave rise to the *Speech of the Envoy*, which is supposed to have been delivered before the Athenian assembly by Hippocrates' son, pleading on behalf of Cos.[46]

The island of Cos, along with the other islands of the Aegean Sea, belonged at that time to the Delian League. Conceived originally after the Persian Wars to prevent the return of the enemy, and led by Athens, the league began as a loose federation of allies but gradually became transformed into an empire. In the process, the allies became subjects—a train of events that later was to be masterfully analyzed by Thucydides. Following the disastrous expedition to Sicily, which left Athens considerably weakened, revolts by the subject cities multiplied, encouraged by the activity of the Lacedaemonian fleet in the Aegean and by the aspirations of the barbarians to regain control over the cities of the Asiatic coast. Cos therefore found itself at the center of the theater of operations, risking pillage at the hands of the enemy. In 412–411, in particular, the island was the victim of a raid by the Spartan naval commander Astyochus, as Thucydides recounts: "On his voyage along the coast he landed at the Mereopid Cos. The city was unfortified and had collapsed in an earthquake which was certainly the greatest one that can be remembered. He sacked the city, the inhabitants of which had fled to the mountains, over-ran the country, and made off with everything in it except for the free men, whom he let go."[47]

While dealing harshly with the allies of Athens, Astyochus took care to treat the inhabitants of Cos gently, in the hope that they might eventually be brought back into the Spartan camp. The island remained, however, under Athenian domination, and served as a naval base for the fleet setting out to put down the rebellion on Rhodes.[48] Alcibiades, having rejoined the Athenian fleet at Samos following his exile, "forced the people of Halicarnassus to contribute large sums of money and fortified Cos. After doing this he appointed a governor for Cos, and, since it was nearly autumn, sailed back to Samos."[49] Alcibiades' actions must be seen as implying more mistrust than confidence with regard to Cos. Moreover, according to Diodorus of Sicily, he pillaged the island on this occasion, bringing the booty back to Samos, and then again in 408 to provide for the needs of his soldiers.[50]

It was in this atmosphere of tension between Athens and Cos that Hippocrates spoke to the Athenians, through his son Thessalus, to plead the case of his threatened homeland. The *Speech of the Envoy* is notable for its moderate tone. But it warned the Athenians against an unrestrained imperialism and against the temptation to settle differences by resort to arms. It even brandished the threat, in the case that negotiations should fail, of appealing for the help of other peoples, particularly that of the Thessalians. Thessalus's mediation seems not to have had any effect, however. If another work contained in the Hippocratic Collection, the *Address from the Altar*, is to be believed, Hippocrates did in fact call upon Thessaly to come to the aid of Cos.[51] In this pathetic appeal for help from an imploring Hippocrates, the accusations of imperialism brought against Athens in the *Speech of the Envoy* for having abused its superiority and deprived the inhabitants of Cos of their liberty are given more forceful expression.

Hippocrates seems therefore to have kept close ties with Cos despite his departure for Thessaly. Even so, he never returned to his native island.

The Death of Hippocrates

After a long career, begun on Cos and carried on in northern Greece, Hippocrates died at Larissa, in Thessaly, at an advanced age. Some biographers put this at 85, others at 90, 104, and even 109—which leaves a fairly wide range of possible dates for his death, between the years 375 and 351.[52] His tomb stood between Larissa and Gyrton, a city to the north.[53] Literary tradition has preserved an epitaph, the authenticity of which is impossible to determine. It emphasizes the bonds between Hippocrates and Thessaly: "Here lieth Thessalian Hippocrates, by descent a Coan, sprung from the immortal stock of Phoebus. Armed by Health he gained many victories over Disease, and won great glory not by chance, but by science."[54]

The best-known biography relates that a swarm of bees, whose honey had therapeutic properties, long made their home on his tomb. Nurses brought children suffering from ulcerations of the mouth to the tomb, rubbing their sores with this honey.[55]

Hippocrates, Hero-Healer

Known only as a physician during his lifetime, Hippocrates became famous in death as a healer of heroic dimensions.

On his native island of Cos he was the object of a public hero-cult, with sacrifices made each year on the day of his birth.[56] The birthday of every deceased person was normally the occasion of a family celebration at which homage was rendered to the departed relative. But what is remarkable in the case of Hippocrates is that this private observance gave way to a public ceremony. It is not known with certainty when exactly his cult was instituted. It must have existed in the first century B.C., when bronze coins appeared on Cos bearing the image of the bald and bearded head of Hippocrates.[57]

After his death, Hippocrates was fated to be thought of in tandem with Heracles. A coin from Cos, preserved in the antiquities collection of the Bibliothèque Nationale in Paris,[58] shows, on the reverse side, Hippocrates seated on a folding chair and, on the front, Heracles with his club. In the popular mind, on Cos, the "divine Hippocrates," who "cleansed the earth and sea . . . of beastly wild diseases,"[59] had thus become the equal of Heracles, who was believed to have purged the earth and the sea of monsters.

The hero-healer was also brought into closer relation with the great healing god of Cos, Asclepius. On island coins bearing the portrait of Hippocrates there appears on the flip side a staff around which is coiled a snake. This is the staff of the god of medicine, with one of his pets wrapped around it: pictured in shrines to the god, and attributed a healing power, it has remained the emblem of the physician since antiquity. Recall, too, that in the mosaic of the imperial era displayed at the Cos Museum, a young Asclepius disembarking on the island is received by the elderly Hippocrates. There is no ancient evidence, however, of syncretism between the cult of Asclepius and that of Hippocrates.

The worship of Hippocrates after his death took unexpected forms. Lucian, a Greek author of the imperial period, reports that a doctor named Antigonus possessed a bronze statue of Hippocrates a cubit high, which he worshipped by offering annual sacrifices.[60] This private cult seems to have been modeled after the public cult of the hero Hippocrates that the inhabitants of Cos celebrated every year on the anniversary of his birth.

Hippocrates even became a healer of souls in the afterlife. His bust appears in a funereal context at the end of the first century A.D. The Hippocrates of Ostia was found in the necropolis of Isola Sacra, in a tomb erected by the court physician Marcus Demetrius (first century A.D.) to the members of his family. The inscription on the pillar that served as the base of the bust is taken from the beginning of the *Aphorisms*, modified for funereal purposes. The phrase "Life is short" is duly engraved upon it; but instead of the expected contrast ("the Art is long"), the inscription continues, "but long is the time that we pass beneath the earth, etc."[61]

The Portraits of Hippocrates

The bust of Ostia depicts an old man, bearded and bald. Hippocrates' baldness is confirmed by biographical writings.[62] As this bust, currently judged the most authentic of all those known, was discovered only in 1940, until then imaginations were stimulated by other plastic representations. In particular, the very large statue of a long-haired man, found in 1929 in excavations of the Odeum at Cos and now held in the museum of the town, was taken to be the most authoritative image of the physician of Cos. This man bears no resemblance to either the bald, elderly man of the bust of Ostia or, for that matter, the head of Hippocrates pictured on the coins of Cos. It was necessary, then, to renounce what turned out to be too seductive an attribution. By contrast, thanks to the discovery of the bust of Ostia, several marble studies that had been believed to be portraits of the philosopher Carneades have been reattributed to Hippocrates.[63]

If our acquaintance with busts of Hippocrates is relatively recent, the portrait of Hippocrates on the coins of Cos has been familiar since the sixteenth century. Small bronze coins from the Roman era show on their face the portrait of a bald and bearded man. Here the identification with Hippocrates is assured by the first two Greek letters of the physician's name. Two other types of bronze coins represent Hippocrates seated on the reverse side. In this case, the identification is authenticated by the presence of his entire name.[64]

In all these representations, the head of Hippocrates is uncovered. Biographers say, to the contrary, that Hippocrates was pictured with his head covered by a *pilos*; that is, by a felt cap—thus Sganarelle's famous chapter on hats!—or otherwise by his *himation*, or cloak. And they record the many explanations that have been proposed to account for this detail. The most complete version is that of the *Life* according to Soranus:

In many portraits he is represented with the head covered, either, according to some, by a *pilos*, sign of the nobility of his origin, like Ulysses, or, according to others, by his cloak, and among those who give this second version, some say that it is out of decency, because he was bald, others on account of the fragility of his head, others to show that it is necessary to protect the region of thought, others as proof of his love of travel, others as proof of obscurity in his writings, others to manifest that it is necessary, even when one is in good health, to protect oneself against what is harmful; others say that in order to prevent his hands from being hindered in operations, he placed on his head the part of his cloak that fell all around [him].

Of this type of portrait, which the biographer claims was fairly common, no ancient trace has been preserved. The sole representation of Hippocrates with his head covered is a very famous Byzantine miniature of the fourteenth century in a Hippocratic manuscript presently held in the Bibliothèque Nationale in Paris.[65] Hippocrates is represented there from the front, with his bald head covered by the right part of his *himation*. Seated on a throne, like a Christ in majesty, he holds in his hands a book in which the beginning of the *Aphorisms* can be read: "Life is short, the Art long, opportunity fleeting." In executing his portrait, the miniaturist must have been guided by the information contained in the *Life* of Hippocrates according to Soranus. This text was readily accessible to him: he found it at the head of the manuscript that he was given to illustrate. In any case, what the painter wished to capture in this portrait of Hippocrates was not Hippocrates the practitioner, but Hippocrates the teacher and author.

Later Hippocratic Legends

Before turning to Hippocrates the teacher and author, it needs to be noted in closing this brief account of his life that, although the historical figure of Hippocrates did not cease to occupy a place in the imagination of men, at Cos and elsewhere, the image of the man himself yet became singularly blurred over time, passing into legend.

This image was initially distorted by a pseudo-Hippocratic literature that took liberties with the chronology of the physician's life. One letter from

Hippocrates on the human constitution is addressed to King Ptolemy. The author of this falsehood did not realize that such a thing was chronologically impossible. When Ptolemy I (Soter), the founder of the Ptolemaic dynasty in Egypt, came into power, Hippocrates had already been dead for several decades. Just the same, the letter enjoyed a great success, as the sizeable number of medieval manuscripts in which it was later reproduced (some thirty or so) testifies.

Chronological constraints were sometimes disregarded entirely. In the French romance of the Holy Grail, written in the early thirteenth century, Hippocrates learns of the resurrection of Lazarus by Jesus Christ. It had not been forgotten, of course, that Hippocrates was a physician. But this single fact came to be embroidered without regard for either time or place. Hippocrates no longer treats the Macedonian king Perdiccas, but the nephew of the emperor Augustus Caesar; Caesar expresses his thanks by causing two life-size gold statues to be erected atop the highest point in Rome. It was no longer remembered that Hippocrates had refused the offer of the Persian king Artaxerxes. He was imagined instead to have treated the son of the Persian king Antonius. And to top it off, Hippocrates came to be portrayed as the victim of the treachery of a beautiful young woman from Gaul with whom he had fallen in love. On the pretext of a romantic rendezvous, she succeeds in suspending him in a basket in the position of a criminal about to be delivered to the executioner, and so exposing him to the ridicule of passersby. It should be noted that in medieval tradition a similar misadventure befalls Virgil. The scene must have made an impression on the popular mind for it to have been pictured by artists of the period on ivory tablets.

Imagination thus came to be wholly detached from reality. Occasionally, however, popular tradition has influenced scholarly sources in surprising ways. In the course of conducting research at Cos at the beginning of the present century, a historian of medicine had the happy idea of inquiring what memories of Hippocrates yet survived among the people of the island. He collected five stories and published them in a learned journal.[66] Here is one of them:

One day, a young shepherdess came across Hippocrates during one of his walks through the countryside. To her greeting he replied with this greeting: "Good day, maiden!" But when, shortly afterwards, the same shepherdess met him again on her way back and greeted him, he replied with this greeting: "Good day, woman!" She turned red with shame. Hippocrates' companion asked him why he had called the shepherdess "woman," when just before he had called her "maiden." Then Hippocrates said that the first time a maiden had passed by and so he called her "maiden," and that afterwards it was a woman who came back and so he called her "woman." Hippocrates' response piqued the curiosity of his companion to the point of anger. He cried out to the shepherdess to stop. She stopped and waited for them, frightened. Then they questioned her and, in tears, she confessed these things: she was a girl in the first instance; but as she was coming back from the cowshed that belonged to them, the son of the shepherd of this cowshed lay in wait for her next to a stream and raped her. Then the companion questioned Hippocrates, for he wished to know how he had inferred that she had been deflowered. Upon which Hippocrates said to him: "By her gait! For the gait of a maiden is one thing and the gait of a woman something else." And so his companion was filled with admiration.

It did not occur to the scholar, while commenting with great seriousness on this anecdote, to compare it with another anecdote, much more anciently attested, having already appeared in the work of an author of the first century A.D. But this time the credit for skillful diagnosis redounds not to Hippocrates, but to Democritus:

Athenodorus in the eighth book of his *Walks* relates that, when Hippocrates came to see him, he ordered milk to be brought, and, having inspected it, pronounced it to be the milk of a black she-goat which had produced her first kid; which made Hippocrates marvel at the accuracy of his observation. Moreover, Hippocrates being accompanied by a maidservant, on the first day Democritus greeted her with "Good morning, maiden," but the next day with "Good morning, woman." As a matter of fact the girl had been seduced in the night.[67]

THREE

Hippocrates and the School of Cos

Hippocrates' activity in the field of medicine was not restricted to practice. He also taught.[1]

In the absence of any public institution dedicated to the training and recruitment of physicians, the transmission of medical knowledge still normally occurred during Hippocrates' time within families. It was within his own family, as we have seen, that the physician of Cos himself was trained. Hippocrates was neither the Father of Medicine nor the founder of the Coan school, but he did manage to confer an exceptionally lustrous reputation upon this school through his teaching.

The Transmission of Medical Knowledge in Homeric Greece

The most ancient literary records contain information about the transmission of medical knowledge in Greece.

From the time of Homer, medicine was an art that was taught. The good centaur Chiron, who inhabited the mountaintops of Pelion ("crowned with foliage") in Thessaly, had taught Asclepius, the prince of Tricca, how to prepare the lenitive balms that were applied to wounds. Asclepius transmitted this knowledge to his two sons, Podalirius and Machaon. One of them, Machaon, was later to apply these balms to the wound of blond Menelaus at Troy.[2] It was also Chiron who imparted knowledge of these soothing remedies to Achilles, who was originally from Phthia in the south of Thessaly. Achilles, for his part, taught them to his friend Patrocles.[3]

This Chironian myth was still vividly alive in classical Greece. Pindar evoked Chiron's teaching to Asclepius at the beginning of one of his poems in honor of a great prince, Hieron of Syracuse, who was ill:

> If I were permitted to utter the prayer
> in everyone's mind, I would wish that Chiron,
> son of Philyra and sovereign Kronos,
> a friend of mankind, now dead and gone,
> were living still and that he ranged
> the ridges of Pelion, even as he was
> when he raised Asklepios, the gentle hero, craftsman
> in remedies for the limbs of men tormented by disease.[4]

In Pindar, who evokes the gorges of Pelion, the myth of the healer-hero remains rooted, as in Homer, in the geography of Thessaly. The first traces of medical teaching in Greece are therefore attested in continental Greece, in Thessaly. In the intervening years, medical tradition was not wholly lost in the region. One family of physicians among the Magnetes, a people who lived on Pelion, claimed to descend from Chiron, just as Hippocrates' family spoke of itself as issuing from Asclepius.[5] But the leading medical centers of classical Greece were to develop elsewhere.

The Transmission of Medical Knowledge in the Greek City-States

With the advent of urban civilization, medical teaching was to be circumscribed within the more restricted framework of city life. It was thus that, according to Herodotus, the most illustrious physicians during the sixth century were those of Croton in southern Italy and, after them, those of Cyrene, a Greek colony in Libya.[6] It is rather surprising that Herodotus does not mention doctors from Cos or Cnidus among the celebrated centers of the age. Could it be that these places were too close to Halicarnassus, Herodotus's native city? Once again, local rivalries may explain the historian's silence.[7]

This teaching, localized in the cities, still remained strongly influenced by the structures of family and aristocracy. In the family of the Asclepiads, at Cnidus as at Cos, knowledge was transmitted from father to son. There was no medical instruction organized by the city-state, nor titles authorizing the exercise of the profession as in our own time. There existed no "alternative" medicine, because there was no official medicine. Hippocrates of Cos was, as we have seen, the student of his father Heraclides and of his grandfather, also named Hippocrates. Instruction and training of the most renowned physicians of classical Greece continued to be provided, therefore, within the great families of the period.

Hippocrates Teaches Medicine to His Sons

Hippocrates carried on the family tradition by initiating his two sons, Thessalus and Dracon, in the art of medicine. If they did not acquire a prestige comparable to that of their father, neither were they unworthy of him.

The better known of the two is Thessalus. According to Hippocratic tradition, he served as physician to the expedition of the Athenians to Sicily (415–413), his father remaining in Thessaly. He then returned home to marry and raise a family.[8] According to Galen, "He was away travelling most of the time, given that he was in the service of the king of Macedonia, Archelaus."[9] This Archelaus was the son of Perdiccas II, the very Perdiccas whom Hippocrates is said to have treated. The information we have about Hippocrates and his family, when it is drawn from a reliable source, hangs together reasonably well, and probably has a firmer basis in fact than a cursory examination would suggest. In Socrates' eyes, Archelaus was the classic tyrant. Nonetheless, he was able to attract to his court many scholars and poets, of whom the most famous was Euripides. Thessalus died, like his father, far from Cos. But while Hippocrates was buried far from his native land, his son's ashes were brought back to the island of his birth, as a funereal inscription of the fourth century found at Cos indicates: "You who are worthy of your ancestors [son of Hippocrates], the fatherland, O Thessalus, received you after your death."[10]

Less is known about Dracon. According to Hippocratic tradition, he was sent to the Hellespont by his father during the plague years of 419–416, when Thessalus went to Macedonia.[11]

The Sons of Hippocrates Perpetuate the Family Tradition

Thessalus and Dracon both carried on the family tradition by teaching medicine to their sons, whom they both named after their father, the boys' grandfather. In choosing this name they continued another tradition, the great Hippocrates (Hippocrates II) having already been named after his grandfather (Hippocrates I). Henceforth, however, the name enjoyed a prestige that could only help advance the career of its bearer. Hippocrates III, as he came to be called, was the son of Thessalus, and Hippocrates IV the son of Dracon.[12]

The Relations of the Asclepiads of Cos with Macedonia

The fourth Hippocrates, son of Dracon, was physician to Roxane, the wife of Alexander the Great. He thus continued the privileged relations between his family and the kings of Macedonia. These ties, if tradition is to be credited, were inaugurated by his grandfather, the great Hippocrates, with the Macedonian king Perdiccas, and sustained by his uncle Thessalus with Perdiccas's successor, Archelaus.

In the meantime, other physicians from Cos practiced in the Macedonian court under Philip and Alexander: Critobulus of Cos was celebrated for having extracted an arrow from Philip's eye when the king was wounded at the battle of Methone in 354, and for having successfully treated the injury, so that no deformity resulted. This anecdote, recounted by Pliny,[13] strangely resembles one of the case studies preserved in the treatise *Epidemics V*: "The man struck in the eye was hit in the eyelid, and the point penetrated some distance, though the barb stuck out. His eyelid was cut and everything removed. Nothing bad; the eye survived and became quickly healthy. There was vigorous bleeding of an adequate amount."[14]

Alexander's doctor was also a member of the family of Asclepiads of Cos, named Critodemus. This relative of Hippocrates treated Alexander when he was wounded during an attack on a fort in India. Here is what Arrian says: "Some authorities recorded that Critodemus, a physician of Cos, of the family of the Asclepiads, drew out the arrow from the wound, cutting the part it had struck."[15]

Thus, from Perdiccas II through Archelaus and Philip to Alexander, several generations of Asclepiads of Cos must have visited the court of the Argive kings and practiced there. The relations between the Argive kings and the Asclepiads are explained in part by ancient bonds of hospitality: "[W]e had an ancestral guest-friendship with the kings of the Heraclids," Thessalus says in the *Speech of the Envoy*.[16]

To return to the grandson of the great Hippocrates who was physician to Roxane, he came to a tragic end in 310, the victim of his fidelity to Alexander's wife, for he was assassinated by Cassandros, the son of Antipater, together with Roxane and the crown prince, Alexander IV.[17]

The tragic end of an Asclepiad and the last-born of the Argive dynasty marked the rupture of the Asclepiads with the Macedonian court. There is no record of a Coan physician subsequently being present at this court.

Hippocrates' Disciples in the Family of the Asclepiads

Hippocrates transmitted his knowledge not only to his sons but also to other inhabitants of Cos who, like him, belonged to the family of the Asclepiads. Among the list of his disciples there appears the name of a certain

Thymbraeus, with no further details given.[18] This Thymbraeus is known in fact for another reason, for he had the rather unusual idea of giving the name Hippocrates to his two sons. They are the Hippocrates V and VI of the Byzantine encyclopedia *Suda*. This source tells us that these two Hippocrates were the sons of Thymbraeus, that they came originally from Cos, that they belonged to the same family as the great Hippocrates, and that they wrote works about medicine.[19] It appears then that their father, a relative and disciple of Hippocrates, was so strongly impressed by the teaching of his master that he suffered from what might be called Hippocratomania. Lucky for him: thanks to this illness his name survived in human memory, albeit only fleetingly.

The impact of the great Hippocrates' teaching on the Asclepiads of Cos may be measured still more fully by the fact that there existed a seventh Hippocrates, likewise a physician belonging to the same family, the son of Praxianax.[20] Prior to his famous ancestor, only one Hippocrates was known in the family from the time of its founding by Asclepius and Podalirius; after him, there were indeed five more.

Opening of the School to Disciples Outside the Family

Hippocrates did not only exercise a profound influence upon the family of the Asclepiads. Through his teaching he gave an exceptional luster and unequaled diffusion to the Coan tradition of medicine.

This diffusion was favored by a veritable revolution that occurred in the transmission of medical knowledge. Communicated at first only within the restricted circle of the Asclepiads, it came to be taught to students drawn from outside the family. "In time," says Galen, ". . . the art came to be customarily imparted not only to kinsmen but to those outside the family. . . . Hence the Art [was] no longer exclusive to the Asclepiad family."[21] When exactly did this opening up take place? Was it prior to Hippocrates or did it date from his time? No evidence exists to help us decide this question. One is tempted to see in the Calydonian youth whom Hippocrates' ancestor Nebros raised in his household a disciple from outside the family. But there is no reference in the corpus to the medical abilities of this native of Calydon as an adult.[22] The fact remains that this opening up of the school, even if it occurred before Hippocrates, acquired an unprecedented scope from his time on. Plato well attests to this when he remarks in his *Protagoras* that it was possible to study medicine with Hippocrates for a fee.[23]

Role of The Oath

The opening up of teaching could not have occurred without the master first obtaining guaranties on the part of the disciple from outside the family of the Asclepiads. These guaranties are very precisely specified in the famous work *The Oath*, which begins:

I swear by Apollo Physician, by Asclepius, by Health, by Panacea, and by all the gods and godesses, making them my witnesses, that I will carry out, according to my ability and judgment, this oath and this indenture. To hold my teacher in this art equal to my own parents; to make him partner in my livelihood; when he is in need of money to share mine with him; to consider his family as my own brothers, and to teach them this art, if they want to learn it, without fee or indenture; to impart precept, oral instruction, and all other instruction to my own sons, the sons of my teacher, and to indentured pupils who have taken the physician's oath, and to nobody else.

This oath, with its detailed contract of association, evidently was not taken by the members of the family of the Asclepiads. For them, the teaching of the son by the father took place naturally, without any need to sign a contract or pay money. This oath was taken instead by pupils who did not belong to the family, at the moment when they elected to receive instruction from the master. The contract specified the duties of the new student and offered moral and financial guaranties to the teacher. The student paid a fee and undertook, in case of hardship, to provide for the material needs of his teacher. The guaranties extended also to the teacher's direct descendants, since the student undertook to teach medicine, if necessary, to the sons of his teacher without either oath or contract. In exchange, the new disciple had the privilege to receive instruction and to transmit it free of charge to his own sons. It is clear that the essential role of the *Oath* was to preserve the interests and privileges of the family possessing medical knowledge from the moment it was made available to others. Thus the famous oath, which has justly been credited with an exemplary value by virtue of the ethical undertakings it contains in its second part, can really only be understood in a specific social context in a particular era. The *Oath* is closely tied to the revolution represented by the opening up to outsiders of a school of medicine whose teaching was originally reserved for the members of a single family.

Why did such an opening occur? According to a *Commentary on the Oath* attributed to Galen, Hippocrates decided to make instruction available to strangers owing to an insufficient number of family members willing to carry on the medical tradition of Cos, and drafted the *Oath* to this effect.[24] This explanation deserves to be taken seriously. The Asclepiads of Cos were well aware of the example of their relatives on the neighboring island of Rhodes, where the medical tradition had died out.[25] One of the *Oath's* clauses reveals precisely this preoccupation with assuring the transmission of medical knowledge within the family. The adopted disciple, in the case of the premature death of his teacher, must see to the instruction of the teacher's sons without requiring payment of them. Paradoxically, the welcoming of foreign students into the family could serve to perpetuate the familial tradition. It is also possible that the reputation of the physicians trained in the family of the Asclepiads brought about this enlargement; in any case, the renown of Hippocrates favored it, if it did not actually cause it to occur.

The Disciples of Hippocrates Outside the Family of the Asclepiads

Of all the disciples of Hippocrates who did not belong to the family of the Asclepiads of Cos, the one who remained the closest to it was Polybus. This Polybus (who is not to be confused with the historian of the Hellenistic period, Polybius) married the master's daughter, as we have seen, when Hippocrates departed for Thessaly.[26] We possess a treatise by this disciple, preserved among the works attributed to Hippocrates, called *Nature of Man*.[27]

In addition to the two sons and two disciples already mentioned, Thymbraeus and Polybus, biographical writings cite ten other names: Philion, Dexippus, Apollonius, Praxagoras the Elder, Archipolis, Tumulicus, Menale, Syennesis, Poliarchon, and Bonos.[28]

Of this list, the most famous disciple was Dexippus of Cos. When the satrap of Caria, Hecatomnus, summoned him to treat his two children, who were desperately sick, Dexippus accepted on the condition that Hecatomnus put an end to the war between Caria and Cos.[29] This confirms that doctors were able to play a political role on occasion. Hippocrates was therefore not the only physician to intercede on behalf of his country. Dexippus left a work on medicine that has come down to us only in the form of indirect accounts.[30] Galen mentions Dexippus several times along with another of Hippocrates' disciples, Apollonius.[31]

Hippocrates' disciples obviously were not all originally from Cos. The case of Syennesis is interesting in this regard. He was originally from Cyprus.[32] He therefore furnishes an example of a disciple who seems to have been attracted from fairly far away by the reputation of Hippocrates. His oriental origins—

Cyprus being to the east of Cos—suggest that in all likelihood he became a disciple of Hippocrates while the master was still resident on Cos. A fragment of one of the works of Syennesis, a brief statement concerning blood vessels, is cited by Aristotle and preserved in a Hippocratic treatise.[33]

The number and importance of Hippocrates' pupils justifies the traditional term "school," so long as it is understood that during this period the existence of a teaching community did not necessarily imply a common set of doctrines shared by its disciples, as was later to be the case with the medical sects of the Hellenistic and Roman eras. Medical knowledge during the classical era was not built up into a system any more than philosophical knowledge was. In the fifth century, "school" referred to a localized center in a city where a teacher dispensed instruction to his sons and disciples within the framework of a familial (and sometimes secular) tradition. In this sense, there did indeed exist a school of Cos distinct from the school of Cnidus.

The School of Cos and the School of Cnidus

Each of the two branches of the family of the Asclepiads seems to have had its own traditions. Among the Asclepiads of Cnidus, as among the Asclepiads of Cos, education was transmitted from father to son. Ctesias, the physician and historian of Cnidus, clearly refers to this shared family tradition in a most interesting passage concerning the use of hellebore: "In my father's and grandfather's time, one did not [as a rule] give hellebore, for neither the mixture, nor the measure, nor the weight according to which it was to be administered, was known. When one did prescribe this medicine, the patient was prepared as [one would] before running a great risk. Among those who took it, many succumbed. Now the use of it seems more sure."[34]

The manner in which this Asclepiad expresses himself about his father and his grandfather clearly indicates that the transmission of medical knowledge was local and familial. Each of these schools had its stars, more or less well known, with Euryphon being to Cnidus what Hippocrates was to Cos.[35] But it is not certain whether education was organized in the same way in the two cities. The Cnidian school produced a collective work for which there was no equivalent in the school of Cos. In fact, we know from a very ancient account that this work, entitled *Cnidian Sentences*, was written by several authors.[36] Nothing of the sort is attested at Cos. No doubt there also existed at Cos a community of doctors.[37] But we have no knowledge of a fundamental work jointly compiled at an early date by the doctors of the school of Cos, as was the case at Cnidus.[38]

With regard to the relations between these two medical communities, antiquity has preserved certain accounts that make mention of a rivalry. Not all of them are equally reliable. No credit is to be given to the tradition according to which Hippocrates burned the contents of the archives of Cnidus.[39] By contrast, a very detailed account has come down to us from Galen about an argument between an Asclepiad of Cnidus and an Asclepiad of Cos: "Those who reproached Hippocrates for reducing the dislocation of the joint of the hip, arguing that the bone immediately came back out again, were first of all Ctesias of Cnidus, his relative—indeed he himself belonged to the family of the Asclepiads—, and following Ctesias certain others as well."[40]

More generally, Galen speaks of a rivalry between the two branches of the Asclepiad family at Cos and Cnidus. According to him it was a healthy rivalry.[41] This, of course, does not exclude debate. Galen, in fact, interprets the argument made by the author of the *Regimen in Acute Diseases* against the *Cnidian Sentences* as an attack by Hippocrates himself on the doctrine of the Cnidians.[42]

Over the last few decades, the question of schools of medicine has given rise to a dispute among classics scholars, the passion and virulence of which is apt—rightly enough—to raise a smile among outsiders to the debate. It has even divided scholars who were personally close, as during the time of the Asclepiads. Some went so far as to deny the very existence of these schools. Just as their existence was being called into question, the inscription about the Asclepiads of Cos and Cnidus that we noted earlier in connection with Hippocrates' relations with Delphi[43] came to light. Since the inscription revealed—what was not known previously—that there existed an "association" (*koinon*) of the Asclepiads of Cos and Cnidus, certain specialists drew the conclusion that the existence of two distinct medical schools had to be regarded as doubtful. Others believed that the school of Cos was a guild rather than a school—a simple professional association of doctors. Such inferences rest on a confusion between the familial and professional.

Hippocratic Oath *versus Asclepiad Oath*

The distinction between the familial and the professional is plain if one compares the two oaths, the famous Hippocratic *Oath* and the oath of the Asclepiads at Delphi.[44] Though they are comparable, the two oaths are not to be confused, because they did not have the same function. The oath of Delphi, instituted by a decree of the association of the Asclepiads of Cos and Cnidus, was intended to protect the common religious privileges enjoyed by the members of a great family descended from Asclepius, whether they belonged to the Coan or the Cnidian branch. The purpose of the medical oath, by contrast, was to protect the transmission of medical knowledge in each of the two branches from the moment when teaching was made available to students from outside the family. These two oaths were therefore not sworn by the same persons. The oath taken at Delphi was reserved for actual members of the family of the Asclepiads of Cos and of Cnidus; that is, to those who belonged to the family through male descent. This group of people was both broader and more narrow than that of the medical schools: broader to the extent that not all authentic Asclepiads were doctors; narrower since not all doctors belonging to the schools of Cos and Cnidus were authentic Asclepiads. The medical oath, on the other hand, was intended to be taken by those who did not belong to the Asclepiad family but who wished to become pupils.

This difference may be illustrated by two specific examples. Thessalus, son of Hippocrates, was an Asclepiad by male descent. To take advantage of his father's teaching, he had no need to take the medical oath. But in going to Delphi, he had to take an oath to enjoy the privileges reserved to his family. Polybus, on the other hand, was obliged as Hippocrates' son-in-law and disciple to take the medical oath in order to enter the school of Cos, since he did not belong to the family by male descent. But for just this reason it was impossible for him to take the oath at Delphi and so share the religious privileges reserved for authentic Asclepiads. In wishing to construe the *koinon* mentioned in the inscription of Delphi as an association of physicians, one confuses precisely what the decree issued by this *koinon* wished to distinguish: true Asclepiads—that is, those who belonged to the family by male descent, whether they were medical doctors or not—from false Asclepiads—that is, doctors who assumed the title of physician while not belonging to the family.[45] Such doctors might have been tempted to call themselves Asclepiads in the broad sense, either because they studied with actual Asclepiads in the school or because they were servants of an art of which Asclepius was the god.[46] Abuses of this sort probably worked to multiply the number of disciples by association. And it was the multiplication of such abuses that in all likelihood forced the association of the Asclepiads of Cos and Cnidus to issue the decree instituting the Delphic oath.

Far from being a professional association devoted to bringing together physicians of diverse backgrounds, the association of the Asclepiads of Cos and Cnidus was a tribal organization anxious to preserve the religious privileges attaching to the family. On the familial and religious level, the ties remained close between the authentic Asclepiads of Cos and Cnidus, despite their belonging to two different cities. But on the medical level, these same Asclepiads could enter into competition with each other, to the extent that they had to defend the local center to which they belonged against external rivals. To take a specific example, Hippocrates of Cos and Ctesias of Cnidus, as members of the Asclepiad family, both belonged from birth to this association. On the medical level, however, Ctesias was the first to criticize Hippocrates for the way in which he set a dislocated hip joint.[47] It may be that the fame of Hippocrates of Cos had offended his relatives in Cnidus.

The Apogee of the School of Cos

One would like to know what influence Hippocrates' departure from his native city had on the fate of the medical school of Cos, and also on the development of medical education in general.

His arrival in continental Greece must have encouraged the spread of the medicine of Cos, just as the arrival of Democedes in Athens had contributed to the fame of the physicians of Croton. In Thessaly, Hippocrates probably trained other students. The *Speech of the Envoy* describes him as sending his disciples to different parts of Greece during the plague years of 419–416. But no account makes a distinction between the pupils whom he trained at Cos and those he was later to train in Thessaly. The new experience of Hippocrates and his students proved to be decisive for certain aspects of Hippocratic medicine. Clinical observations were enriched and diversified. We know, for example, that the individual cases collected in the *Epidemics* were not prior to the Thessalian period. The influence of various factors peculiar to each city upon the state of health of the population was henceforth better measured: the position of the city with respect to prevailing winds, the quality of the local water, the nature of the soil, the regimen of the inhabitants. A treatise such as *Airs, Waters, Places*, intended specially for itinerant physicians, would never have been written if it were not for this exposure of Hippocrates, his sons, and certain of his disciples to a vaster and more diverse world than that of a modest island of the Dodecanese.

The Medical Tradition at Cos after the Departure of Hippocrates

Hippocrates' departure did not shut down the medical school at Cos itself. The master took care to assure its continuity in naming Polybus as his successor.[48] The instruction that he had dispensed at Cos prior to his leaving continued to bear fruit, at least indirectly, for his disciples carried on the tradition of transmitting medicine from father to son. A fine example of the continuity of Hippocratic teaching at Cos is provided by the fact (if traditional accounts are correct) that Praxagoras, the most celebrated of the Asclepiads of Cos after Hippocrates, was the grandson of Praxagoras the Elder, who was himself a disciple of Hippocrates.[49]

Regarding the permanence of medical tradition in the family of Hippocrates of Cos, epigraphy has quite recently supplied us with a welcome surprise. A fragmentary inscription of the third or second century B.C., discovered at Cos, reveals the existence of a new Hippocrates, son of Thessalus, physician of Cos. His name appears in an honorary decree issued by an (unknown) city as a reward for his services. The translation reads:

Since Hippocrates, son of Thessalus, physician of Cos, does not cease to furnish every [kind of] help and usefulness, and in public for the people and in private for anyone among the citizens, the people have decreed: that Hippocrates of Cos be commended for the concern and benevolence that he shows for the people; that he be crowned at the theater during the Dionysia with a crown of gold, for his excellence and for his benevolence; that the agonothetes [directors] of the musical competition see to the proclamation of the crown.[50]

Which Hippocrates does this refer to? It is known that Thessalus, the son of the great Hippocrates (Hippocrates II), himself had a son whom he named after the boy's grandfather. The inscription is obviously too recent for it to refer to this Hippocrates III, son of Thessalus. The Hippocrates of the inscription is probably a younger descendant belonging to Thessalus's branch. In this case there is yet another Hippocrates to be added to the line of the great Hippocrates, one who likewise practiced medicine. Up until the discovery of this inscription, seven physicians named Hippocrates belonging to the family of the Asclepiads of Cos were known, according to the census published in the *Suda*, the historical encyclopedia of the Byzantine era. The new inscription adds an eighth to the list.

It also attests to the continuation of the medical tradition of the family of the Asclepiads of Cos in the Hellenistic period, and to the reputation that the physicians of Cos still enjoyed during this period. Certain cities continued to call upon doctors native to the island to hold the office of public physician, as several other honorary decrees preserved in inscriptions of the third and second centuries B.C. confirm. These were chiefly cities near the island of Cos, on neighboring islands or on the Carian mainland.[51] But other more distant cities are mentioned as well, such as Delos and Delphi, and above all the cities of Crete.[52] It is clear that during this period the fame of the sanctuary of Asclepius at Cos could work only to the advantage of doctors coming from that island. For inscriptions extolling their merits were exhibited in the sanctuary, even in the case of decrees issued by cities outside Cos.[53] By contrast, the physicians of Cnidus do not figure in the inscriptions of the Hellenistic period, which suggests that medicine at Cnidus experienced an early decline.[54]

The medical tradition of Cos could still boast a celebrated representative during the imperial era. This was Xenophon, the physician to the emperor Claudius who is mentioned by Tacitus. Like Hippocrates, he belonged to the Coan branch of the Asclepiads. The emperor Claudius himself referred to this family background in a speech in which, referring to the history of Cos, "he gave the names" of the members of the family of Asclepius who had brilliantly cultivated the art of medicine on the island, and "the epochs at which they had all flourished."[55] This is splendid testimony to the fact that in the imperial period an educated person might be expected to know of not only Hippocrates but all the other great physicians of the Asclepiad family of Cos, and to be able to situate them chronologically. There was still therefore a quite general awareness of the existence of a family tradition. This latest Asclepiad does not appear to have remained faithful to the prescriptions of *The Oath*, however. When Agrippina, having had a plate of poisoned mushrooms served to Claudius, saw that the poison was not acting swiftly enough, she summoned Xenophon, whose complicity she had managed to obtain: "He, it is believed, under cover of assisting the emperor's struggles to vomit, plunged a feather, dipped in a quick poison, down his throat: for he was well aware that crimes of the first magnitude are begun with peril and consummated with profit."[56]

The fact remains that this Xenophon, though he had left his homeland, remained devoted to it and interceded to defend its interests, exactly as Hippocrates had done. Moreover he shared with Hippocrates the rare privilege of being pictured on the coins of Cos.[57]

But despite the survival of medicine on the island of Cos during the Hellenistic period, and even during the Roman era as well, the evolution of the Hippocratic school eludes our grasp, particularly with the replacement of the old city of Astypalaea in the west of the island by the new Hellenistic city to the east. To what extent did the family of the Asclepiads, who had given the first impetus to medicine on Cos, continue to exercise its influence on this tradition, above all after Hippocrates' departure for Thessaly? Not all physicians of Cos were Asclepiads, quite obviously; and not all were necessarily trained in the tradition of the Asclepiads. In any case, the school of Cos lost its primacy at the same time that the world of city-states gave way to that of the great Hellenistic kingdoms and their capitals, Alexandria and Pergamum. Neither of the two great physicians of the Hellenistic period, Herophilus and Erasistratus, were natives of Cos, nor did they practice there; they practiced instead at Alexandria, which became the leading medical center of the age.[58] It was henceforth with Alexandria, and no longer with Macedonia, that the physicians of Cos enjoyed privileged relations. While Praxagoras of Cos was Herophilus's teacher, Herophilus himself—and this is symbolic of the passing of medical leadership from Cos to Alexandria—was the teacher of Philinus of Cos.[59] A page in the history of medicine had been turned. Hippocrates, however, was to remain a great presence by virtue of his work, which the scholars of the library at Alexandria endeavored to assemble and comment upon.

Writings in Search of an Author

Some sixty medical writings in the Ionian language have been passed down to us by tradition under the name of Hippocrates. They can be read in the monumental ten-volume edition published in the nineteenth century by Émile Littré, containing Greek text with French translation.[1] Despite the progress made by Hippocratic philology over the last one hundred years, the Littré edition has not yet been entirely superseded.

Between what is known of the life of Hippocrates and this immensely ample and rich body of work, there remains a gap that modern scholarship will probably never manage to fill. For all these treatises cannot possibly have been written by one man.

A Collection of Writings Both Heterogeneous and Homogeneous

To suppose that everything that has been attributed to Hippocrates by tradition could actually have been written by him ignores the fact that, despite the undeniable unity of this set of treatises, which stems from the rational spirit of a medicine freed from all traces of magic, there is nothing homogeneous about the work as a whole. It is for this reason that it is referred to today as the Hippocratic Collection or the Hippocratic Corpus.

Many things argue against a single author. An examination of the various treatises reveals differences in vocabulary, indeed contradictions among doctrines; and it is clear from the few ancient accounts we possess regarding the question of authorship that certain treatises are not from the master's hand. In fact, the oldest account we have concerning the author of a document preserved among the Hippocratic works points us not in the direction of Hippocrates, but toward one of his disciples. This account is of some importance, because it comes from Aristotle. In his *Historia animalium*, the philosopher cites a long description of blood vessels that he attributes to Polybus.[2] This description is found in the Hippocratic treatise entitled *Nature of Man*.[3] This work ought therefore to be attributed to Polybus, Hippocrates' disciple and son-in-law, and not to Hippocrates. Now this is the treatise that presents the famous theory of the four humors—blood, phlegm, yellow bile, and black bile—which throughout the history of Western thought since Galen has been considered the cornerstone of Hippocratic teaching. If Aristotle is right, what was due to the disciple was wrongly attributed to the master.

In the same passage of the *Historia animalium*, Aristotle also cites a brief description of blood vessels that he attributes to Syennesis of Cyprus.[4] This description is likewise found in the Hippocratic Collection.[5] And this Syennesis was also, as we have seen, a disciple of Hippocrates.[6]

Thus it turns out that the only two passages in the Hippocratic Corpus to which a name can be attached with confidence, thanks to the existence of an ancient and reliable account, do not come from the master, but from two of his disciples. In a certain sense, this is disappointing. One would have hoped that Aristotle had cited a passage by the master himself. But in another sense it is reassuring, since Aristotle directs our attention in any case to persons close to Hippocrates.

While we must guard against the illusion that what is attributed by tradition to Hippocrates was actually written by him, we must not surrender to the convenient and fashionable skepticism that regards these writings as having come to be grouped together only by the purest chance. An important core of treatises is doubtless due to Hippocrates and his circle—to what is traditionally called the school of Cos. But it is now accepted that other treatises long associated with this primary core have their source outside Hippocrates and his school.

Diverse in origin, the Hippocratic treatises are also diverse with respect to date of composition. Most of them, to be sure, are contemporaneous with Hippocrates; but some date from the time of Aristotle, or even later. The diversity of the corpus derives also from the various audiences aimed at by the treatises, as well as from substantive discrepancies among the treatises themselves. Certain treatises are addressed to a broad readership composed of both specialists and lay people; others are aimed chiefly at a specialist readership. Some writings take the form of notes or memoranda originally reserved for the personal use of the physician or physicians of a school; others—practical manuals, or handbooks, in effect—are only compilations based on various treatises, some preserved, some lost. The *Aphorisms* is undoubtedly the most famous of these manuals. As for the subjects considered, they are varied to the extent that Greek doctors were generalists, rather than the sort of specialists who were typical of Egyptian medicine.[7] Surgery and gynecology, in particular, were not yet separate specialties. But this does not mean that specialist treatises were not composed during this period: two large parts of the Hippocratic corpus are constituted by surgical treatises and gynecological treatises.

The disparate character of this collection was further accentuated by the hazards of textual transmission, beginning with its initial compilation during the Hellenistic period and carrying on through the medieval manuscripts that serve as the basis for the modern edition. Works that originally formed a whole, or at least a group, came to be separated into distinct treatises. For example, the series of *Epidemics* currently comprises seven books, numbered I to VII. But this ordering systematically breaks down into three incontestable groups: *Epidemics I* and *III*; *Epidemics II, IV,* and *VI*; and *Epidemics V* and *VII*. This breakdown was favored by the way in which these works were transmitted, in the form of papyrus scrolls, each work being transcribed on a separate scroll. It was also favored by the various transpositions, accidental or deliberate, that were liable to occur through repeated copying. Conversely, treatises that today form a group or a series were in fact originally composed as distinct works. The series of four books on diseases entitled *Diseases I, II, III,* and *IV,* for example, is contrived. The treatises do not follow one another and were written by different authors; one of them, *Diseases II,* is itself composed of two originally distinct parts.[8]

To try to organize and master this body of work, scholars have aimed first at separating the wheat from the chaff by searching for those works that could have been written by Hippocrates' own hand. There exists therefore a Hippocratic question, just as there exists a Homeric question.

The Hippocratic Question

From the Hellenistic and Roman periods until the present, Hippocratic criticism has been largely concerned with determining which works were written by Hippocrates himself. The modern tendency, however, has been to minimize the problem of the origin of the treatises and to study them on their own terms.

The debate over the question of authorship has been all the more lively as the evidence has been scarce and sometimes ambiguous.

The most ancient account that can be relied upon is that of Plato in the *Phaedrus*. There Plato refers to Hippocrates' method for knowing the nature of the body.[9] This account has been used since antiquity. Galen claimed to see in it a reference to the treatise on the *Nature of Man*, or, more precisely, to that part of the treatise he judged to be authentic.[10] By contrast, in the nineteenth century, Littré thought he had definitively demonstrated that the treatise alluded to by Plato was *Ancient Medicine*,[11] and made it the touchstone by which all the treatises personally composed by Hippocrates could be identified. But his demonstration was not unanimously accepted. The very interpretation of Plato's text, it must be admitted, has been the source of bitter dispute among scholars. When Plato has Hippocrates say that it is not possible to know the nature of the body without knowing the whole, what did he understand by this "whole"? Scholars disagree. Was it a matter of knowing the universe, as the majority supposes, or of knowing the whole formed by the object in question, as a minority believes? Depending on the interpretation adopted, one inclines either to a view of medicine as philosophical (*Regimen*) or meteorological (*Airs, Waters, Places*) in nature, or to a view of medicine as resting on a knowledge of the body in the totality of its constitutive elements or of its types of constitution (*Nature of Man* or *Ancient Medicine*). After all is said and done, Plato's account brings no clear light to bear upon the identification of authentic writings. The only conclusion that emerges from it with certainty is that Hippocrates' method was already famous enough during his lifetime that one of Socrates' interlocuteurs could refer to it as something well known.

The Hippocratic question acquired new life at the end of the last century with the publication of a papyrus. In 1890, the British Museum acquired a papyrus of the first or second century A.D. containing the remnants of thirty-nine columns that summarized the theories of certain Greek physicians. It was assigned the classification number 127, but traditionally has been referred to as the *Anonymus Londinensis*.[12] What aroused excitement was the fact that from the end of the fifth column there was a rather long statement of the causes of disease according to Hippocrates. Here is a translation of part of this statement:

Hippocrates says that breaths [*physai*] are causes of disease, as Aristotle has said in his account of him. For Hippocrates says that diseases are brought about in the following fashion. Either because of the quantity of things taken, or through their diversity, or because the things taken happen to be strong and difficult of digestion, residues are thereby produced, and when the things that have been taken are too many, the heat that produces digestion is overpowered by the multitude of foods and does not effect digestion. And because digestion is hindered residues are formed. And when the things that have been taken are of many kinds, they quarrel with one another in the belly, and because of the quarrel there is a change into residues. When however they are very coarse and hard to digest, there occurs hindrance of digestion because they are hard to assimilate, and so a change to residues takes place. From the residues rise gases, which having arisen bring on diseases. What moved Hippocrates to adopt these views was the following conviction. Breath [*pneuma*], he holds, is the most necessary and the supreme component in us, since health is the result of its free, and disease of its impeded passage. . . . On this theory, when residues occur, they give rise to breaths, which rising as vapour cause diseases. The variations in the breaths cause the various diseases. If the breaths are violent [many], they produce disease, as they also do if they are very light [few]. The changes too of breaths give rise to diseases. These changes take place in two directions, towards excessive heat or towards excessive cold. The nature of the change determines the character of the disease. This is Aristotle's view of Hippocrates.[13]

At the beginning of the passage, as at the end, this explanation of illnesses according to Hippocrates is expressly attributed to Aristotle. Now we know from Galen that the theories of the ancient physicians were recorded in a collection of several books, attributed to Aristotle but in fact written by one of his disciples, Meno. There is therefore every chance that the ultimate source of this statement may have been the same collection by Meno. In theory at least, then, the papyrus preserves a valuable account concerning Hippocrates since its source is almost contemporaneous with the physician of Cos. But when specialists became aware of the actual contents of this account, there was surprise on all sides. Only one treatise in the Hippocratic Collection—*Breaths*—affirms that all diseases are caused by winds inside the body. At the time of its discovery, this treatise was generally taken to be the work of a second-rate Sophist, indeed of a mere gossipmonger. The revelation caused a scandal, forcing scholars to scramble to save face. The similarities and differences between the theories of the Aristotelian Hippocrates and those of the author of *Breaths* were minutely scrutinized with great ingenuity. Contradictory conclusions were drawn from this comparison. Some scholars stressed the differences, and denied that the new document concerned the treatise *Breaths*, arguing instead that the authentic treatise by Hippocrates of which Meno spoke had been lost. That did not prevent them from characterizing the lost treatise: it displayed some resemblance to the *Breaths*, of course, but it was obviously much more rich—*Hippocrate oblige*! Others accepted that the *Breaths*, either in its current form or in some more developed form, was the treatise attributed to Hippocrates by the Aristotelian school. But they explained this away by denouncing a gross error on the part of Aristotle's disciple: Meno had committed the crime of lèse-majesté in attributing to the great Hippocrates the work of his grandson Hippocrates, the son of Thessalus.

It is clear that as much imagination as learning was exercised on both sides. But, despite the contradiction of the two positions, at bottom they achieved the same result. The reputation of the great Hippocrates had been saved, along with that of the scholars themselves, who were spared the embarrassment of seeing their judgment regarding the *Breaths* called into question. *Amicus Aristoteles sed magis amica veritas!*

Less well known, but perhaps more important, were the criticisms directed at Hippocrates by doctors who either were his contemporaries or came after him by a generation or two. We have already had occasion to cite one of these charges, brought by his younger kinsman Ctesias the Cnidian. According to Galen, Ctesias had been the first to reproach Hippocrates for his method of setting a dislocated hip, arguing that the dislocation recurred shortly afterwards.[14] Now Galen recalls this polemic in connection with the Hippocratic treatise *On Joints*, which lays out the procedure for setting such dislocations.[15] As the two surgical treatises *On Joints* and *On Fractures* were written by the same author, this external evidence raised the possibility that the group formed by these two texts might be due to Hippocrates himself. In any case, there emerges from these two treatises a strong personality, brimming with lucidity and humanity. Here at least are two works that do not appear unworthy of the image that one is likely to form of Hippocrates on other grounds.[16]

Another criticism was brought against Hippocrates by a man who, after Hippocrates himself, was the most famous physician of the fourth century— Diocles, a native of Carystus in Euboea. His criticism did not have to do with the quarrel over setting dislocations of the hip, for in this matter Diocles sided with Hippocrates. Like him, Diocles performed the procedure.[17] Moreover he knew the treatise *On Joints*. Galen tells us that he borrowed a sentence from it and used it in slightly modified form in his own treatise *On Bandages*.[18] But it was in connection with fevers that Diocles took issue with Hippocrates. According to Galen, Diocles reproached him for having admitted three kinds of fever—quintans, septans, and nonans—in addition to the four traditionally recognized—continuous fevers, quotidians, tertians, and quartans: "To which signs and to which humors will you say that the quintan, septan, and nonan periods correspond? You will not have any [to cite]."

Diocles' criticism is to be understood with reference to the theory of the four humors, to which only four sorts of fevers could correspond. This quadripartite classification of fevers had already been advanced by Polybus in his *Nature of Man*.[19] But the treatise in the Hippocratic Collection that proposes a classification including fevers of greater duration, up to nine days (nonans), is book I of the *Epidemics*, and it is precisely in his commentary on this passage that Galen mentions Diocles' criticism.[20] This external evidence invites us therefore to suppose that Hippocrates was the author of *Epidemics I* (and consequently of *Epidemics III* as well, since this is by the same author). On this assumption, his disciple Polybus later simplified and systematized the master's teaching by making the various kinds of fevers correspond to the four kinds of humors.

Such in any case are the oldest external accounts that can be adduced as bearing upon the Hippocratic question. All of them go back to medical sources prior to the Hellenistic period.

It goes without saying that the further removed in time one is from Hippocrates, the less likely it is that solid arguments can be found for distinguishing the works of Hippocrates from those produced by members of his circle or by other writers. But this did not prevent the Hippocratic question from being debated with great gusto during and after the Hellenistic period. The work of Galen, from the second century A.D., is teeming with references to quite passionate disputes on the subject. The physician of Pergamum himself even wrote an entire treatise, unfortunately lost, entitled *On the Authentic and Illegitimate Writings of Hippocrates*. A telling example of Galen's style is the way in which he reasons in connection with the authorship of the treatise *Nature of Man*. His solution is complicated, and depends on a thoroughly subjective notion of what was worthy or unworthy of Hippocrates, particularly in the field of anatomy. The first part, in his view, containing the statement of the doctrine of the four humors, is authentic, and actually constitutes the basis of Hippocrates' teaching. Galen vehemently inveighs against uneducated commentators who cast doubt upon its authenticity. The last part, on regimen, or diet, he takes to be due to Hippocrates' disciple Polybus. By contrast, the middle part, which contains a description of blood vessels, he judges to be lamentably poor, unworthy of Hippocrates, even of Polybus.[21] But Galen has simply forgotten that Aristotle had earlier cited this description of blood vessels, attributing it to Polybus. And ever since the discovery of the *Anonymus Londinensis* it has been known that the first part of the treatise was likewise attributed to Polybus within the Aristotelian school.[22] Galen's Hippocrates is frankly puzzling at times. What is more, one of the treatises that Galen is fondest of citing and considers typically Hippocratic—the treatise on *Nutriment*—was later shown to be a work dating from after Hippocrates' time that was influenced by Stoicism.

Even so, one should not reject out of hand all of the information contained in the writings of Galen, particularly his *Commentaries* on Hippocrates and his *Glossary* of rare words in the Hippocratic treatises. It suffices to read the preface to the *Glossary* or to skim the *Commentaries* to realize that thanks to the diligence of his predecessors he had at his disposal a greater amount of material than we do.[23] The philological tradition of annotating or commenting upon Hippocrates goes back very far indeed. Erotian, a physician contemporary with Nero, had edited a Hippocratic glossary a century before Galen, of which we possess a reworked and simplified version. Although the oldest Greek glossaries that we have are due to the textual labors of Erotian and Galen, they were hardly the first of their kind. They take their place in a long and rich tradition going back as far as the Hellenistic period at Alexandria, to the third century B.C. The references of Galen and Erotian to their predecessors give us some idea—a more precise idea than one might suppose, actually—of the Alexandrian philologists who endeavored to explicate Hippocrates, and of the Hippocratic works that they annotated and commented upon.

All of this brings us back to Herophilus and his disciples. Herophilus wrote a book against Hippocrates' *Prognostic*, or, at the least, formulated criticisms of it.[24] Here again we have a treatise that external evidence suggests is to be attributed to Hippocrates. There is no question that philological inquiry into the works of Hippocrates grew out of the circle around Herophilus. His disciple Bacchius of Tanagra (ca. 275–200 B.C.) was the first great glossator of Hippocrates.[25] Bacchius also edited and commented upon certain of his treatises.[26] From what can be reconstructed of his *Glossary*, originally in three books, we have some idea which treatises were attributed to Hippocrates in Herophilus's circle at Alexandria—nearly twenty in number. It does not come as a surprise to find listed there *On Joints*, *Epidemics I* and *III*, and the *Prognostic*, which the most ancient accounts assign to Hippocrates. Figuring most notably among the other works attributed to him are treatises that modern critics assign to the school of Cos, in particular the *Aphorisms*.[27] This list obviously is not exhaustive, because Bacchius's work has not come down to us. Since it has had to be reconstructed essentially on the basis of the numerous (more than sixty) references to his predecessor made some three hundred years later by Erotian in his own *Hippocratic Glossary*, Bacchius may have known more treatises than we are sure he did know.

It is to Erotian (first century A.D.) that we owe the most ancient list that has come down to us of the works judged authentically Hippocratic. This is worth citing because it gives a precise statement of the contents of the corpus prior to Galen, at the time of Nero, and moreover because it supplies a logical classification of the treatises whose order was later to be adopted by a famous edition of the late sixteenth century, due to Foës:

Among the authentic treatises of Hippocrates, some are semiotic, others are "physical" [relating to nature] and etiological, others relate to the art; and among the therapeutic works, some are dietetic, others surgical, and there are works totally mixed. . . .

Here are the semiotic works: *Prognostic, Prorrhetic I; Prorrhetic II* (though this treatise is not by Hippocrates, [as] we shall show elsewhere); *Humours.*

Etiological and "physical" works: *Breaths; Nature of Man; Sacred Disease; Nature of the Child; Places and Seasons* [= *Airs, Waters, Places*].

Therapeutic works:

—those bearing upon surgery: *Fractures; Joints; Ulcers; Injuries and Traits; Wounds of the Head; In the Surgery; Mochlicon* [= *Nature of Bones* and *Mochlicon*]; *Haemorrhoids and Fistulas;*

—those bearing on regimen: *Diseases I* [= *Diseases I* and *Diseases II*]; *Diseases II* [= *Diseases III, Sevens* (?), and *Internal Affections*]; *On Ptisane* [= *Regimen in Acute Diseases*]; *Places in Man; Diseases of Women I–II; Nutriment; On Sterile Women; On Waters* [= *Use of Liquids*];

—mixed treatises: *Aphorisms; Epidemics*: VII books;

—treatises relating to the art: *Oath; Law; Art; Ancient Medicine.*

The *Presbeutikos* and the *Epibomios* show the man more as patriot than physician.[28]

This list includes all the treatises already known to Bacchius in the Hellenistic period. It adds many others—so many in fact that the total has doubled, increasing from about twenty to forty or so. One of the chief novelties of Erotian's list, by comparison with that of Bacchius, is that it incorporates treatises whose authorship had been attributed not to the school of Cos but to the Asclepiads of Cnidus; namely, the works on *Diseases* and *Diseases of Women*. With Erotian, then, we find attributed to Hippocrates most of the major treatises that form what today we call the Hippocratic Collection. He even knew a surgical treatise that has not come down to us: *Wounds and Traits*. Just the same, his list is not as long as the one we currently have. It is missing some twenty titles by comparison with the treatises transmitted in medieval manuscripts under the name of Hippocrates. In particular, Erotian did not attribute to Hippocrates, or did not know, two important treatises of philosophical medicine, *Regimen* and *Fleshes*, in addition to the *Letters*.[29]

The optimistic confidence of ancient times, when the majority of treatises transmitted under the name of Hippocrates were attributed to him personally, was to be challenged by the critical skepticism of the modern period. In Erotian's time, the proportion of those writings judged authentic (as opposed to those judged "bastard," as they were called) was at least two-thirds, since the entire collection of writings attributed to Hippocrates never exceeded some sixty treatises or so. If one now compares this proportion with that found for example in Littré, whose work represented an important stage in the history of Hippocratic scholarship during the nineteenth century, one finds the proportion dramatically reduced. Of the sixty or so treatises that make up the Hippocratic corpus, Littré attributed no more than eleven to Hippocrates: *Ancient Medicine, Prognostic, Epidemics I* and *III, Regimen in Acute Diseases, Airs, Waters, Places, On Joints, On Fractures, Mochlicon, Oath, Law.*[30]

Modern scholarship has shown itself still more skeptical than Littré on the Hippocratic question. For example, his attribution of *Ancient Medicine* to Hippocrates rests only on an interpretation of Plato's ambiguous account in the *Phaedrus*. Even if one restricts oneself to the least ambiguous ancient accounts (Ctesias of Cnidus regarding *On Joints*; Diocles of Carystus regarding *Epidemics I*; Herophilus regarding the *Prognostic*), one runs into difficulties. Terminological analysis seems to rule out the possibility that all these treatises might be by the same author, unless a major change in Hippocrates' style is assumed. It is easy to see, then, why the Hippocratic question should have come to an impasse, and why scholars sought henceforth to reason on the basis of groups of treatises rather than of authors.

The situation is essentially this. One set of treatises forms the original core of the collection and is due to the school of Hippocrates, known as the school of Cos. This was the state of the corpus during the Hellenistic period, at the time of Bacchius in the third century B.C. Other treatises then came to be added to this core, issuing notably from the Cnidian branch of the Asclepiads, known as the school of Cnidus. Erotian's list, drawn up during Nero's reign in the first century A.D., corresponds to this intermediate stage in the development of the corpus. Finally, still other treatises of unknown provenance were subsequently added to this secondary body of Hippocratic works, yielding the Hippocratic Collection as it was transmitted by the medieval manuscripts we now possess.[31] Naturally this sketch oversimplifies matters to some degree, and fails to account for the various smaller changes undergone by a collection of writings that was perpetually subject to modification and whose history in large measure escapes us. Nonetheless, by grouping the treatises under these three heads it is possible to form a rough impression of the evolution of the *Corpus Hippocraticum* as a whole.[32]

Outline of the Principal Hippocratic Treatises

The primary set of treatises is traditionally assigned to the school of Cos. To this set belongs the well-defined group of surgical treatises. It includes thoroughly finished treatises that masterfully and meticulously describe different wounds to the head, particularly those caused by thrown weapons, and their treatment, with a very precise description of trepanation (*On Wounds in the Head*), for example, as of the different methods for setting and treating dislocations or breaks while respecting the natural conformity of the limbs and avoiding uselessly spectacular procedures for reducing fractures (*On Fractures* and *On Joints*). Alongside these works intended for publication are found less polished treatises—notebooks summarizing the results of practice that were written in a pithy style and meant to serve as manuals: *In the Surgery* lays down the general rules concerning operations and dressings in the doctor's office; the *Mochlicon* (which derives its title from the Greek word for a surgical instrument—a "lever"—used to set dislocated bones) is an abridged and revised version of *On Fractures* and *On Joints*.

Another coherent group attributed to the school of Cos is constituted by the *Epidemics*. These treatises, as we have seen, appear to be related to the activity of Hippocrates and his disciples during the Thessalian period.[33] Their division into three subgroups (I and III; II, IV, and VI; V and VII) is unanimously accepted. These subgroups were written at different times over a period that lasted from the last decade of the fifth century to the middle of the fourth century B.C.[34] Such treatises grew out of the experience of doctors who traveled and practiced in different cities, more or less far removed from their native countries, where they stayed for one or more years. In their original form, which is fairly well preserved in *Epidemics I* and *III*, these treatises recorded on a year-by-year basis the seasonally predominant diseases in a given place, with reference to the prevailing climatic conditions. They may have also included general propositions drawn from such observation, on the one hand, and, on the other, clinical descriptions of particular diseases with their day-by-day development scrupulously noted. To this group of *Epidemics*, terminological analysis suggests that several other treatises may be added. One treatise, *Humours*, has especially close ties to this group, particular to the subgroup of *Epidemics II, IV* and *VI*.[35]

The treatise on *Airs, Waters, Places* is likewise to be located among the works inspired by the practice of the itinerant physician, being expressly aimed at the physician who has just settled in an unfamiliar city. An introductory section reviews the various external factors that the doctor must observe to understand diseases, to anticipate them and to treat them successfully: first, the orientation of places with respect to winds; next the waters used by their inhabitants; and, finally, the local climate. This first section continues with an ethnographical discussion in which the author, applying his medical method to the study of peoples, famously compares Europeans and Asians: their physical and moral differences are explained mainly by climate and geography, and secondarily by political organization and customs; more than this, in rejecting any explanation by divine intervention, the author expounds a rational ethnography. The importance accorded to climate, and above all the rejection of all arguments from divinity, reappear in a brief but remarkable treatise called *The Sacred Disease*. Probably written by the same author, it opens with a sharp attack denouncing physicians who attributed the different forms of the sacred disease, epilepsy, to various gods and who claimed to know how to treat it by magical processes—interdicts, cleansings, and incantations. It goes on to show that this illness is no more sacred than others, and that, to the contrary, it is explained by natural causes, the onset of the crisis being triggered by a change in the winds.

No matter how important climatic factors may have been for an itinerant physician, it remained necessary for the practitioner who found himself summoned to a patient's bedside to know how to interpret the symptoms presented in order to understand the nature of the disease, and to forecast its evolution for the purpose of treating it. This is the subject of the celebrated *Prognostic*, which deals with the favorable or unfavorable signs to be observed in connection with acute diseases: it is here, by the way, that one encounters the still classic description of the patient's visage (later known as the "Hippocratic facies"), altered by disease and foretelling death. As for the therapy indicated in the case of acute diseases, it is the subject of the treatise bearing this very title, *Regimen in Acute Diseases*. The author begins by expounding at length upon the use of decocted barley, or ptisane (which explains why this treatise was formerly called *On Ptisane*),[36] in addition to other beverages, and baths. Throughout the treatise, the physician is warned against making abrupt changes to the patient's customary regimen.

The final group of works to be mentioned in connection with the core set of Coan treatises is one whose aphoristic form was to assure Hippocratic knowledge widespread diffusion over the centuries. The *Aphorisms*, which lead off with the most famous maxim of the entire Hippocratic Collection ("Life is short, the Art long"), contain a host of extremely rich propositions on the various aspects of the medical arts, on prognosis, on the influence of seasons and ages, on therapeutics (chiefly evacuation and diet)—all this in an entirely unsystematic way, although some of the aphorisms can be grouped together. Of all the Hippocratic treatises, this was to be by far the most read, the most cited, the most published, and the most commented upon. The *Precepts*, which dates from a later period, is a sort of analytical encyclopedia of Hippocratic prognosis. As for the oath, it was probably taken, as we have seen, by medical students in the school of Cos who were bound by a contract of indenture and received instruction in exchange for a fee, at a time when the school was forced to open itself to members from outside the family of the Asclepiads.[37]

To the primary treatises issuing from Hippocrates' own circle there came to be added a secondary set of treatises of Cnidian origin.[38] The oldest attestation of the existence of a Cnidian medical school is found in the Hippocratic Collection itself. It is in the preamble to the *Regimen in Acute Diseases* that mention is first made of a Cnidian work written and then revised by a group of physicians—the *Cnidian Sentences*. It is mentioned in the first sentence, in fact, and there in a polemical context. Galen, who attributed the *Regimen in Acute Diseases* to Hippocrates himself, interpreted this preamble as an attack by the master of Cos against the Cnidians, which is to say against his relatives, the Asclepiads of Cnidus. It was thus, too, that Littré judged the matter in the nineteenth century. The present atmosphere of skepticism surrounding the Hippocratic question inclines us to greater circumspection. There is no positive ground on which to attribute the treatise to Hippocrates himself. On the other hand, there is no positive reason for withholding credit for authorship from him. There is every reason to believe, however, that the treatise belongs to the school of Cos: it makes up part of the most ancient core of the corpus, since it was already known to Bacchius. Its author criticizes the *Cnidian Sentences* on several counts: insufficient observation of symptoms for establishing a genuine prognosis; overly precise reckoning of the different kinds of diseases; cursory treatment favoring medication based on purgatives, typically milk or whey, while neglecting diet. But several other treatises in the corpus, whose similar wording shows they derive in whole or in part from a common model, display affinities with what direct or indirect accounts tell us about the *Cnidian Sentences* and Cnidian medicine.[39] These nosological treatises, such as *Diseases II*, *Diseases III*, and *Internal Affections*, may reasonably be regarded as Cnidian in origin or as relying upon Cnidian material. The recommendation to drink purgatives having a milk or whey base, criticized by the physician of Cos, indeed appears in both *Diseases II* and *Internal Affections*.[40] As for the Cnidian subdivision of diseases, regarding which Galen gives us very specific information, this corresponds to what one finds in the *Internal Affections*. Its author distinguishes, exactly as do the Cnidians, four kinds of jaundice, four kinds of kidney disease, three kinds of tetanus, and three kinds of consumption.[41] Related to this group of nosological treatises are the gynecological treatises, which also exhibit similar wording among themselves: *Nature of Women* and the complex set made up by *Diseases of Women (I–II)* and *Barrenness*.[42] The kinship among these four treatises is visible particularly in their expository structure. They are constituted, for the most part or in their entirety, of a succession of notes about different diseases or varieties of diseases. These notes are composed in conformity with a fairly constant schema consisting of three fundamental parts—description of symptoms, prognosis, treatment—to which are sometimes added lists of remedies. The nosological treatises do not all necessarily date from the same period, for innovations can be detected from one treatise to another through a comparison of similar wording, especially with respect to the etiology of diseases. Nonetheless, this group, taken as a whole, preserves evidence of a rather closed medical tradition that is not guided by the experience of the traveling physician, as is the case with the *Epidemics*. The authors are interested less in individual diseases than in diseases as things to be codified and subtly subdivided into varieties; the diseases themselves are described as entities generally independent of place and time, and fairly often even of the nature of the patient. Nor do these treatises contain the sort of general remarks about medical method and art that one finds in the treatises of the school of Cos. Their authors seem to have shied away from the controversial new thinking of the Sophists on the arts. But symptoms are described in great detail, and here for the first time in the history of medicine one finds a description of auscultation. Considered in its entirety, this group of treatises represents a more traditional approach to medicine than that of Cos.

Finally, treatises independent of both the school of Cos and the school of Cnidus came to further enlarge the collection. These writings are for the most part absent from the list drawn up by Erotian. The most important ones are medical treatises that display a philosophical bent. They assert that a knowledge of the constitutive elements of human nature is a necessary condition of medicine. These primary elements, it is held, coincide with those of the universe. The two major philosophical treatises that do not figure in Erotian's list are *Fleshes* and *Regimen*. Their method is comparable, but their conceptions of humanity and of the universe are different. *Fleshes* moves from a cosmology of three elements (aether, air, earth) to expound an anthropogenesis—that is, a theory of the original formation of the different parts of the human body—on the basis of the mixture and transformation of the primary elements of the universe. *Regimen* retains only two elements, water and fire. One of the peculiarities of this treatise is that it presents the oldest surviving formulation in Greek literature of the micro/macroscopic theory. Man, it holds, is "a copy of the whole."[43] As a consequence, the anatomy and physiology of the treatise depend more on this analogy than on observation. Thus it is that the belly is imagined to be enveloped by three "circuits," on the model of the three revolutions of moon, sun, and stars about the earth. These two treatises are contemporaneous with Hippocrates. More recent is another philosophical treatise, *Sevens*.[44] Like the *Regimen*, it establishes a correspondence between man as microcosm and the universe as macrocosm; but it is distinguished by its ambition to explain everything by the number seven.

Two treatises known to Erotian and contemporaneous with Hippocrates reacted vigorously against this philosophical style of medicine. One of them, *Nature of Man*, certainly belonged to the school of Cos. The author of this treatise was, as we have seen, Hippocrates' disciple Polybus. In a famous preamble, he criticizes the monist philosophers, who held that human nature is constituted by a unique primordial element, whether it be air, fire, water, or earth. The other treatise is *Ancient Medicine*. Its author denounces physicians who wish to break new ground in explaining diseases by means of simplifying postulates such as the hot, the cold, the moist, and the dry. He inverts the requirements of philosophical medicine in asserting that all positive knowledge about human nature, far from being prior to medicine, must flow from medicine itself. In these two treatises, medicine appears as an autonomous science that posits itself in opposition to philosophy.

Among the treatises not mentioned by Erotian but contained in our medieval manuscripts, some are plainly quite late. The treatise *The Heart*, for example, displays an anatomical knowledge far superior to that of Hippocrates' time; its precision in describing this organ was to remain unrivaled until the sixteenth century, in fact. But relatively recent authorship is not in all cases a sign of discontinuity. Three late ethical treatises, *Decorum*, *Precepts*, and *Physician*, advocate a medical ethic that descends directly from the Hippocratic ideal: respect for the patient and abhorrence of charlatans. In the words of one of these treatises: "For where there is love of man, there is also love of the art."[45]

The Hippocratic Collection is so ample and so diverse that no classification can account for the whole of it. The classification into three sets of writings presented here is unquestionably the least bad method, for it corresponds better than any other with what can be concluded about the historical formation of the corpus, the most ancient core of which unarguably issues from Hippocrates and his disciples. If the third set is by its very nature heterogeneous, the first two, formed respectively by the writings of Cos and Cnidus, are relatively homogeneous. This does not mean that it would be a simple matter to specify the origin of all the treatises in detail. The skepticism that has triumphed in our time with regard to the Hippocratic question has also carried the day with regard to the distinction between the treatises of Cos and those of Cnidus. Some scholars deny any such distinction exists.

But beyond the differences and contradictions to be found among the various writings that make up the Hippocratic Collection, a certain unity yet manages to emerge, with respect to both medical practice and to the rational approach to disease and treatment they advocate. And without wishing to ignore these differences and contradictions, we may speak from now on of the "Hippocratic physician" in the broad sense of the phrase—indeed, for the sake of convenience, of "Hippocrates"—without thereby prejudging the question of authorship. The name Hippocrates signifies in fact two things. It signifies, first of all, Hippocrates the historical figure. But it also stands for the work that has been bequeathed to us under his name. For as long as this collection of medical manuscripts has been known, this ambiguity in the use of the name has been constant. It cannot really be gotten away from. The essential thing is that we are aware of it.

PART II

The Physician in the Practice of His Art

FIVE

The Physician and the Public

The practice of medicine in Hippocrates' time exhibits fundamental similarities with its practice today. The duty of the physician, then and now, is to help the patient fight disease in order to regain health. But medical practice in classical Greece also displays serious differences by comparison with modern practice. These differences relate both to the particular conditions of the medical profession in antiquity and to the agonistic character of Greek civilization.

Medicine and Theater

Since the physician's trade was not licensed by official qualifications regulating access to the profession, the physician had to make his mark at once if he was to succeed. The first condition of success, it goes without saying, was competence. But he also had to prove his eloquence before a public that was sometimes large and in any case fond of verbal jousting. This was necessary at various important moments of his career, for instance if he sought a municipal post as public physician, or if, as a traveling doctor, he arrived in a new city unfamiliar to him. But it was also necessary in the everyday practice of his trade. Whether he received patients in his office or made the rounds of his patients in their homes, the physician was never alone with the patient. The patient's entourage of family and friends, together with other curious on-lookers, made up a public before which the physician was obliged to perform, above all if he carried out a surgical procedure or if he engaged in oral argument with a rival physician. What would otherwise have been a private conference with the patient therefore became transformed into a face-to-face encounter with the public. This transition from the closed to the open, which the ancient Greek love of public performance virtually required, gave the art of medicine in classical Greece a rather different character than that to which we are accustomed today, and lent it an atmosphere verging on spectacle, in which even the private physician was a public man. In the practice of his art, the physician was always on stage.

Some physicians sought to profit from theatrical effects so that, by astounding the public, they might mask their incompetence. The Hippocratic physicians, to their credit, denounced such excesses and placed the interest of the patient before the effect produced on the spectator. But though they repudiated the histrionic methods of other practitioners, they did not neglect the arts of oratory and acting, mastery of which was essential for the purpose of winning the confidence of the patient, his family and friends, and the rest of the public. One Hippocratic author compared inept doctors to the "extras," or nonspeaking players, of tragedy: "Such men in fact are very like the supernumeraries in tragedies. Just as these have the appearance, dress, and mask of an actor without being actors, so too with physicians; many are physicians by repute, very few are such in reality."[1] This amounts also to saying that able physicians were genuine actors.

The Public Physician

Several exceptional circumstances could bring a physician into direct contact with a vast public. One of them, the selection by a city of a public physician, is completely unknown in modern society.

The office of public physician existed from the sixth century B.C. Only one example from this period is known, but it is famous. It involved Democedes of Croton, whose brilliant career we have already briefly looked at.[2] With the fifth century, accounts regarding public physicians become more numerous. Here we are still dealing with literary texts. It is necessary to wait until the fourth century to find engraved on stone the honorary decrees issued by cities in honor of public physicians.[3]

The presence of public physicians is well attested in classical Athens. In Aristophanes' comedy *Acharnians* (425 B.C.), Dikaiopolis, a brave Athenian weary of the war with Sparta and the privations it entailed, decides to conclude a separate peace with the enemy. He then opens outside his door a small market, into which flows—for his consumption alone—all the food and produce of which his fellow citizens have been deprived for so long. Surrounded by so much bounty, he scoffs at all the warmongers and starving people. A poor Athenian laborer comes to ask him for a little "balm of peace" to soothe his eyes, which ache from crying. "Away, scoundrel!" cries Dikaiopolis. "I am not the public physician. . . . Go to Pittalus's and do your sobbing there!"[4] This passage implies that Pittalus was himself a public physician. He is mentioned a second time in the course of the play, when the wounded general Lamachus has himself carried to Pittalus and confides himself to his "healing hands." In the comedy *Wasps*, produced three years later, this same doctor continues to excite the imagination of Aristophanes. The elderly Philocleon advises a man whom he has beaten up, and who subsequently returns to accuse him of battery, that he should go instead to Pittalus's office. We may conclude, then, that this Pittalus was public physician at Athens and that he practiced there longer than Democedes. Despite Aristophanes' mockeries, he must have given satisfaction to the Athenians since they could have gotten rid of him after a year. Almost a decade later, in 415–413, Hippocrates' son Thessalus was recruited as public physician at Athens to participate in the Sicilian expedition, if the *Speech of the Envoy* is to be believed.[5] Owing to the generosity of his father, as we have seen, he served the city without demanding a salary.

Why Were There Public Physicians?

One wonders why the institution of public physician came into being. According to some, it was due to a general shortage of doctors in ancient Greece. By means of this institution, cities assured themselves of the services of at least one physician who would be permanently available for a year or longer.[6] It is true that there were not many medical schools. The few reputable ones could be counted on the fingers of one hand: Croton, Cyrene, Cos, and Cnidus. But while this explanation may be valid for certain small cities, the situation of the large cities appears to have been different.

To read the works of Hippocrates, one does not have the impression that physicians were rare in the large cities of the classical era. It seems rather to have been the reverse. In Larissa, the most important city of Thessaly, several doctors could be found gathered at the bedside of a single patient. This is what emerges from a passage in *Epidemics V*: "In Larissa Hipposthenes seemed to the *physicians* to have peripleumonia. But that was not it."[7] Here the author criticizes the diagnosis of medical colleagues who evidently did not belong to the Hippocratic circle. Competition must have been lively. A doctor making house calls had to face the possibility that a rival who was short of clients might show up looking to supplant him by impressing the patient's family and friends with fabulous claims of prognosis.[8]

If physicians were numerous, it was probably because it was not necessary to come from a medical family or to graduate from a reputable school in order to become established. All that was needed was an office and a sign, if one is to trust the anecdote told about the orator Antiphon in Plutarch's *Lives of the Ten Orators*: "But while he was still busy with poetry he invented a method of curing distress, just as physicians have a treatment for those who are ill; and at Corinth, fitting up a room near the market-place, he wrote on the door that he could cure by words those who were in distress; and by asking questions and finding out the causes of their condition he consoled those in trouble. But thinking this art was unworthy of him he turned to oratory."[9]

Antiphon, no doubt, did not exactly pretend to be a physician. But this example shows that anyone was free to set up an office. This was truly a free-market medicine, as opposed to the state-run medicine of Egypt.[10] And while Egyptian physicians were liable to legal sanctions (including the death penalty in the case of mistakes in the supervision of traditional treatment),[11] medicine in the Greek cities was subject to no penalty other than the loss of reputation.[12] Under these circumstances, it is understandable that Hippocratic authors should rather often have expressed a certain bitterness at seeing their profession disparaged because ignoramuses and charlatans styled themselves as doctors.[13]

The institution of public physician, at least in the large cities, ought therefore to be explained less by the shortage of physicians than by the desire of cities to assure themselves of the services of a competent practitioner. It was Democedes' reputation that explains his "transfer" from Aegina to Athens, for example.

A Qualifying Examination before the Popular Assembly

How was the recruitment of a public physician conducted? As surprising as it may seem to the modern mind, the choice was not left to specialists of the art.

"I had always heard and observed that states that wished to be healthy elected a board of health, and also that generals for the sake of their soldiers took physicians out with them," says Xenophon in the *Cyropaedia*.[14] In democratic cities such as Athens, this choice was made by the whole of the citizenry, brought together in popular assembly. Imagine if we elected doctors today as we elect our political representatives! The fact remains that in ancient Greece the business of selecting technical experts in the art of medicine was left up to an assembly of lay people. It needs to be remembered, of course, that this election took place in a coherent democratic system in which all technical experts, including shipbuilders and other artisans, were chosen by the assembled people. Voices were raised at the time, however, and that of Socrates in particular, against the dangers of a system that confided the choice of specialists to the judgment of nonspecialists.

The most vivid and suggestive details we have concerning the post of public physician are given by Plato in the *Gorgias*. Candidates presented themselves before the assembly of the people, which is to say before a large audience, at least theoretically, since the assembly was composed of all citizens.[15] Each candidate delivered a speech aimed at favorably impressing his listeners. Each one probably had to reply to various questions as well. Socrates may be referring to the content of this sort of candidate address when he says to one of his interlocutors, Callicles:

> Isn't it so in all cases, especially if we attempted to take up public practice and called on each other, thinking we were capable doctors? I'd have examined you, and you me, no doubt: "Well now, by the gods! What is Socrates' own physical state of health? Has there ever been anyone else, slave or free man, whose deliverance from illness has been due to Socrates?" And I'd be considering other similar questions about you, I suppose. And if we found no one whose physical improvement has been due to us, among neither visitors nor townspeople, neither a man nor a woman, then by Zeus, Callicles, wouldn't it be truly ridiculous [to seek such a post]?[16]

The candidate therefore had to furnish proof of his ability by citing the cases of successful treatment he had to his credit. Socrates does not seem to contemplate any other necessary conditions, apart from the candidate's good health. For the ancients, a sick doctor was a bad doctor. If he was incapable of treating himself, how would he be able to treat others?

But the candidate had also to describe his training and name the teacher who taught him medicine. This can be concluded *a contrario* from the ridiculous speech that Xenophon puts in the mouth of a candidate for the post of public physician. Socrates is making fun of the young Euthydemus, who has just announced his intention of becoming a statesman without studying politics:

> This exordium might be adapted so as to suit candidates for the office of public physician. They might begin their speeches in this strain:
> "Men of Athens, I have never yet studied medicine, nor sought to find a teacher among our physicians; for I have constantly avoided learning anything from the physicians, and even the appearance of having studied their art. Nonetheless I ask you to appoint me to the office of a physician, and I will endeavor to learn by experimenting on you."[17]

A candidate who spoke in this way would succeed only in provoking a roar of laughter on all sides. Xenophon's caricature in any case shows what was expected from the job talk of a serious candidate: it was supposed to answer all questions about the applicant's training.

However neither the health, nor the record of service, nor the competence of the candidate was sufficient. Oratorical talent was required as well if one was to be able to charm the crowd and win it over from one's rivals. This is what we are given to understand by another passage from Plato, who puts this speech in the mouth of Gorgias:

And I maintain that if an orator and a doctor came to any city anywhere you like and had to compete in speaking in the assembly or some other gathering over which of them should be appointed [public physician], the doctor wouldn't make any showing at all, but the one who had the ability to speak would be appointed, if he so wished.[18]

It goes without saying that to Plato's way of thinking this argument does not tell in favor of the rhetoric of the Sophist. According to him, it is an "art of illusion," which is capable of impressing a crowd only because of the crowd's incompetence. Nonetheless, the anecdote well shows that a physician absolutely had to be trained in the oratorical arts if he wished to pass the examination required of a public physician.

The Hippocratic Physician Was Also an Orator

No speech of candidacy for the post of public physician is found in Hippocrates. The works transmitted under his name nonetheless contain an oral literature.

Alongside the treatises written expressly for publication, there exist others that were intended initially to be spoken. This is the distinction that is implied by a Hippocratic author's use of either the term "write" or "speak" in describing his work. In the treatises originally meant to be delivered as speeches, the first person singular of declarative verbs ("I declare," "I assert," "I hold," and so forth) testifies to the vehement desire of a speaker to earn the approval of his audience. The fact that both written and oral literature have a place in the Hippocratic Collection should not come as a surprise. It is a faithful reflection of the habit of the time. The author of *Ancient Medicine* speaks at the outset of his treatise of "All who, on attempting to speak or write on medicine," thus confirming that doctors were not only authors but orators as well.

Courses and Discourses

Among the treatises meant to be delivered orally in the first instance, two groups can rather readily be discerned: on the one hand, a group of didactic presentations—"courses" of private lectures, in effect—addressed to students and specialists; and on the other hand, a group of rhetorical presentations—

public speeches, or "discourses"—intended for a broader audience.[19] These two types of presentations are distinguished first of all by their length. The discourses are briefer than the courses. Whereas the physician in his role as academic lecturer does not hesitate to go back to clarify an idea he has introduced previously, as a public speaker he dares not repeat himself, for fear of straining the patience of his listeners. These two types of presentations are also distinguished by their style. Although a lecturer certainly cannot afford to neglect oratory, this is not his chief purpose, for he is addressing himself to an audience that is well versed in medical subjects. An orator, by contrast, finds himself faced with a larger public than the lecturer: the less knowledgable it is, the more susceptible it will be to sparkling displays of eloquence. Here the interest in producing rhetorical effects is necessarily greater, though the physician's primary aim remains to state and defend a medical argument.

In introducing lecture courses, the physician contented himself with a fine phrase or two before turning to the main part of his subject. Thus the author of *Generation / Nature of the Child* declares at the outset, "Law governs everything," and then gets on at once with the business at hand: "As for the seed of man, it comes from every humour that is found in the body."[20] He may even take up his subject directly, with no preamble at all: "Whoever wishes to pursue properly the science of medicine must proceed thus," the author of *Airs, Waters, Places* announces straight off, signaling that he is addressing himself to physicians and, more particularly, to those who travel from city to city.

In the ceremonial discourses, by contrast, the statement of the argument is prefaced by a long introduction that piles up general ideas and brilliant phrases in order to capture the attention of his audience and to win its approval. The most characteristic discourse in this regard is the treatise on *Breaths*. Before stating his thesis, that all diseases arise from a single cause, namely air, the author opens with a preamble on what it means to be a doctor and on the nature of medicine. This long prologue, which the author himself describes as an hors d'oeuvre, was to remain very famous, particularly for one of its first formulas regarding the experience of the doctor: "For the medical man sees terrible sights, touches unpleasant things, and the misfortunes of others bring a harvest of sorrows that are peculiarly his." This sentence, which defines with great effect the difficult but generous duty of the physician, enjoyed considerable celebrity, not only in medical circles but also in the political, philosophical, and religious thought of late antiquity. It is cited by a number of authors, Christian and pagan alike—among them Plutarch, Dio Chrysostom, Lucian, Origen, Eusebius of Caesarea, Gregory of Nazianzus, Isidore of Pelusium, Simplicius, and Eustathius, to cite only the best known.

This same treatise contains some truly bravura passages. The most famous is the one praising the power of the wind, which, while invisible, works visible wonders in the universe. Here are the opening lines: "It is the most powerful of all and in all, and it is worth while examining its power. A breeze is a flowing and a current of air. When therefore much air flows violently, trees are torn up by the roots through the force of the wind, the sea swells into waves, and vessels of vast bulk are tossed about. Such then is the power that it has in these things, but it is invisible to sight, though visible to reason."[21]

This passage was to inspire the Latin poet Lucretius. In his poem *On Nature*, he describes a storm while insisting on the invisibility of the wind's force.[22] In the Renaissance, Rabelais also had it in mind when, in his *Third Book*, he praises the "pantagruélion"—that is, hemp ("herbe")—used especially to weave sails: "By means of this herb, invisible substances are visibly arrested, caught, detained, and as it were imprisoned. . . . Thanks to it by retention of the waves of the air, the stout cargo ships, the ample cabined barges, the mighty galleons, the ships holding a thousand or ten thousand men, are launched out of their stations and driven forward at the will of their commanders."

The antithesis between the visible and the invisible as applied to the air and the mention of seagoing vessels are a reminder of the praise of air in the Hippocratic treatise. Rabelais knew the text perfectly, being a physician himself and a publisher of Hippocrates' works.[23]

Medicine and Sophistry

Stylistic studies of the medical discourses, even of the courses, bear the mark of the influence exercised by the Sophists, and by one in particular, Gorgias.

Born at Leontini in Sicily, Gorgias came to Athens for the first time in 427 as part of an embassy sent by his native city. The virtuosity of his eloquence impressed the Athenians, hard though they were to impress in such matters.[24] Gorgias systematically sought to construct antitheses, which he embellished through the use of sophisticated balancing devices, the opposed parts of a sentence having the same length and ending in the same sound. His success was such that he traveled throughout Greece giving lessons in rhetoric, for which he was paid great sums.

Certain medical discourses preserved in the Hippocratic corpus show signs of being influenced by Gorgias's rhetorical style. This is perhaps the reason why some ancient sources hold that Gorgias had been Hippocrates' teacher.[25] The discourse entitled *Breaths*, in particular, displays striking similarities with

Gorgias's *Encomium of Helen*, both for its eulogistic element, its technique of composition, and its style. These points of resemblance have led modern scholars to suppose that the author of *Breaths* was not a physician, but rather a Sophist or a kind of centaur, half physician, half Sophist, who has sometimes been called (anachronistically) an "iatrosophist."[26] This is probably an error of perspective. Rhetoric was not incompatible in Hippocrates' time with an authentic medical education.

To be sure, the Hippocratic physicians did not hide their contempt for the "art of bad speech,"[27] which is to say for bad rhetoric, which conceals ignorance under the veil either of a glib delivery[28] or of fine appearances,[29] which criticizes the discoveries of others without proposing anything new and slanders the knowledgable before the ignorant.[30] And while of course they might confess to lacking a polished command of public speaking, this was the purest form of coquetry, the confession coming at the end of a brilliant speech.[31] To the contrary, these physicians were keenly aware that rhetoric was an indispensable means for establishing their credibility in the eyes of the public.

Verbal Wrestling Matches

On which occasions did physicians deliver discourses before a large audience?

Aside from the qualifying examination of an applicant for the post of public physician before the popular assembly of a city, one of the occasions on which a physician might address himself to a large group was upon his arrival in a city unknown to him. The coming of a new doctor in a city must have been a bit like the arrival of a Sophist, an event that attracted a crowd of experts and curious onlookers, above all if the doctor was famous. To acquire a clientele, the new doctor had immediately to make a good impression upon this mixed group of listeners. He was likely, too, to be confronted by colleagues who were already established there and who would come to argue with him. In these circumstances, or in other similar situations, real sparring matches were liable to take place.

Regarding the conditions under which these competitions unfolded, one of the Hippocratic discourses, *Nature of Man*, provides us indirectly with valuable information in its polemical preamble, where the author denounces the ignorance of his adversaries:

The fact that, while adopting the same idea, they do not give the same account, shows that their knowledge is at fault. The best way to realize this is to be present at their debates. Given the same debaters and the same audience, the same man never wins in the discussion three times in succession, but now one is victor, now another, now he who happens to have the most glib tongue in the face of the crowd. . . . But in my opinion such men by their lack of understanding overthrow themselves in the words of their very discussions.[32]

This passage makes it clear that these debates were apt to oppose two orators exactly as two wrestlers were matched against each other, and this before a crowd that played the role of referee. The metaphor of the wrestling match, in which the winner had to triumph three times in a row, well captures both the agonistic quality and the spectacle of these debates. The arguments employed ressembled the holds used by opponents to take each other down. The same wrestling metaphor is found in the work of the earliest of the Sophists, Protagoras, who is said to have been the first to invent "knockdown" arguments. All this suggests that one should not necessarily think of the physician's discourses as speeches delivered before a receptive audience. Whether in the public square of the city or at the municipal wrestling ground, the palaestra, he had to confront a passionate and unruly crowd of spectators, opponents from various walks of life, fellow physicians, gymnastics teachers, and athletic trainers,[33] as well as soothsayers and local charlatans.[34]

The most formidable of these adversaries may well not have been the doctors or those who called themselves doctors, despite the liveliness of the professional disputes. The most formidable were rather certain Sophists who "made an art of vilifying the arts," in particular that of medicine. It was vital for the physician to triumph over such adversaries. One Hippocratic discourse, the treatise *The Art*, is entirely devoted to the refutation of these vilifiers of the medical art and to the justification of medicine: "[T]he present discourse will oppose those who thus invade the art of medicine, and it is emboldened by the nature of those it blames, well equipped through the art it defends, and powerful through the wisdom in which it has been educated."[35] This, of all the discourses in the Hippocratic Collection, speaks most directly to the question of rhetorical contest.

Eristic Dialogues

In order to immediately establish himself, confronted with an adversary, it was not enough that the physician was glib, and so able to drown his opponent in a flood of words. It was necessary, too, that he know the art of eristics, which is to say disputation by means of questions and answers. One Hippocratic treatise presents itself explicitly as a manual of medical argument: "Anyone who wishes to ask correctly about healing, and on being asked, to reply and rebut correctly, must consider the following. . . ." Thus the beginning of *Diseases I*. There follows a rather long enumeration of the points to be considered in connection with illness, the patient, and the art of medicine. Then the prologue concludes by restating the initial theme: "When you have considered these questions, you must pay careful attention in discussions, and when someone makes an error in one of these points in his assertions, questions, or answers—for example, if he asserts that something that is many is few, or something large small, or claims that something impossible is possible, or errs in any other way in his statements—then you must catch him there and attack him in your rebuttal."[36]

The treatise presents itself, then, as a handbook aimed at supplying the basic medical knowledge necessary to carry on a debate involving questions, replies, and objections. No doubt the author was persuaded that professional ability was essential to triumph: his treatise is a manual of medicine rather than of rhetoric. There existed, nonetheless, a medical eristics that no physician in classical Greece who wished to succeed could afford to ignore.

The author does not say how and where this form of eristics was played out. It may have been a matter of debating not in the public square, but with a fellow physician at the patient's bedside.

The Physician as a Public Figure

All these examples show that it was necessary for a physician of the fifth century to ally the art of persuasion with the art of medicine. As an important person in public view in a city, even a doctor who had set himself up in private practice was to a large extent a public figure. He was obliged from time to time to speak in front of substantial audiences of varying size, whether arguing against a colleague before the patient's family and friends, or taking part in verbal sparring matches in the public square, or presenting his candidacy for the post of public physician before the popular assembly of the city. Lacking eloquence, and a command of the art of persuasion, a physician could not expect to make a great name for himself.

The Physician in Daily Practice

But under ordinary circumstances in the practice of his art, it is true, the doctor was not concerned with theatrical displays and oratorical exhibitions.

What was expected of him most of all was competence and efficiency. Nonetheless, the way he carried himself—his gestures, his manner of speaking, the way in which he administered treatment—was closely observed by the patient, as by the patient's entourage and the physician's own disciples. Here again, the doctor found himself on stage. It was important for him to be aware of this fact, and to know how to conduct himself with dignity and control.

Several shorter treatises in the Hippocratic corpus advertise themselves as manuals of proper conduct for the practicing physician. Among these are *In the Surgery*, an old work belonging to the group of surgical treatises, and two more recent opuscules, *Physician* and *Decorum*. Various incidental remarks contained in many other treatises also warn against errors to be avoided, and help fill out the picture of the good physician, whether he is at work in his office or making the rounds of his patients at home.

Setting the Stage: The Physician in His Dispensary

The physician who has set up practice in a city naturally needed to have an office at his disposal—a dispensary, where he could receive patients and treat them during regular office hours. The dispensary was to medicine what the tribunal was to justice.[37]

This office was a much larger proposition than the doctor's office we are familiar with today. The needs of the time were different. In the absence of medical specialization, it was both an office for consultation and a surgical hospital, cluttered with instruments (many of them quite bulky) for setting fractures and dislocated bones. It served also as a pharmacy, storing all the ingredients necessary to prepare medicines, and as an outpatient clinic. A great many people regularly passed through: not only were the doctor and his patient surrounded by assistants and students, relatives of the patient probably were present as well, along perhaps with a few bystanders and, of course, other patients who had come to wait their turn to be treated. The modern term "office" is therefore poorly suited to describe such a place. The older term "dispensary," outdated as it may seem to us now, actually comes nearer to describing what must have been the reality of the situation.

The oldest evidence we have relating to the dispensary of a Greek physician is an iconographic document dating from about 470 B.C., which is to say some ten years or so prior to Hippocrates' birth. The document is a perfume vase, now held in the Louvre, known as the Peytel aryballos.[38] How can we be sure that the scene pictured on this vase takes place in a doctor's office? Because we see three cupping glasses hanging against the wall—the distinctive sign of doctors in iconographic representations.[39] The doctor, seated on a chair, holds the arm of the patient with his left hand; with his right hand, he prepares to bleed it at the bend of the elbow; on the floor, beneath the patient's arm, lies a metal basin positioned to collect the blood. To one side, several patients wait their turn: one is seated with his left arm bandaged; two others are standing and also wear bandages, one on the wrist, the other on the left leg.

Literary accounts, on the other hand, begin only with Hippocrates. They contain advice regarding the proper way to set up and organize a medical dispensary. An office must be well situated—that is, protected against drafts—and well lighted, without the sun entering in such a way as to hurt the patient's eyes, however.[40] It is on the subject of light that such treatises are most specific, for it is crucial for operations:

Now there are two kinds of light, the ordinary and the artificial, and while the ordinary is not in our power the artificial is in our power. Each may be used in two ways, as direct light and as oblique light. Oblique light is rarely used, and the suitable amount is obvious. With direct light, so far as available and beneficial, turn the part operated upon towards the brightest light—except such parts as should be unexposed and are indecent to look at—thus while the part operated upon faces the light, the surgeon faces the part, but not so as to overshadow it. For the operator will in this way get a good view and the part treated not be exposed to view.[41]

Artificial light was obtained by means of torches, the illumination from which could be directed more conveniently than natural light, either frontally or obliquely. Oblique light, according to Galen, was used only in treating ocular diseases. It was necessary for the doctor to see clearly without the light hurting the eyes of the patient. Clearly such accounts advised the doctor to seek above all to assure the most favorable conditions for the success of the operation, while also taking into account the patient's suffering and sense of decency.

The physician's dispensary stocked medicines and instruments of every sort. Since doctors served as their own pharmacists,[42] they had to have supplies of medicines on hand, arranged by type. Among these the most frequently used were purgatives. Plato, in fact, indicates in the *Laws* that people went to dispensaries to have purgative substances administered to them.[43] Regarding the preparation and storage of such medicines, the author of *Decorum* gives the following advice: "You must make ready beforehand purgative medicines also, taken from suitable localities, prepared in the proper manner, after their various kinds and sizes, some preserved so as to last a long time, others fresh to be used at the time, and similarly with the rest."[44]

The physician had also chosen and stored in his dispensary all the small instruments necessary for the most common operations: lancets (broad or pointed, straight or curved), cupping glasses (narrow- and wide-necked), cauteries, as well as forceps for pulling out teeth or making the uvula jut out.[45] Everything needed to be maintained in the greatest state of cleanliness, especially all that which was used to treat wounds: sponges, linen rags, compresses, and bandages.[46]

More spectacular were the large instruments, the various "machines" (*mechanai*) used by the physician to set dislocations and fractures: windlasses, levers,[47] and above all what was later called the "Hippocratic bench." This latter was a rather complicated machine, minutely described by the author of the treatise *On Joints*. The description is worth citing, because historically it is very famous: it was recalled by all the great physicians of antiquity, Rufus of Ephesus, Galen, Oribasius, Paul of Aegina, to say nothing of the surgeons of the Renaissance, such as Vidus Vidius:

[I]t is worth while for one who practices in a populous city to get a quadrangular plank, six cubits [2.70 m] long or rather more, and about two cubits [90 cm] broad; while for thickness a span [about 22 cm] is sufficient. . . . Then let there be short strong supports, firmly fitted in, and having a windlass at each end. It suffices, next, to cut out five or six long grooves about four fingers' breadth apart; it will be enough if they are three fingers broad and the same in depth, occupying half the plank, though there is no objection to their extending the whole length. The plank should also have a deeper hole cut out in the middle, about three fingers' breadth square; and into this hole insert, when requisite, a post, fitted to it, but rounded in the upper part. Insert it, whenever it seems useful, between the perineum and the head of the thigh-bone. This post, when fixed, prevents the body from yielding when traction is made towards the feet; in fact, sometimes the post of itself is a substitute for counterextension upwards. Sometimes also, when the leg is extended in both directions, this same post, so placed as to have free play to either side, would be suitable for levering the head of the thigh-bone outwards. It is for this purpose, too, that the grooves are cut, that a wooden lever may be inserted into whichever may suit, and brought to bear either at the side of the joint-heads or right upon them, making pressure simultaneously with the extension, whether the leverage is required outwards or inwards, and whether the lever should be rounded or broad, for one form suits one joint, another another. This leverage, combined with extension, is very efficacious in all reductions of the leg-joints.[48]

This contraption allowed extensions to be obtained that were both powerful and measured, combining the action of winches and levers.[49] Surgeons continued to use it throughout antiquity, while making certain improvements to it. Feet were added, for example, which explains the term "bench," already known at the time of Rufus of Ephesus in the first century A.D.[50] Such a heavy piece of equipment must have been rather costly. As this passage indicates, the machine was recommended only for doctors practicing in large cities.[51] It was of course possible to achieve extensions and counterextensions by other means, for example by using levers, or by applying human force directly.

Thus the stage was set—an imposing scene because of its various instruments, but also because of the order and neatness that reigned over it. This was the physician's operating theater.

Nonspeaking Players: The Physician's Assistants

Before allowing the physician—one might say the protagonist, as the principal actor was known in ancient Greece—to make his entrance on stage, it is appropriate to present first the physician's aides and assistants. They complete the spectacle, in much the same way that the extras who played the nonspeaking roles of Greek theater did. During an operation, an aide might hand instruments to the physician (just as a surgical nurse would in an operating room today), alert and ready to carry out any other orders the physician might issue.[52] But the aide's place was mainly to hold down the patient, since it was not yet known how to put a person to sleep. Thus it is said in *In the Surgery*: "Let those who look after the patient present the part for operation as you want it, and hold fast the rest of the body so as to be all steady, *keeping silence and obeying their superior.*"[53]

The aides are indeed silent actors. They must execute the orders of the physician in silence, exactly as in the theater the guards silently obey the orders of the king. They have a definite role, and become identified with it. The role varies, of course, depending on the nature of the operation. Although in some cases they are restricted to holding the patient in position and presenting to the physician the part to be operated upon, as in the cases of incision and cauterization, for example, they may have a more active role in administering extensions and counterextensions when it is a matter of putting a dislocated joint back into place: "As a rule [in the case of dislocated bones in the foot] two men suffice, one pulling one way and one the other."[54] The aides must be strong enough to do the job. Extension in the case of a fractured leg, according to the same author, requires "two strong men."[55] This was not work for weaklings.

But strength was not everything. More complex procedures required instruction, and called for skill on the part of at least some aides. Two passages in the treatise *On Joints* insist on the necessity of having aides who were well trained. In these cases, the physician's aide does not play a minor role, it is true: he is the one who actually reduces the dislocation. In one case the operation necessarily takes place in the dispensary, because the patient suffering a (forward) dislocation of the hip is laid down on the Hippocratic bench. Once the necessary extensions have been performed with the help of windlasses, this is what the aide must do:

[T]he strongest-handed and *best-trained* assistant available should make pressure at the groin with the palm of one hand, grasping it with the other, and pushing the dislocated part downwards, while at the same time the part at the knee is brought forwards.[56]

This double movement, which consists in pushing downwards and at the same time forwards to put the head of the femur back in place, required strength and dexterity. The other operation, while it concerned the same kind of dislocation, did not involve use of the Hippocratic bench. It was a more spectacular procedure, and had the advantage of being able to be carried out outside the doctor's office. The injured person was suspended upside down by his feet from the crossbeam of his house, his legs being bound by a broad, flexible strap wrapped around them above the knees, with his arms extended along the sides and similarly fastened. At this moment the physician's aide intercedes:

When [the patient] is suspended, let an assistant who is *skilful* and no weakling insert his forearm between the patient's thighs, and bring it down between the perineum and the head of the dislocated bone. Then, clasping the inserted hand with the other, while standing erect beside the suspended patient, let him suddenly suspend himself from him, and keep himself in the air as evenly balanced as possible.[57]

In these two passages the same adjective is used to describe the aide: he must be "well instructed" (*eupaideutos*).[58] From this it may be deduced that certain aides received a sound medical training. These aides are more properly thought of as assistants.

Nevertheless, like the silent characters of the theater, such assistants remained anonymous actors. Neither their exact number—there were generally at least two for surgical operations, though there may have been more—nor their social background is known. Surgical treatises typically were very vague about the identity of those who assisted the physician: "someone," "a man," "another" are words frequently used. The Greek word used to refer to them as a class is *hyperetai*,[59] a term borrowed from the navy. It originally meant "he who rows under orders," but was later enlarged to take in those who worked as assistants in other domains, such as the hoplite's servant who accompanied him into battle.

Were these trained aides slaves attached personally to the physician, or were they free men in his service? The Hippocratic Collection is silent on this point. According to the *Laws* of Plato, both cases were known:

> *Athenian*: [W]e usually speak, I think, of doctors and doctors' assistants [*hyperetai*], but of course we call the latter "doctors" too.
> *Clinias*: Certainly.
> *Athenian*: And these "doctors" (who may be free men or slaves) pick up the skill empirically, by watching and obeying their masters.[60]

This account makes it clear that assistants (whom Plato, like Hippocrates, calls *hyperetai*) might either be slaves or free men.[61] Whatever their social origins may have been, these instructed aides are not to be confused with the physician's pupils (*mathetai*).[62]

Disciples in the Dispensary

The physician's students were present in the dispensary and enjoyed the same status as his sons. They learned by observing the master or possibly by practicing the manipulation of instruments after his example. "Now the things treated in the surgery are perhaps what the beginner should learn," declares the treatise *Physician*.[63] And after having enumerated the instruments necessary for the various procedures carried out there, the author concludes: "These then are the instruments necessary in the surgery, and with which the learner must be proficient."[64]

The Physician Makes His Entrance

Let us now bring on stage "he who acts" (*drôn*)[65]—the actor in the etymological sense of the term. Because it was the physician's role to act, or operate, upon the patient. Before operating, however, he had first to make a favorable impression upon his patient and upon whomever else might accompany him.

For this purpose, the first of the conditions needing to be satisfied was that the physician himself appear to be in good health. It will be recalled that Socrates, kiddingly imagining himself as a candidate for the job of public physician, mentioned this as the basic condition.[66] The treatise *Physician* assigns it priority as well: "The dignity of a physician requires that he should look healthy, and as plump as nature intended him to be; for the common crowd consider those who are not of this excellent bodily condition to be unable to take care of others."[67] Though it is formulated in a late treatise, this idea had to have been very widespread in Hippocrates' time. It had earlier been expressed in Greek theater. The chorus of Aeschylus's *Prometheus Bound*, seeing the hero nailed to a rock for having stolen fire from Zeus, exclaims:

> . . . and like a bad doctor who
> has fallen sick, you have lost heart not finding
> by what drugs your own disease is curable.[68]

The comparison is all the more cruel since Prometheus claimed to be the inventor of medicine. The good physician therefore did not have the right to be sick.

Moreover, to the patient he was to treat and to the patient's entourage he had to present the image of a man who was solemn and dispassionate, lacking in harshness but equally without excessive joviality. On the one hand, "dourness is repulsive to both the healthy and the sick,"[69] but on the other, "a man of uncontrolled laughter and excessive gaiety is considered vulgar."[70] It was always the golden mean that defined the Hippocratic ideal—that proper balance so difficult to attain, situated midway between contrary extremes.

What mattered most, finally, in assuring the prestige and reputation of the physician was the way in which he operated. The good physician had learned his role well; he had prepared himself in advance for everything that needed be done, so that he would not be taken aback by anything unforeseen. This required memory, practice, and self-control. Nothing was left to chance or improvisation. Everything was codified. Precepts, which according to *The Oath* form a part of medical education, were not confined to precepts of moral instruction. They also embraced all the rules that governed the posture and the gestures of the man who operated, down to their smallest details. Some idea of what this amounted to can be had by considering excerpts from the admirable passage in which the author of *In the Surgery* recalls the rules needing to be respected in every operation. First, here is how the physician must operate when he is in a seated position:

As regards himself, when seated his feet should be in a vertical line straight up as regards the knees, and be brought together with a slight interval. Knees a little higher than the groins and the interval between them such as may support and leave room for the elbows. Dress well drawn together, without creases, even and corresponding on elbows and shoulders.

As regards the part operated upon, there is limit for far and near, up and down, to either side and middle. The far and near limit is such that the elbows need not pass in front of the knees or behind the ribs, and for up and down, that the hands are not held above the breasts, or lower than that, when the chest is on the knees, the forearms are kept at right angles to the arms. Such is the rule as regards the median position but deviation to either side is made by throwing forward the body, or its active part, with a suitable twist, without moving the seat.[71]

This passage recreates the spectacle of the ideal physician in the midst of operating: it lays out the scene—in which the two characters, the physician and the patient, appear under a full light—and constructs the space in which the movements of the torso and arms are inscribed, displaying an astonishing sense of the limits not to be exceeded. The author here rivals the vase painter for precision of detail. If one compares this scene with the one presented by the small perfume vase at the Louvre we looked at earlier,[72] one will be surprised by the resemblance. The seated physician, seen in profile on the vase, holds his knees, elbows, and hand in correct position: all these parts are inscribed within the space judged appropriate by the Hippocratic author. As this vase painting is prior to the Hippocratic text, however, it is clear that Hippocrates was not the inventor of this set of conventions, but rather repeated a well-codified tradition that the vase painter had already respected. The fact remains that writing is superior to drawing for transmitting all the details of such a tradition. In the Hippocratic text, the two-dimensional space depicted on the vase—two-dimensional since painters of the sixth century did not yet know how to render perspective—became a three-dimensional space in which lateral movements were taken into account as well.

The Hippocratic text next presents a second scene. Here the physician operates standing up: "If he stands, he should make the examination with both feet fairly level, but operate with the weight on one foot (not that on the side of the hand in use); height of knees in the same relation to groins as when seated, and the other limits the same."[73]

By contrast with the stable and balanced stance of the observing physician, the movements of the operating physician are lighter and more supple, amounting in effect to a medical orchestics—a sort of dance aesthetic for doctors, as it were. The doctor is not only an artisan; he is an artist who operates with his hand.

The Hand of the Artist

The gesture of the physician's hand in preparing to make an incision on the arm of the patient is most elegantly rendered on the vase in the Louvre. The Hippocratic text offers an excellent commentary on this gesture, with the additional advantage that it permits a full view to be had of the hand in its entirety, including the fingers and even the nails:

The nails neither to exceed nor come short of the fingertips. Practice using the finger ends especially with the forefinger opposed to the thumb, with the whole hand held palm downwards, and with both hands opposed. . . . Practice all the operations, performing them with each hand and with both together—for they are both alike—your object being to attain ability, grace, speed, painlessness, elegance, and readiness.[74]

The accumulation of nouns in the last sentence of this quotation calls our attention to the many aspects of the operating gesture that the physician needed to keep in mind. Exactness and precision were paramount: the physician took aim when he made an incision or cauterized, and he had to hit his target. But he also needed to take into account the rhythm of the gesture: quickness was generally required, but in certain cases a slower approach was recommended.[75] Finally, there was an aesthetic dimension: it was necessary that the gesture be agreeable to the eye.

The hand of the artist thus acquired a sort of autonomy. At once precise, efficient, and elegant, it served as a kind of ideal physician's aide. Manual dexterity occupied an important place in Hippocratic medicine. The treatise *Diseases I* gives a glimpse of the role it played in this compact passage:

Dexterity is as follows: when a person is incising or cauterizing, that he does not cut a cord or vessel; if he is cauterizing a patient with internal suppuration, that he hits the pus, and when cutting, the same; to reduce fractures correctly; to return any part of the body that has fallen out of its normal position to that position correctly; what you must reduce forcefully, to take hold of and to press tight, what you must take hold of gently, to take hold of and not to press tight; when bandaging, not to make uneven twists or to apply pressure where you should not; when palpating, wherever you do, not to cause unnecessary pain. These things are [judged to constitute] dexterity.[76]

Among the medical procedures that oblige the physician to display manual dexterity, this passage mentions not only operations such as incision and cauterization, but also the application of bandages and the reduction of fractures or dislocations. The application of bandages, no less than an incision or a cauterization, was a genuinely theatrical moment. As for the reduction of dislocations and fractures, this was sometimes capable of elevating ordinary theater to the level of high drama.

The Bandaging Scene

The application of a bandage is nowadays a minor therapeutic activity. The physician of antiquity, by contrast, accorded it great importance.

The theatrical dimension of this act did not escape vase painters. On the small Louvre vase representing the physician's dispensary, for example, patients are pictured wearing bandages.[77] But the painter has chosen to depict venesection rather than bandaging. The latter operation is represented on an ancient cup also dating from the fifth century, now found in the Berlin Museum.[78] There one sees Achilles, who, as we know from the *Iliad*, had learned medicine from the good centaur Chiron,[79] wrapping a white band around the left arm of his friend Patrocles. The wounded man is seated, his head turned away, while Achilles dresses the wound with one knee on the ground. Both are shown wearing their armor. The scene recalls one of the chief occasions when it was necessary to know how to apply bandages: when wounds were sustained in war.

In the classical period, warriors were no longer versed in medicine as Achilles was, and physicians no longer took part in combat as the Asclepiads Machaon and Podalirius did.[80] But public physicians accompanied the military expeditions of the city where they were recruited to practice, and treated soldiers wounded in battle.[81] As for court physicians, it will be recalled that Ctesias of Cnidus, who served as doctor to Artaxerxes II, treated the Persian king when he was wounded in the battle of Cunaxa.[82]

If the war surgeon does not figure prominently in the *Corpus Hippocraticum*, this is again owing to the hazards of textual transmission. The only major Hippocratic treatise that has been lost, in fact, is one dealing with war injuries.[83] Nonetheless one learns in the corpus that the doctor is advised to participate in military expeditions in order to train himself in performing surgical operations.[84] The application of bandages was a common procedure not only in times of war, however. In times of peace, work–related accidents apart, the need for it arose from the dislocations and fractures that were sustained particularly often by those who exercised at the palaestra.

All this explains the importance that ancient physicians attached to this aspect of surgery. But it does not suffice to account for the degree of refinement that the art of bandaging had achieved by the time of Hippocrates. Indicative of the remarkable attention given by doctors to bandaging is the imbalance between, on the one hand, the relative brevity of the advice given by the author of *In the Surgery* on operations such as bleeding or cauterization, and, on the other, the astonishing length of the passages given over there to binding. Four-fifths of the treatise touch upon this question to one degree or another.

Mastery in the art of bandaging could only be the result of training: the physician should "[p]ractice the rolling with both hands at once, and with each separately."[85] Achilles, on the cup in Berlin, rolls the band with both hands at the same time. But the painter was surely not an artist of bandaging himself: since the two ends of the band are not rolled in opposite directions, his bandage was unlikely to remain in place.

The first thing to be desired was that the bandage be effectively wrapped, neither too loosely nor too tightly. But physicians were not to neglect the aesthetic aspect. It was not easy for a layman to appreciate all the fine points of the art of bandaging. The different patterns created by different types of bands were as subtly codified as the figures of the dance. In some cases each wrapping of the band exactly overlapped the one preceding; in others, it was more or less out of line with the previous wrapping; still other methods of bandaging had evocative or mysterious names, such as the "eye" or the "rhomb."[86] The variety of these figures testifies in any case to the complexity of this part of the medical art, which in the mind of the public must have constituted an important test of the physician's ability and, for certain practitioners, a cheap way of arousing admiration in the patient and other spectators.

Hippocratic physicians, unlike certain of their rivals, did not give in to the temptation of abusively exploiting this theatrical dimension of the art. They pointed out such excesses in others and condemned them. To judge from what the author of *On Joints* says, the bandaging of the nose, because it presented the greatest opportunity for superficial artistry, was the technique most carefully studied by the physician who aimed at sensational effects. The scene is marvelously well sketched:

Now, as I said, those who devote themselves to a foolish parade of manual skill are especially delighted to find a fractured nose to bandage. The result is that the practitioner rejoices, and the patient is pleased for one or two days; afterwards the patient soon has had enough of it, for the burden is tiresome; and as for the practitioner, he is satisfied with showing that he knows how to apply complicated nasal bandages. But such bandaging acts in every way contrary to what is proper.[87]

This condemnation of splendid but useless bandages, associated here with a particular case, becomes a general precept in the treatise *Physician*: "Reject graceful and showy [*theatrikas*] bandages as doing no good, for this sort of thing is vulgar and purely a matter of display, and will often bring harm to the person being treated: the ill person is not looking for what is decorative, but for what is beneficial."[88]

Theatricality was therefore condemned in the name of utility. But it was also condemned in the name of nature. Certain physicians distinguished themselves less by their actual technique of bandaging than by the extraordinary position in which they insisted broken bones were to be bandaged. One physician maintained, for example, that it was necessary to hold a broken arm fixed in the position of the archer. "Where, then, is the advantage of the archer position?" retorts the author of *On Fractures*, adding that "perhaps our theorizer would not have committed this error had he let the patient himself present the arm."[89] While denouncing the ignorance of those who are enamored of sensationalism for its own sake, the author is under no illusion about the success that they are apt to meet with among a clientele fascinated by the novelty of their treatment:

> In fact the treatment of a fractured arm is not difficult, and is almost any practitioner's job, but I have to write a good deal about it because I know practitioners who have got credit for wisdom by putting up arms in positions which ought rather to have given them a name for ignorance. And many other parts of this art are judged thus: for they praise what seems outlandish before they know whether it is good, rather than the customary which they already know to be good; the bizarre rather than the obvious.[90]

A Show-Stealing Scene: Succussion by Ladder

The application of bandages was therefore an opportunity for the sensationalist physician to display his talent before a limited audience. His ability to put on a real show before a large public, on the other hand, was due above all to mechanical devices for reducing dislocations and fractures.

The most spectacular procedure was the one known as *succussion* (or shaking), by means of a ladder. It served—in principle!—to correct deviations of the spine. The humpbacked patient was first firmly attached to a ladder, upside down. Next, the ladder was hoisted into the air from the flat roof of a house or from the top of a high tower, and then suddenly let go, on the theory that the shock produced when it hit the ground would straighten out the curvature of the spine. This was indeed a spectacular procedure. It was also a perilous one. Once again the physician's aides, whose role was to let out the cable in such a way that the ladder fell perpendicularly to the ground, while taking care not to fall over the edge themselves, needed to be well trained. A pulley and winch might also be used, but such equipment was heavier and more costly. It also needs to be kept in mind that an operation of this type could not be carried out inside the physician's dispensary in front of a relatively small audience: it took place in open air before a large crowd. The physical setting rivaled that of a full-scale theatrical performance. The author of *On Joints* takes a dim view of this phenomenon, judging the procedure employed to be ineffective, and denounces the charlatanism of the doctors who used it:

[S]uccussions on a ladder never straightened any case, so far as I know, and the practitioners who use this method are chiefly those who want to make the vulgar herd gape, for to such it seems marvelous to see a man suspended or shaken or treated in such ways; and they always applaud these performances, never troubling themselves about the result of the operation, whether bad or good. . . . For myself, however, I felt ashamed to treat all such cases in this way, and that because such methods appertain rather to charlatans.[91]

Certain physicians appear actually to have staged the ancient equivalent of fairground sideshows—thrilling for the crowd, but dangerous for the patient. They counted on profiting from the admiration of a crowd awed by amazing feats in order to attract new clients, and in this way gain an advantage over their less flamboyant colleagues. But such practitioners were clearly condemned by the Hippocratic author in the name of an ideal that placed the interest of the patient ahead of the reputation of the physician.

Theatricality and the Reputation of the Physician

If the Hippocratic physician inveighed against these theatrical practices, this is also because it was in his own interest to do so. A reputation founded solely on the astonishment aroused by spectacular shows of dubious skill was apt to be short-lived. Indeed, admiration swiftly gave way to dishonor once the ineffectiveness of a particular treatment was discovered. This is the point of the remark with which the author of *On Joints* concludes his discussion of succussion by ladder: "[I]t is disgraceful in any art, and especially in medicine, to make parade of much trouble, display, and talk, and then do no good."[92]

The same physician, in *On Fractures*, after having described an apparatus permitting continuous extension of the leg, issues a stern warning against the inexpert use of grandiose machines that has general implications: "Other mechanisms also should either be well arranged or not used, for it is shameful and contrary to the art to make a machine and get no mechanical effect."[93] The shame which, in case of failure, reflected upon doctors enamored of spectacle was liable therefore to be in proportion to the admiration that they were able to arouse through resort to elaborate theatrical effects.

Is this to say that the Hippocratic physician wholly neglected the dramatic dimension of the therapeutic art? To the extent that it was vital for a physician to look after his reputation, our answer must be qualified. The author of *On Joints* and *On Fractures* surely did not himself contemplate therapeutic method from this perspective. For him, the fundamental question was to know whether the method was both natural and effective. But where a procedure that was spectacular turned out also to be sound, he was not averse to recommending it to colleagues who were inclined to favor a more extrovert style of practice. It is thus that in describing the procedure for reducing a dislocation of the thigh, which consists in suspending the patient upside down from the gable of a house, and after having stressed that this method is "good and correct" because it operates in a regular fashion consistent with the natural disposition of the bones, the author continues: "It is . . . one too that has something striking about it, which pleases a dilettante in such matters."[94]

The Physician on His Rounds

In the normal course of practicing his trade, the physician had occasion to exploit such spectacular methods only rarely. Everyday work was more modest. So long as he remained in his office, however, the physician profited from the imposing setting in which he practiced, with its impressive machines as background scenery. This was no longer the case when he went round calling upon patients who had summoned him to their homes. Entering into a place that he did not necessarily know, and encountering the patient's entourage— family members, neighbors, friends who had come to find out what had happened, all awaiting the physician's arrival with a mixture of hope and anxiety, and, in the case of some at least, simple curiosity—here more than elsewhere he needed to establish his authority right away, so that his onlookers were already filled with respect and confidence by the time he arrived at the patient's bedside.

The precepts regarding the behavior to be observed in these decisive moments are laid out chiefly in the later treatises. But the early treatises pay great attention to them indirectly. Some of them, in fact, are entirely devoted to what was the cardinal test of the physician on his arrival: prognosis.

The rules to be followed by the physician in his house calls arose from the same ethical and aesthetic code of conduct that governed his activities in the dispensary. His visit was to be prepared in its smallest details. Accompanied probably by one or more of his aides and pupils, he went to the patient's home carrying a bag—much as modern physicians used to do until recently—that contained all the tools he would need to handle any imaginable situation. Nothing was more damaging to the reputation of a physician than to be taken by surprise.[95] The treatise *Decorum* breaks down the doctor's visit into its various moments with a stunning precision, as if in slow motion. First comes the moment preceding the actual entrance:

When you enter a sick man's room, having made these arrangements, that you may not be at a loss, and having everything in order for what must be done, know what you must do before going in. For many cases need, not reasoning, but practical help.[96]

Then the entrance itself:

On entering bear in mind your manner of sitting, reserve, arrangement of dress, decisive utterance, brevity of speech, composure, bedside manners, care, replies to objections, calm self-control to meet the troubles that occur, rebuke of disturbance, readiness to do what has to be done. In addition to these things be careful of your first preparation. Failing this, make no further mistake in the matters wherefrom instructions are given for readiness.[97]

Having composed himself before entering, the physician, now that he found himself subject to the scrutiny of others, needed to act quickly and properly. The number and exactness of precepts give some idea not only in what minute detail the physician's role was conceived, as if by a stage director, but also of how many difficulties he was liable to be confronted with, arising in particular from confusion due to the presence of too many assistants or to objections raised by professional colleagues who were not always well intentioned.

Now that the doctor found himself in the presence of the patient and his circle of family and friends, what mattered above all was the prognosis. The author of *Decorum*, continuing with his description of the physician's visit, declares: "[Y]ou must from your experience forecast what the issue [of the illness] will be. To do so adds to one's reputation, and the learning thereof is easy."[98] The importance of prognosis for the physician's reputation could not be stated more plainly than this.

The Prognosis of the Physician and the Prophecy of the Soothsayer

The status of prognosis among physicians in ancient Greece can only be understood by putting it back into the larger context of the social and religious life of the period.

The prognosis of the Hippocratic physician, though it was an act of rationalization that depended on carefully observing even the smallest signs and on taking into account many different factors, showed the influence of a particular heritage connected with traditional forms of prophecy, and of competition with seers and soothsayers. For a modern physician, prognosis—clearly distinguished from diagnosis—consists in forecasting the development and outcome of a disease. For an ancient physician, prognosis had a much wider definition and assumed greater importance. This is shown by the prologue of the treatise taking its name from this very activity, *Prognostic*, in which the able physician and sound prognosis are defined. Here one gets a sense of the feelings of confidence and admiration that an able doctor could inspire in a patient by means of accurate prognosis. The essential part of the prologue reads as follows:

I hold that it is an excellent thing for a physician to practice forecasting. For if he discover and declare unaided by the side of his patients the present, the past and the future, and fill in the gaps in the account given by the sick, he will be the more believed to understand the cases, so that men will confidently entrust themselves to him for treatment. Furthermore, he will carry out the treatment best if he know beforehand from the present symptoms what will take place later. . . . For in this way you will justly win respect and be an able physician. For the longer time you plan to meet each emergency the greater your power to save those who have a chance of recovery, while you will be blameless if you learn and declare beforehand those who will die and those who will get better.[99]

The prognosis of the ancient physician therefore bore upon the past, the present, and the future alike. This definition, which strikes the modern mind as utterly peculiar, is to be understood in terms of the traditional prophecy of soothsayers. The earliest attestation we have of the form taken by prophecy in ancient Greece is found at the beginning of the *Iliad*, in connection with a disease, in fact: plague had fallen upon the Achaean army laying siege to Troy. No one doubted that it was due to the wrath of Apollo. But what was the exact cause of this wrath? The diviner Calchas then revealed in a prophecy the cause of the plague and what could be done to put an end to it. The cause of it was the sin committed against Chryses, a priest of Apollo, by Agamemnon, the leader of the Achaeans, who had refused to return his daughter, even in exchange for a ransom. To end the plague, it was necessary that Chryses's daughter be given back to him without ransom and that an expatiatory sacrifice be performed in honor of Apollo. Calchas's prophecy clearly did not bear solely upon the future, which is to say upon the development and end of the plague, but also upon its past, upon its cause. This total dimension of prophecy, which embraced temporality as a whole, is confirmed by the way in which Homer introduces the seer before having him utter his prophecy:

> . . . and among them stood up
> [C]alchas, Thestor's son, far the best of the bird
> interpreters,
> who knew all things that were, the things to come
> and the things past.[100]

It is remarkable how closely this definition in Homer of the best soothsayer coincides with the definition in Hippocrates of the best physician. Medical prognosis was thought to resemble prophecy, since human knowledge bears upon the past, present, and future, while being distinguished from it to the extent that prognosis had its origin not in signs sent by the gods but in symptoms presented by the condition of the patient.

No doubt being able to predict the future remained the essential thing. This emerges plainly from the preamble to the *Prognostic*: it is the forecast of the future of the disease that interests the patient and that allows the physician to take further precautions against it. But the physician always considered it a real success to be able to announce the past and the present in discovering, without the patient's telling him, the nature of the ills from which the patient suffered or continued to suffer. Specific examples of this particular aspect of prognosis are reported elsewhere in the Hippocratic Collection. Thus, in connection with patients who experience pain in their joints, the author of *Prorrhetic II* makes a prognosis about the present state of the disease: "If these people appear to have a poor colour, ask whether they have pains in the head; they will say they do."[101]

One of the criticisms directed against the Cnidian school by a member of the school of Cos was precisely its failure to attend to this part of prognosis bearing upon past and present: the ancient Cnidians had in large measure neglected to teach "what the physician should know besides, without the patient's telling him."[102]

In discovering the past and present of a disease, and announcing its future evolution and ultimate issue, the Hippocratic physician therefore resembled the soothsayer, although he stood fundamentally apart by virtue of the rational method that grounded medical prediction, and did not make any attempt to conceal his sarcasm in speaking of such diviners and seers.[103] But in the minds of ordinary people, the resemblance must have seemed all the more natural since they were accustomed to hearing in the theater of mythic physicians or physician gods who were seers as well: Apollo of Delphi, in particular, was both a physician and a seer.[104] The words of the human physician who uttered a prognosis could therefore easily become words of prophecy in the public mind, arousing astonishment and admiration.

Spectacular Prognostications

Physicians understood this, and did not fail to seek ways to make a name for themselves by means of extraordinary prognostications that were worthy of prophecy. "There are reports of physicians making frequent, true and marvellous predictions, predictions such as I have never made myself, nor personally heard anyone else make," declares the author of *Prorrhetic II* at the outset of the treatise, which is devoted entirely to prognosis. He gives a whole series of examples, the first of which are as follows:

A person seems to be mortally ill both to the physician attending him and to others who see him, but a different physician comes in and says that the patient will not die, but go blind in both eyes. In another case where the person looked in a very poor state, the physician that came in foretold that he would recover, but be disabled in one arm; to another person who was apparently not going to survive, one said that he would recover, but that his toes would become black and gangrenous.[105]

One sees here how a physician who was short of clients made predictions that were reassuring and surprising at the same time, in order to win the confidence of the patient and his entourage, and to supplant rival colleagues. In desperate cases he played on two quite human feelings at once, the longing for hope and fascination before the unexpected.

Such extraordinary prognostications were condemned by the Hippocratic physician who reported them in *Prorrhetic II*: "I, however, shall not prophesy anything like this; rather I record the clinical signs from which one must deduce which persons will become well and which will die, and which will recover or die in a short or a long time."[106] In singling out spectacular prognoses, which he denounces by the term "divinations," the author makes it clear that he likens them to the oracles of soothsayers. He condemns them because they do not rest on observation of the signs of disease. If he warns against such ostentatious prognostications, this is because they can be turned against their authors: "I advise you to be as cautious as possible not only in other areas of medicine, but also in making predictions of this kind, taking into account that when you are successful in making a prediction you will be admired by the patient you are attending, but when you go wrong you will not only be subject to hatred, but perhaps even be thought mad."[107]

While ruling out the use of predictions of this sort in his own practice, however, as well as warning against the dangers they carry for the reputation of the practitioner, the Hippocratic author admits that they can be made, so long as they are founded on medical knowledge: "But anyone who desires to win such successes should make predictions only after learning about all these details; it is indeed possible from what is written to foretell death, or madness, or good health."[108]

In sum, the position of the author of *Prorrhetics II* with regard to extraordinary predictions matches that of the author of *On Joints* with regard to spectacular operations. In both treatises, the Hippocratic physicians accept compromise with the partisans of theatrical methods, if necessary, so long as the methods used to produce astonishment on the part of their audience are in contradiction neither with the interest of the patient nor with the requirements of the medical art.

Correct Prognosis and Just Admiration

What Hippocratic physicians sought most of all was accuracy in prognosis. For nothing could more effectively help build a lasting reputation than a clear and precise prognosis that turned out to be correct.

It was by means of such prognoses that the physician "will justly win respect and be an able physician," as the author of the *Prognostic* notes in his prologue. If the author feels the need to qualify the phrase "win respect" by the adverb "justly," this is because ordinarily in the Hippocratic Collection the feeling of astonishment or admiration was what ignorant charlatans elicited by means of disreputably spectacular methods. For the Hippocratic author it was a question of admiration for the knowledge of the true physician—this admiration going hand in hand with the confidence that would subsequently be placed in him by the patient. From Plato's *Gorgias* we know how difficult it was for a physician to win the patient's confidence.[109]

The pride felt by the Hippocratic physician whose prognosis proved to be correct comes through in even the most objective accounts. Here, for example, is a case study relating the fate of a naval commander, part of whose hand was crushed by the ship's anchor:

Inflammation developed, gangrene, and fever. He was purged moderately. Mild fevers and pain. Part of the finger fell away. After the seventh day satisfactory serum came out. After that, problems with the tongue: he said he could not articulate everything. Prediction made: that *opisthotonos* [a type of tetanus] would come. His jaws became fixed together, then it went to the neck, on the third day he was entirely convulsed backward, with sweating. On the sixth day after the prediction he died.[110]

In keeping with the practice followed in these case studies, the development of the illness is narrated with reference to the number of days that had passed since the onset of the condition. The moment when a prognosis that subsequently turned out to be accurate was actually made was of such importance, however, that it was treated as a new starting point from which the days of the illness were to be counted all over again. The day of the patient's death was in fact calculated from the time of the prognosis, and not from the beginning of the illness.

The physician's satisfaction was surely still more keen if his prognosis was borne out in spite of going against the generally accepted forecast. This scenario is attested in another case study written by the same author:

At the siege of Datum [358–357 B.C.], Tychon was struck in the chest by a catapult. Shortly later he was overcome by a raucous laughter. It appeared to me that the physician who removed the wood left part of the shaft in the diaphragm, and the patient thought so. The physician gave him an enema towards evening and a drug by the bowel. He spent the first night in discomfort. At daybreak he seemed to the physician and others to be better. Prediction: spasms would come on and he would die quickly. On the subsequent night, discomfort, sleeplessness. He lay on his stomach for the most part. Convulsions began with daybreak the third day and he died at midday.[111]

Although the case is reported here without commentary, the details are precise enough to allow the scene of the prognosis to be reconstructed. The Hippocratic author, who was not the physician attending the injured man, had the courage to make a pessimistic prognosis that was opposed not only to the opinion of his colleague but also to the prevailing consensus. Now we know how perilous it was for a physician to find himself alone against everyone else. The author of *On Joints* confesses that he very nearly lost his reputation in a dispute of this kind.[112] It is easy then to imagine the physician's satisfaction, and relief, when his prognosis came true in spite of the contrary opinion of practitioners and laymen alike—with the patient's death.

The discretion of the physician in this case is nevertheless remarkable: the facts are left to speak for themselves. Another Hippocratic author displays somewhat less restraint in making a prognosis that was every bit as awkward from the point of view of the patient: "[I]f a convulsion does occur in such a patient, death is to be expected—this is a splendid prognosis to make."[113] To be sure, the translation of this passage renders only the aesthetic aspect of such things. For to the Greek mind the beautiful was also the good. An elegant prognosis was also a good prognosis, one that was sure to be realized. Leaving aside the fact that the two things coincided in this case, the fact remains that its beauty was thought to eclipse the sad fate of the patient.

Speed of Prognosis; Prognosis at a Distance

The skill of the good physician did not consist only in making a correct prognosis on seeing the patient for the first time. It was necessary, too, that the prognosis should be made rapidly. Deliberateness in examination seems not to have been valued. When the author of *The Art*,[114] in his defense of medicine, declares that slowness in the examination of hidden illnesses is the fault not of those who treat them, but due to the nature of the patient and of the illness, it is obvious that he is replying to an accusation of unwarranted delay brought against the physician. In the best case, an immediate verdict could be delivered, which would have the effect of calming the impatience of the patient's entourage and possibly of preempting rivals as well.

This is the reason provision was made in certain cases for prognosis at a distance, prior to laying hands upon the patient. This method is plainly attested in the surgical treatise *On Wounds in the Head*:

> The first thing to look for in the wounded man is whereabouts in the head the wound is, whether in the stronger or weaker part, and to examine the hair about the lesion, whether it has been cut through by the weapon and gone into the wound. If this is so, declare that it is likely that the bone is denuded of flesh and injured in some way by the weapon. One should say this *at first inspection, without touching the patient*. It is while handling the patient that you should try to make sure whether the bone is denuded of flesh or not.[115]

In this passage, it is explicitly recommended that the physician make a preliminary prognosis about the present state of the wound and its apparent degree of seriousness, before even touching the injured man. It hardly seems likely that such a prognosis could have been useful for purposes of medical investigation, since the physician was obliged to determine if what he asserted was in fact the case by touching the patient immediately afterwards. This form of prognosis appears therefore to have been justified only by the physician's desire to give the patient and his entourage immediate proof of his competence, in predicting from a distance what would then be confirmed by close examination, and thus preparing the way for an initial success.

This method of prognosis at a distance was applied not only in the presence of an injured person. When the physician arrived at the bedside of a patient suffering from acute illness, he needed also to begin by observing remotely visible signs. The order in which the author of the *Prognostic* states his recommendations suggests as much: "In acute diseases the physician must conduct his inquiries in the following way. First he must examine the face of the patient, and see whether it is like the faces of healthy people, and especially whether it is like its usual self. Such likeness will be the usual sign, and the greatest unlikeness will be the most dangerous sign."[116] After observing the face, the physician will observe the position of the patient in his bed, the movements of his hands, his breathing, his perspiration—everything that can be detected by remote examination. It is only from the moment when the examination must focus on the hypochondrium that the physician draws near to the patient to palpate him.

Prognosis of Incurable Cases and Refusal of Treatment

In some cases, the observation of the sick or injured person from a distance, prior to intimate examination, constituted a decisive moment for the physician as well as for the patient, the importance of which may be difficult for the modern mind to grasp. For a prognosis based on remote observation could lead the physician to take the critical decision of not treating a patient he judged to be incurable.

This decision, which may seem shocking to a modern sensibility, was not something exceptional in ancient medicine. In Egypt it was actually an integral part of prognosis. Egyptian medical writings were divided into three parts: semiology, prognosis, therapeutics. The middle part dealing with prognosis often contained an indication whether the patient should be treated or not. The situation was rather different in Greek medicine. Although the Cnidian nosological treatises exhibit similarities with their Egyptian counterparts so far as the expository schema of an illness is concerned, the part having to do with prognosis typically did not address the question of whether or not to treat it, with two exceptions. One involved a condition of the lung. Following the description of symptoms, this prognosis is given: "If the hair is falling out of the head, which is already on the point of becoming bald from the disease, and if, when the patient spits on to coals, his sputum has a heavy odour, [say] that he is about to die before long. . . . When the case is such, do not treat this patient."[117] The other involved a female complaint, the formation of a uteral mole: "As far as possible do not treat such a case; and if one treats it, give warning."[118]

These are the only two such passages to be found in the Cnidian nosological writings. Otherwise a treatment is indicated, even when the illness is called "mortal." The prohibition against treatment is therefore entirely exceptional in the Cnidian tradition, by contrast with Egyptian medicine.

Nonetheless there exist other accounts in the *Corpus Hippocraticum* about this practice, which cast a shadow on the reputation of Greek medicine. In the case of injuries, one Hippocratic physician,[119] who otherwise gives sensible recommendations that modern practitioners would approve, suggests not assuming responsibility for treatment if the injured person is unconscious and cannot actively take part in the treatment. Such a person, whose only fault was being unconscious and so unable to assist the physician, was unfortunate indeed!

Already by Hippocrates' time voices were being raised against practices of this sort, reproaching physicians who "undertake cases which would cure themselves, [whereas] they do not touch those where great help is necessary."[120] It is true that such criticisms seem to have been motivated less by a desire to defend the rights of the patient than to attack medicine and to show that it was not a science. "If the art existed," these opponents contended, "it ought to cure all alike."[121]

The vehemence with which the Hippocratic author of *The Art* refutes these critics comes as rather a surprise. He frankly accuses them of ignorance and madness: "For if a man demand from an art a power over what does not belong to the art, or from nature a power over what does not belong to nature, his ignorance is more allied to madness than to lack of knowledge."[122]

We should make a special effort to understand what moved the author to speak out so violently against a position that seems to us today to be justified. For the Hippocratic physician, it was indeed a question of life or death—of medicine. It needs to be kept in mind that the prohibition against treating incurable cases belonged in his view to the very definition of the medical art. At the outset of his treatise he declares: "First I will define what I conceive medicine to be. In general terms, it is to do away with the sufferings of the sick, to lessen the violence of their diseases, and to refuse to treat those who are overmastered by their diseases, realizing that in such cases medicine is powerless."[123]

This definition is not lacking in either greatness or subtlety in its first part, where the author has the patient in mind, and where he makes a distinction between complete and relative healing. But the prohibition that comes at the end is troubling.

The Hippocratic author was not alone in antiquity in holding this view, however. Plato subscribes to it in the *Republic*, and actually generalizes it. Comparing the able sea pilot with the good physician, he argues that this refusal to undertake the impossible is valid for all the arts: "[Like a] first-rate captain or doctor, for example, [a clever craftsman] knows the difference between what his craft can and can't do. He attempts the first but lets the second go by."[124]

In the Hellenistic era, this opinion was shared by Herophilus, one of the two most famous physicians of the period. When asked for his definition of the perfect physician, he replied: "He who is capable of distinguishing between the possible and the impossible."[125] Galen, in the Roman era, adopted the very same language of the Hippocratic treatise on the medical art in maintaining that the physician must not treat patients overcome by illness.[126]

This prohibition against treating those cases judged incurable rests finally on theoretical presuppositions that seem foreign to the modern mind. One was asked to suppose, in effect, that the art of medicine was wholly known and that its field of application was limited once and for all, as though it were altogether ruled out that progress might be made in devising new methods of treatment that could push back the limits of what was curable. The domain of the incurable, lying outside the art, became instead a sort of taboo justified in the name of reason. Are we to regard this as a rationalization of the ancient conception according to which a prohibition against treatment could be explained by the belief that the patient had been condemned by divine will? The various texts we have are so different that it is hard to say.

In any case, this view of the incurable as standing outside the physician's field of investigation did indeed function in effect as a taboo among medical practitioners. One of the great physicians whose work is preserved in the Hippocratic Collection felt the need to justify his dwelling on cases that were judged incurable, in particular ones involving people who had been permanently disabled by the failure to reduce a dislocation backwards of the thigh:

One might say that such matters are outside the healing art. Why, forsooth, trouble one's mind further about cases which have become incurable? This is far from the right attitude. The investigation of these matters too belongs to the same science; it is impossible to separate them from one another. In curable cases we must contrive ways to prevent their becoming incurable, studying the best means for hindering their advance to incurability; while one must study incurable cases so as to avoid doing harm by useless efforts.[127]

Evidently, then, there were differences of opinion among Hippocratic physicians on the issue of curable versus incurable. Not all endorsed the theoretical requirements of the author of *The Art*. Some believed in the possibility of progress in medicine.[128] Others did not bother themselves with theory. One even went so far as to see in hopeless cases the best opportunity for providing evidence of audacity in treatment: "In any of the dangerous diseases you take on, you must accept some degree of risk: for if you are lucky, you will make the patient well, but if you fail, he only suffers what was likely to have happened anyway."[129] By his boldness, this practitioner must have seemed a daredevil in the eyes of the learned theoreticians of the age, who knew well how to decide between the curable and the incurable.

In practice, at the moment when he had to decide whether or not to give up treating a patient, the physician found himself faced with a dilemma from which it was very difficult for him to escape. The author of *On Fractures* states this dilemma very clearly in the case of compound fractures of the femur or humerus, from which he says very few patients recover: "One should especially avoid such cases if one has a respectable excuse, for the favourable chances are few, and the risks many. Besides, if a man does not reduce the fracture, he will be thought unskilful, while if he does reduce it he will bring the patient nearer to death than to recovery."[130]

This was a terrible moment for the physician: he had entered into an impossible role—committed himself to an unwinnable battle—and so had now to contrive a way out for himself, an honorable retreat. In a flash, immediately upon making a first prognosis about the condition of the patient, he had to make a second prognosis regarding his own situation. Could he withdraw without doing harm to his reputation or not? The precarious position of the physician in antiquity consisted in just this: as a public figure he was the prisoner of the judgment of the public—a public that was sometimes demanding, ignorant, and unpredictable, capable of making or unmaking reputations, and of hurling against the physician the supreme accusation: "He does not know the art!" It does not come as a surprise, therefore, that in the *Gorgias* Plato should have imagined a physician judged by a tribunal of children who in the end prefer a cook to him.

The paradox is that at a time when the responsibilities of the physician were not yet codified by law, and professional malpractice went unpunished, the medical practitioner risked a harsher and more irrational penalty than any legal sanction—social censure. To avoid its consequences, the physician was obliged on occasion to resort to cunning, to resign himself to "noble flight." In surrendering himself to so untheatrical a gesture, a gesture so at variance with the heroic ideal, the physician may seem to have fled from the battle against illness, throwing down his arms in the face of danger and uncertainty.

But such flight was indeed noble because it was justified by a higher ideal. The real grandeur of the physician consisted in just this. If the author of *On Fractures* elected to shirk responsibility in certain cases, it was in the last analysis less out of concern for his own reputation than for the well-being of the patient. Intervention risked bringing the patient "nearer to death than to recovery." But that would have been contrary to the ethic that until our own day has continued to be the glory of the Hippocratic physician and the true source of his nobility—an ethic whose object is neither the reputation of the physician nor even the art of medicine, but, quite simply, the patient.

SIX

The Physician and the Patient

Who were the patients whom the Hippocratic physician treated? What was the relation between physician and patient in the Hippocratic Collection?

Slaves and Free Men

Reading the account given by Plato in the *Laws*, one wonders whether in Hippocrates' time slaves who fell ill were treated by the same doctors as free men. There Plato contrasts a free medicine, available to free men, with a slave medicine in which physicians' assistants, who may themselves have been either free men or slaves, treated slaves. According to Plato, these two medicines were distinguished not only by the social origin of their patients but also by the medical methods applied:

> *Athenian*: . . . we usually speak, I think, of doctors and doctors' assistants, but of course we call the latter "doctors" too.
>
> *Clinias*: Certainly.
>
> *Athenian*: And these "doctors" (who may be free men or slaves) pick up the skill empirically, by watching and obeying their masters; they've no systematic knowledge such as the free doctors have learned for themselves and pass on to their pupils. . . . A state's invalids include not only free men but slaves too, who are almost always treated by other slaves who either rush about on flying visits or wait to be consulted in their surgeries. This kind of doctor never gives any account of the particular illness of the individual slave, or is prepared to listen to one; he simply prescribes what he thinks best in the light of experience, as if he had precise knowledge, and with the self-confidence of a dictator. Then he dashes off on his way to the next slave-patient, and so takes off his

master's shoulders some of the work of attending the sick. The visits of the free doctor, by contrast, are mostly concerned with treating the illnesses of free men; *his* method is to construct an empirical case-history by consulting the invalid and his friends; in this way he himself learns something from the sick and at the same time he gives the individual patient all the instruction he can. He gives no prescription until he has somehow gained the invalid's consent.[1]

In this passage, Plato's intent is not to faithfully describe the state of medicine during his time, but to set up a contrast between the good physician and the bad physician that he could then use to bring out the differences between the good legislator and the bad legislator. His account must be used with caution, therefore, since the broader purpose to which it is put slants, to some degree, the picture he presents. Nonetheless, Plato was not at liberty to construct so selective a view of everyday life that it was wholly at variance with daily reality. The text above can certainly be regarded as providing us with reliable information about how medicine was organized during the classical period, so long as we are careful to make allowances for its role as part of a larger argument. According to Plato, physicians had available to them assistants, slaves and free men both, whom they trained on the job. These assistants might from time to time treat a clientele that was composed for the most part of slaves, whether in their master's dispensary or on a visiting basis. As for the physicians themselves, they had learned their trade from their fathers and generally had a clientele of free men and women, though Plato indicates that they were known to treat slaves as well.

If one now compares Plato's text with those that bear upon the subject in the Hippocratic corpus, one meets with no major contradiction, but the accounts given there cast a quite different light. In Hippocrates, one does not find physicians' assistants ministering to a particular clientele. The only instance of a physician delegating his powers occurs in a later treatise that mentions not a physician's assistant, but rather a student, and an advanced one at that, whom the physician left behind in a patient's home to supervise the proper dosage of medication and possibly also to complete the treatment, but in any case to inform the physician of what went on in the interval between his visits.[2] When the physician's assistants are mentioned, it is clear they are strictly assistants and nothing more, working under the orders of the physician. Even so, the silence of Hippocratic authors on this point should not cause us totally to doubt Plato's account. The physician's assistants surely were allowed to treat slaves from time to time. However, in saying that these assistants were also called physicians, Plato played upon a confusion that may have existed in the mind of part of the public, but certainly not in medical circles. The Hippocratic writings never confuse the two.

Plato also helped give currency to the popular notion of the true physician's clientele. It was necessary, for the purposes of his argument, that the authentic physician, who was himself a free man, treat free persons. The inattentive reader may allow himself to be carried away by the neat antithesis between slave medicine and free medicine. But Plato recognized, in spite of himself as it were, that the clientele of the authentic physician was not exclusively composed of free persons, noting that the physician treated patients of free status "most of the time"—which is to say that sometimes he treated slaves as well. Interpreted in this way, Plato's account does not contradict that of the Hippocratic Collection, according to which physicians treated not only free persons but also slaves.

The *Epidemics* provide a great deal of information about the clientele of the Hippocratic physicians. These treatises contain more than 450 individual cases. Some of them are anonymous; others are individualized in various ways that make it possible fairly often to determine the social origins of the patients mentioned. In the case of some, the first name is given: these are free men. Others are designated by their connection with a proper name: these belonged to the family of a free man (daughters or sons) or to his household (manservants or maidservants). Several patients are expressly referred to as "slave of so-and-so" or "manservant [maidservant] of so-and-so." Here is one example among many: "The foot of Aristion's female slave spontaneously ulcerated in the middle of the foot on the inner side. The bones became corrupted, separated and came off little by little, eroded. Diarrhea developed; she died."[3]

Details are sometimes given about these slaves: one slave is branded;[4] one maidservant is newly bought;[5] another maidservant has just had a child.[6] It is not possible to give a precise accounting of the number of slaves treated nor to calculate the exact proportion between slaves and free persons in the clientele of the Hippocratic physicians. One of the difficulties has to do with an ambiguity of the Greek word used: the same term *pais* can mean either "child" or "slave." But it is clear that Hippocratic physicians treated the slaves they were summoned to treat, which is to say when the slaves' masters were willing to pay for consultation and treatment.

Considerate masters must have sought treatment for their slaves in case of illness. Two accounts by Xenophon confirm this. In the *Oeconomicus*, the master of the house, speaking to his wife, tells her that one of her chores is to look after the health of the slaves:

"One of the duties that fall to you, however, will perhaps seem rather thankless: you will have to see that any servant who is ill is cared for."

"Oh no," cried my wife, "it will be delightful, assuming that those who are well cared for are going to feel grateful and be more loyal than before."[7]

Here, it is not specified who will administer the treatment. The second account, by contrast, states that the doctor was called. In the *Memorabilia*, Socrates gets Diodorus to acknowledge that he spends money on his slaves in order to make him admit that, a fortiori, he must help a friend in need, for a friend is worth several slaves. One of the occasions when a master spends money on his slaves is precisely when they fall ill:

"And further [Socrates continued], if one of your servants is ill, do you take care of him and call in doctors to prevent him dying?"

"Indeed I do."[8]

These two accounts paint rather a rosy picture. Some masters surely did not pay much attention to the health of their slaves. The case of the newly bought female slave mentioned by the author of *Epidemics IV* is revealing in this regard. Her new master, after the fashion of Xenophon's Diodorus, summons a doctor who cures the slave of a lump in the groin and restores her periods. It may be doubted whether her former master was as kind, for it had been seven years since this woman had her period.

The Hippocratic physician, whether he was called to a slave's bedside or to that of a free man, made no distinction between the two. The slave, for him, was no less a patient than the free man. The proof of this is that the physician observed the development of the slave's illness with the same care as that of the free man. The example of the branded slave is especially significant. Bad slaves who ran away were branded; probably they did not fetch high prices at auction. But it should not be inferred from this that the case of such a slave was therefore taken lightly by the Hippocratic physician. Here is the study relating one such illness: "The branded slave [at] Antiphilus'[s], who had caustic crisis on the seventh day, biliousness and delirium, had the same evacuation on the third day after the crisis. He spat up blood. He survived and had a later relapse. It is likely that the first crisis was around the setting of the Pleiades. And after the setting of the Pleiades he was bilious to the extent of madness. A crisis about the ninth day, without sweating."[9] It is clear that the sick slave was closely monitored by the physician over a fairly long period. Otherwise the chronology of the illness could not have been noted with such precision. And if the physician felt the need to mention in his report that the patient was a slave who had been branded, it was in order to identify the patient, not to call attention to his social background.

On the rare occasions when a Hippocratic physician considered slaves as a group distinct from free persons, it was not at all, as it was for Plato, to assert the superiority of free persons over slaves. The reference to slaves as a separate category of persons was made solely from a medical point of view. In the course of a long epidemiological description concerning a winter cough accompanied by various complications, among them throat infections, the physician of *Epidemics VI* made a distinction between free and slave women: "Women did not suffer similarly from the cough. . . . I attributed this to their not going out as the men did and because they were not otherwise susceptible like the men. Two free women got quinsy, and that was of the mildest sort. Slave women got it in a more extreme way, and those with very violent cases died very quickly. But many men got it; some survived, some died."[10]

The distinction between free and slave women sharpens the epidemiological analysis by introducing a difference within the category of women as opposed to that of men. While free women were spared quinsy for the most part, slave women were hit hard by it. The reason for this was that slave women, on account of their work, had to go outdoors more often than free women, and thus, like men, were exposed to the disease. A similar sort of difference in ways of life is noted by the author of *Airs, Waters, Places* when he makes a distinction between free and slave women among the Scythians. Having explained the low fertility of the (free) Scythian women by their inactivity and their stoutness, this author adds: "A clear proof is afforded by their slave-girls. These, because of their activity and leanness of body, no sooner go to a man than they are with child."[11] The difference between free women and slave women, even when it was apparent from their physical appearance, derived in the last analysis from their way of life and not from nature.

When it came to treating slaves, then, there was little difference between the theory and practice of Hippocratic physicians. They treated slaves exactly as they did free persons and made no distinction between the natures of the two. They thus minimized the social divisions stressed by Plato in his picture of Greek medicine. The humanism of the Hippocratic physicians makes them seem more modern than Plato.

Trades of Patients: Poor and Rich

This Hippocratic humanism was to survive in the medical tradition of the following centuries. An honorary decree of the first century B.C. issued by a city in Laconia praised a public physician for having treated slaves and freemen alike.[12] The same physician was also praised for having cared for both the poor and the rich. In earlier times, this praise might have been bestowed upon Hippocratic physicians.

Humble artisans accounted for a part of their clientele. This much is plain from the information about the trades of certain patients given by the authors of the *Epidemics*. Reference to a trade was relevant in the case of work accidents. Thus, as we saw previously, the skipper of a large ship had part of his hand crushed by its anchor during the course of repairs.[13] A cobbler stabbed himself in the thigh above the knee with his awl, while sewing the sole of a shoe, and died two days later.[14] A carpenter suffered a fractured skull;[15] a potter fell from atop his kiln.[16] An injured patient's trade was judged relevant when the nature of his professional activity had an effect on the subsequent manifestation of illness. If the author of *Epidemics IV* mentions in connection with a coughing epidemic that a young vineyard worker was paralysed in the arm he used to tie up grape vines, this is because he had noticed that this cough was liable to be accompanied by paralysis of the limb customarily used in working.[17] But a trade was sometimes mentioned only to identify the patient or to facilitate his identification.[18] Looking at the *Epidemics* as a group, a whole series of trades can be seen to come back to life. For the most part these were artisanal trades practiced in towns. To the ones already cited— shoemaker, carpenter, potter—can be added fullers, a stonecutter, a mine worker, a cook, and a shopkeeper.[19] There were also trades associated with the countryside, such as vinedresser, gardener, groom;[20] and those with the sea, represented by the ship's skipper. The world of sport is represented by a boxer and a wrestling master.[21] And, finally, there is mention of a more intellectual profession: schoolmaster.[22] Most of these trades were humble, which suggests that the Hippocratic physician did not disdain to treat clients who were not wealthy. Among those patients whose trade is indicated, some undoubtedly were slaves. This is the case, for example, with those who are designated both by their trade and by their attachment to a master, such as Menander's vinedresser, Cleotimus's shoemaker, Palamedes' groom.[23] But one also goes inside the homes of small artisans of free status: for example, that of the "leatherworker" whose wife suffered from a chronic strangury except during childbirth.[24]

It was on the basis of such examples, drawn from the *Epidemics*, that Galen gave the prospective physician the following advice: "You will treat the poor at Crannon, at Thasos and in the other cities."[25] The physician of Pergamum had an interest in giving credence to this hagiographic view of Hippocrates as a physician of the poor in order to denounce the avarice of certain of his colleagues, whom he accused of being drug peddlers rather than real doctors. But this view distorts what must have been the real situation. While there is evidence that poor persons were among the clients of the Hippocratic physicians, to make Hippocrates into a minister to the poor requires passing over in silence the fact that he treated wealthy clients as well.

Hippocratic physicians seem to have acted as family doctors in certain cases. This becomes apparent if one compares the various references to treatment of members of a single family that are scattered throughout the *Epidemics*. The two families most frequently mentioned are those of Timenes and of Apemantus in Perinthus. Timenes' family comprised several households: in addition to Timenes' own home, where a son had been sick, there was the household of his sister, in which a slave had fallen ill, and a third household, that of his niece, who herself had been a patient along with a slave.[26] Apemantus's family probably also consisted of three households: Apemantus and his wife were both patients, as was the wife of Apemantus's brother, and the young slave belonging to Apemantus's sister.[27] It is true that we possess no information regarding the social status of these two families. But comparison of the proper names of these patients with inscriptions and other documents supplies indirect evidence of the wealthy background of part of the Hippocratics' clientele. At Thasos, one of the patients mentioned in the *Epidemics* is Antiphon, son of Critobulus.[28] Now it is known from a municipal decree, preserved in stone, that this Antiphon was a theor of Thasos under the oligarchy around 410.[29] The theors at Thasos were important magistrates who were recruited from the most prominent families. Here then is an example of a patient who must have belonged to one of the great families of the city. At Larissa in Thessaly, where Hippocrates resided and where he died, the Hippocratic physicians were probably in contact with the illustrious and powerful family of the Aleuadae, from which the tyrants of the city were recruited. Among the names of the inhabitants of Larissa mentioned in the *Epidemics*, it is possible to identify with a high degree of confidence several members of this great family: Dyseris, Simus, and Echecrates.[30] The name Aleuas, mentioned without any indication of his native city, quite naturally seems to refer to the same family.[31] Other names have been connected with other leading families of Larissa without much justification, it is true; but Palamedes of Larissa, whose eleven-year-old groom was struck by a horse in the forehead, must surely have been a well-to-do landowner.[32] Let us recall, too, the privileged relations of Hippocrates' family with the royal family of Macedonia, which several of his descendants served as court physicians.[33] Reverting to the example of Democedes, whose salary as court physician was higher than what he was paid as public physician at Athens, it seems fair to conclude that physicians belonging to Hippocrates' family, or to his entourage, did not neglect either the material side of their practice or their relations with a wealthy clientele—any more than Hippocrates himself did. But however this may be, there reigns throughout the oldest writings in the Hippocratic Collection an aristocratic silence on the question of the physician's salary. If there were no external evidence on this point, one might indeed wonder whether physicians ever received even a meager tip in exchange for their help.

The Physician's Fees

In fact, all physicians were paid fees for the services they rendered. "[Physicians] earn their fee when (for instance) they have cured their patients," says Aristotle.[34] The image of an often greedy physician appears in Greek literature from before the time of Hippocrates. Even Asclepius, who is supposed to have been the ancestor of the physician of Cos, was unable to resist the temptation of money, if Pindar is to be believed:

> But even wisdom feels the lure of gain—
> gold glittered in his hand, and he was hired
> to retrieve from death a man already forfeit:
> the son of Kronos hurled and drove the breath,
> smoking from both their chests.[35]

This picture of the divine physician, intent upon gain, was to outrage Plato, who accused poets of slandering the gods.[36] Nor were human physicians spared. Heraclitus railed against the perversity of those who tortured their fellow man and then charged him for it: "[D]octors . . . who cut and cauterize and wretchedly torment the sick in every way are praised—they deserve no fee from the sick, for they have the same effects as the diseases."[37]

In Hippocrates' time, complaints about the high cost of health care were heard in the theater, too. Euripides, speaking through the mouth of a humble laborer, declared that only the rich could afford to summon a doctor: "In times like these, when wishes soar but power fails, I contemplate the steady comfort found in gold: gold you can spend on guests; gold you can pay the doctor when you get sick."[38]

The link between the lure of money and the practice of medicine was jokingly underlined, *a contrario*, by Aristophanes in the last of his comedies, dating from the beginning of the fourth century: "What doctor is there now left in town?" laments an old Athenian. "There's no money to be offered, so there's no medicine practiced."[39] The old man makes a direct connection between fees and medicine: no payment, no medicine.

The demands of physicians in respect both of salary and services worked to create a gap between rich and poor. The poor, who had to work to earn their livelihood, had neither the leisure nor the means to seek treatment, while the rich, who had both time and money, could afford the luxury of looking after their health. Plato forcefully noted this difference in the *Republic*.[40] A more discreet echo of the Platonic text is met with in the Hippocratic Collection, where an author proposes two treatments for a single disease, one long and involved, for those who had the time to be taken care of in this way, and a briefer regimen for the mass of people pressed for time by the need to make a living.[41] What the Hippocratic physician is recommending here, in effect, is a two-track system of medicine, even though he is very careful to avoid raising the question of salary.

It was in reaction to the perceived greed of physicians that the noble ideal of the *Precepts* came to be defined: "I urge you not to be too unkind, but to consider carefully your patient's superabundance or means. Sometimes give your services for nothing, calling to mind a precious benefaction or present satisfaction. And if there be an opportunity of serving one who is a stranger in financial straits, give full assistance to all such. For where there is love of man, there is also love of the art."[42]

These fine maxims date from after the time of Hippocrates; however there is no reason to doubt that they carried on a Hippocratic tradition. A physician belonging to the Asclepiad clan surely could count on a wealthy clientele, from whom he received payment commensurate with his reputation in exchange for treating the members of prominent families, and even their household slaves. This would have allowed him also to serve a humbler clientele, adopting a sliding scale of fees calculated in accordance with the more modest means of these patients. Moreover, as we know from Plato, our earliest source of information about Hippocrates, he made money from teaching medicine.

On the evidence of Plato and later sources, we are justified in forming an image of Hippocrates as an active physician who directed the work of a sizeable medical staff and also taught medicine on a salaried basis, and as an elite practitioner catering to a wealthy clientele who was nonetheless generous enough not to neglect the needs of a rather less favored class of patients, nor balk at sending his son at his own expense to serve as public physician on the Athenian expedition to Sicily. Everything considered, this is the picture more of a charitable aristocrat than of a selfless minister to the poor.

Women

The Hippocratic physician treated both women and men. The list of patients given in the *Epidemics* leaves no doubt on this point. The physician was frequently called to the bedside of women suffering from genital tract disorders. To go back to the case of the two families of Timenes and Apemantus, one notes that of the eight people treated, free persons and slaves, four patients were male—Timenes' son, the slave of Timenes' niece, Apemantus, and the slave of Apemantus's sister—and four were female—Timenes' niece, the female slave of Timenes' sister, the wife of Apemantus, and the wife of Apemantus's brother. One notes, too, that specifically female complaints attracted the attention of Hippocratic physicians.[43]

The importance accorded gynecology by Hippocratic authors does not mean that women willingly called upon a doctor in connection with ailments of an intimate nature. Evidence to the contrary emerges from the theater of Hippocrates' day as well as from the Hippocratic treatises themselves. When the young women of the choir of Euripides' *Hippolytus* learn of Phaedra's mysterious illness, they ask each other what could be responsible for it, observing that, among other possible causes, "Unhappy is the compound of women's nature";[44] then, a bit later, the nurse, addressing Phaedra in the presence of the choir, says to her:

> If you are sick and it is some secret sickness,
> here are women standing at your side to help.
> But if your troubles may be told to men,
> speak, that a doctor may pronounce upon it.[45]

This passage clearly indicates two things. First, that doctors were men: no woman could claim the title of physician during Hippocrates' time. Second, that women hesitated to entrust themselves to the care of men for specifically female ailments, preferring to help each other by sharing their experience: the young women of the choir can advise Phaedra because they have experience of childbirth. Herodotus had earlier testified to such reluctance, which he put down to modesty, in recounting how much Queen Atossa had hesitated before being treated by the physician Democedes for a lump in her breast.[46] Physicians, for their part, deplored such reticence, for it could have grave consequences for women's health:

Sometimes women themselves do not know what ails them before they have experienced maladies arising from their periods and they are older. Then, necessity and time teach them the cause of their maladies. Indeed sometimes, among women who do not know the source of their ailments, maladies become incurable before the physician has been correctly informed by the patient with regard to the origin of the ailment. In fact, modesty prevents them from speaking even if they do know, and owing to inexperience and ignorance they regard that as shameful.[47]

But this lack of communication between physician and patient was coupled with a certain inexperience on the part of the physician with the specific details of women's ailments. This is emphasized by the same Hippocratic author, who adds: "At the same time, physicians commit the error of not informing themselves exactly of the cause of this disease and of treating it as if it were a masculine disease. . . . There is a great difference for treatment between the diseases of women and those of men."

A sense of modesty therefore led women to turn not only to friends, but also to women who had assisted them in childbirth. While there were no female doctors in the classical period, midwives were well known. Socrates' mother is a famous example. To credit Plato's Socrates, only older women who had had experience of childbirth and who could no longer have children themselves were authorized to exercise this function. In addition to their personal experience, they were familiar with a kind of popular medicine, part pharmacology, part magic, relating to all aspects of childbirth—even abortion. Socrates says: "And then it is the midwives who have the power to bring on the pains, and also, if they think fit, to relieve them; they do it by the use of simple drugs, and by singing incantations. In difficult cases, too, they can bring about the birth; or, if they consider it advisable, they can promote a miscarriage."[48]

The Greek term used by Plato to refer to midwives—the noun *maia*, 'little mother', which is applied to old women in general and to nurses in particular—clearly indicates that theirs was less a profession than a rather vaguely defined activity. Midwives, according to Socrates, were also the most expert procuresses. They also figure, though rarely, in the Hippocratic Collection. Although there were not yet any female doctors in Hippocrates' time,[49] midwives were by then referred to by a term that was directly connected with the idea of caring—the noun *akestris*, literally, 'healer', or the nominative participle *he ietreuousa*, 'she who treats'. Midwives were valued for their experience even by doctors. The author of *Fleshes*, who maintains (within the framework of a septenary theory) that a child can be born at seven months, calls for support upon the testimony of midwives: "Someone who lacks experience might wonder whether a child can really be born in seven months, but I have seen it myself, and often. If anyone wishes proof, the matter is easy: let him go to the midwives that attend women who are giving birth and ask them."[50]

This passage also reveals that a physician might sometimes be present at childbirth. Physicians and midwives must have worked together at least in the case of difficult deliveries or abortions. In fact, one Hippocratic physician gives a prescription—whether for abortion or delivery, he does not say—that assumes the presence of a midwife: "She who treats is to open the uterine orifice gently, proceed slowly, and draw out the umbilical cord at the same time as the foetus."[51]

To get around the wall of silence that women must have observed in many cases, the Hippocratic physician was sometimes obliged to obtain information indirectly. One physician tells us how he came to learn of a woman who had become pregnant without wishing to: "A woman of my acquaintance possessed a highly valued singer, who had intercourse with men: she could not become pregnant, lest she lose her value. This singer had heard what the women said among themselves: for a woman to become pregnant, the seed must not come out, but must stay inside. Having heard these things, she noted them and always remembered them. So when she realized that the seed was not coming out, she confided in her mistress, and word made its way to me."[52] We will come back later to the rest of this account and what the physician found out.[53] What matters for the moment is the manner in which women spoke among each other of their ailments, and the fact that the physician was alerted to what had happened by accident, owing to an indiscretion.

All of this implies that the physician needed to demonstrate a great deal of tact and discretion in treating a woman who had entrusted herself to his care. Vaginal examination was a particularly sensitive matter. Did the doctor conduct the examination personally or did he leave it to a woman? It depended on the doctor, and perhaps on the era as well. According to the oldest sections of the gynecological treatises, the doctor performed the examination himself. Thus in the case of a woman who was unable to conceive, though her periods were normal, he was advised to determine by means of digital inspection of the vagina whether there was an obstacle: "You will know if with the finger you touch the obstacle."[54]

In the more recent sections, however, the doctor does not perform the digital examination himself, but relies instead upon a woman. Among the causes of a spontaneous abortion in the third or fourth month, the author mentions the worn condition of the womb: "One will recognize these various conditions in questioning the patient precisely; but for the worn state of the uterus, it is necessary that another woman touch the uterus when it is empty, for otherwise the thing would not be apparent."[55]

To become familiar with the other causes, the author is instructed to question the patient closely; but for the digital examination of the vagina, he is to turn to a woman for assistance, or, failing that, to allow the patient herself to conduct the examination.[56] This shows that certain physicians made it an absolute duty to respect a woman's sense of modesty.

Foreigners

The Hippocratic physician's clientele may possibly have also included foreign patients who found themselves in the city where he practiced. Here once again the case studies recorded in the *Epidemics* are our main source of evidence. The author of *Epidemics I* treated at Thasos a foreigner named Hermippus who was a native of Clazomenae, a city on the coast of Asia Minor known mainly as the home of the philosopher Anaxagoras, a contemporary of Hippocrates.[57] We know, too, that, in some unspecified city, the physician of *Epidemics IV* treated the servant of "the man from Attica."[58] The *Precepts*, a later treatise, counsels the physician to display philanthropy in treating foreigners and the poor.[59] Similarly, according to inscriptions, some physicians were publicly rewarded by foreign cities for having treated their nationals in the physicians' own cities. Thus it was that a Coan physician named Philistus, son of Nicarchus, was honored by a decree of the city of Samos for having treated Samians staying at Cos, whether or not they were there in an official capacity.[60]

It sometimes happened that barbarians were present in Greek cities. This was particularly the case with slaves. One of the cases recorded in *Epidemics V* expressly refers to a slave patient as a non-Greek: "The slave woman: after a potion she evacuated a little bile above, and choked; passed much below. She died that night. She was a barbarian."[61]

The Hippocratic physician had no scruples about taking on the case of this woman; neither the fact that she was a slave nor that she was a barbarian deterred him. It must be emphasized, however, that this reference to a non-Greek patient is unique in the *Corpus Hippocraticum*. Even so, it cannot be used to contradict passages in the biographical writings where Hippocrates is said to have refused to go to a barbarian country to end a plague, or to serve as physician to the court of the king of Persia. There is no contradiction in these cases, because the care freely given by a Greek physician to a barbarian slave in a Greek city had nothing to do with the decision of a Greek physician whether or not to practice abroad, be it in a barbarian land in Europe or in Asia. What this exceptional case goes to show is that whatever information the Hippocratic Collection may have to provide about the practice of medicine, it has to do with the practice of medicine in Greek cities and nowhere else.

To summarize our discussion of the patients whom the Hippocratic physician observed or treated, within the context of the life of the Greek city in which he practiced, we may say that the physician cared—to be sure, for a fee—for men and women, citizens and foreigners, free persons and slaves, Greeks and non-Greeks. The Hippocratic physician regarded the patients who came before him, first and foremost, as human beings. Of this humanism we have tangible evidence in the form of the very vocabulary employed: the Greek word *anthropos*, which means "human being," is repeatedly used in the writings of the Hippocratic Collection to refer to the patient. This is a sign that other distinctions—of sex, of social status, or of racial origin—were secondary, and that what counted before everything else was the relation between physician and patient, no matter who the patient was.

Theoretical Foundations of the Physician-Patient Relationship

The physician had duties toward the patient that were commensurate with the nobility of an art whose purpose seems to have been linked in Greek thought from the very first to the survival and happiness of humanity. The purpose of medicine was to fight, as far as the resources of nature and man permitted, against one of the main causes of the unhappiness of the human condition—sickness and disease. As Hesiod had long before said, "There are diseases for people during the day, and others in the night that wander under their own power, bringing evils to mortals secretly because Zeus the Planner took out their voice."[62] At the same time, medicine must try to preserve or restore what the Greeks regarded as the supreme good and as something divine: health. Its praises were sung in Hippocrates' time in this celebrated hymn by the poet Ariphron of Sicyon:

Health! The most venerable of the blessed divinities, would that I might pass the rest of my life with thee! Would that thou might be a benevolent companion to me in my house! If there is, in fact, any charm in wealth, or in children, or in the royal power that makes man equal to a god, or in the desires that we pursue with the secret nets of Aphrodite, or any other pleasure or repose come from the gods may so appear to [us in] our tiredness, it is in thy company, blessed Health, that everything flourishes, that the company of the Graces shines; but without thee, there is no happiness.[63]

The medicine that dispelled illness and brought health also fell, according to the Greeks, under the category of arts of salvation. Already in the myth of Prometheus, brought to the stage by Aeschylus, medicine was one of the arts discovered by the kindhearted thief to save men from the annihilation planned for them by Zeus.[64] But it was above all with the philosophers of the fourth century, Plato and Aristotle, that this art of salvation became a paradigm for political thought: medicine was taken as a model of disinterestedness, which the politician must follow, for its object was to secure the advantage not of the physician, the one who practiced the art, but of the patient, the one to whom the art was applied.[65]

The main part of the Hippocratic Collection was composed between the time of Aeschylus's *Prometheus Unbound* and the time when the philosophers were writing. On the subject of the duties of the physician toward the patient, the lofty ideals of the Hippocratic treatises are altogether exemplary; and on the relations between the physician and the patient, their humanity is also quite exceptional. And so it is not surprising that, having first made a deep impression upon contemporaries, they should have become the bible of the physician over the course of succeeding centuries. In our own day, despite the progress of medical science, which has once and for all turned its back on Hippocrates, they still possess a freshness and a topicality for specialists; more broadly, they offer rich grounds for reflection for anyone who wishes to become acquainted with the earliest roots of humanism, even if this is considered in its modern form, the doctrine of human rights.

The Hippocratic message concerning the foundation on which rest the relations between physician and patient may be summed up in a famous maxim of *Epidemics I*: "As to diseases, make a habit of two things—to help, or at least to do no harm."[66] Here Hippocrates clearly asserts, prior to Plato and Aristotle, that the purpose of medicine is to protect the interests of the patient. But the physician's unique point of view serves to lend nuance to what was to become a more dogmatic position with the philosophers. Because the injunction to "do good" represents an ideal that the physician cannot always attain, he adds "or at least do no harm." Failing to be useful, the physician must not worsen a patient's condition through an untimely intervention. It is this dimension of human concern that constitutes the originality of Hippocratic thought. Even when the practitioner allows himself to reflect in general terms about medicine, in a way that prefigures the philosophers, his vision preserves the special richness of lived experience. The best example is found in the preamble to *Breaths*:

There are some arts which to those that possess them are painful, but to those that use them are helpful, a common good to laymen, but to those that practise them grievous. Of such arts there is one which the Greeks call medicine. For the medical man sees terrible sights, touches unpleasant things, and the misfortunes of others bring a harvest of sorrows that are peculiarly his; but the sick by means of this art rid themselves of the worst of evils, disease, suffering, pain, and death. For medicine proves for all these evils a manifest cure.[67]

In this passage, where sincerity of tone is allied with brilliance of style, it is clear that the author of *Breaths* was the first, before either Plato or Aristotle, to enunciate the conception of a medical art useful to the one who is treated and not to the one who treats. But the abstraction of this idea is not incompatible with the author's evocation of the reality of medicine—not only of the misfortunes of the patient, but also of the inconveniences of a trade from which the physician, in exchange for the good he has done for others, reaps only unpleasantnesses. It was this latter aspect of the text that the nineteenth-century French physician Charles Daremberg, a leading expert on the Hippocratic Collection, had in mind when he declared: "Hippocrates painted in a single stroke the sad spectacle which the physician witnesses every day and all the disgust he must overcome, all the ingratitude that awaits him as his reward for so much vigilance and concern."[68]

The Discretion of the Hippocratic Physician in the Face of Pain

This complaint on the part of the physician regarding his own condition is, however, exceptional in the treatises of the collection. Everywhere else discretion is the rule with respect to all that is frightful and painful, not only for the physician but also for the patient. The almost total silence regarding the pain of the one being operated on, whether in the case of common procedures such as venesection and cauterization, or in the case of more dangerous ones such as trephination, is surprising. After all, these patients were not operated on under anaesthesia. It is all the more surprising since the Hippocratic Collection is filled with their pain, and sometimes, too, with their anguished cries. One of the words used to refer to pain (*odunè*) occurs more than seven hundred times in the treatises. But it almost always signifies the pain felt by the patient on account of his illness. This pain interested the physician insofar as it was a meaningful symptom for establishing the diagnosis or prognosis of the illness. The pain of the patient when he was being operated on was of another kind: it was a necessary evil that did not enter into the language of signs and symptoms. The Hippocratic author noted only that which was useful, which is why the patient's pain during the course of operations was generally not mentioned. Here, for example, is the description of an operation that we have already noticed because of the introduction it gives to the physician's assistants: "Let those who look after the patient present the part for operation as you want it, and hold fast the rest of the body so as to be all steady, keeping silence and obeying their superior."[69] In this operation, the voice of the physician, who gives orders, is contrasted with the silence of his aides, who carry them out. But nothing is said about the pain and cries of the patient whom they are holding down, immobilized—as if he had been gagged, or put to sleep!

One has really to root around in the recesses of the vast library constituted by the Hippocratic Collection to uncover evidence of the patient's suffering during operations. The clearest mention appears in a late treatise, *Physician*, where the desire to ease the patient's pain guides the rhythm of the operation itself:

> In surgical operations that consist in incising or cautery, speed or slowness are commended alike, for each has its value. In cases where the surgery is performed by a single incision, you must make it a quick one; for since the person being cut usually suffers pain, this suffering should last for the least time possible, and that will be achieved if the incision is made quickly. However, when many incisions are necessary, you must employ a slow surgery, for a surgeon that was fast would make the pain sustained and great, whereas intervals provide a break in its intensity for the patients.[70]

The Duties of the Physician Toward the Patient

If the painful condition of the physician and that of the patient were often omitted as a matter of authorial discretion, the rules of conduct for physician and patient are, by contrast, plainly specified. For the most part, obviously, these amount to an ethic of the practitioner. But there also existed an ethic of the patient.

The fame of *The Oath* derives from its second part, which lays out the principal duties of the physician toward the patient and his entourage:

> I will use treatment to help the sick according to my ability and judgment, but never with a view to injury and wrong-doing. Neither will I administer a poison to anybody when asked to do so, nor will I suggest such a course. Similarly I will not give to a woman a pessary to cause abortion. But I will keep pure and holy both my life and my art. I will not use the knife, not even, verily, on sufferers from stone, but I will give place to such as are craftsmen therein. Into whatsoever houses I enter, I will enter to

help the sick, and I will abstain from all intentional wrong-doing and harm, especially from abusing the bodies of man or woman, bond or free. And whatsoever I shall see or hear in the course of my profession, as well as outside my profession in my intercourse with men, if it be what should not be published abroad, I will never divulge, holding such things to be holy secrets. Now if I carry out this oath, and break it not, may I gain for ever reputation among all men for my life and for my art; but if I transgress it and forswear myself, may the opposite befall me.

Although originally the entire oath was taken only by disciples from outside the family of the Asclepiads, and not by the sons of the master, it is plain that the medical ethic contained in this second part applied to everyone—master, sons of the master, and disciples. And so it is not unreasonable that the oath as a whole, diverted from its initial purpose, should later have come to be uttered by physicians in general. In uniting lofty ideals with solemnity of tone and economy of expression, it singlehandedly raised pagan morality to new heights. The *Oath* was later taken over in its entirety by the Christians, who limited themselves to replacing the pagan divinities, called upon at the outset as witnesses, with God and Jesus Christ. A Christian version of the *Oath* survives, in fact, in a medieval manuscript.[71]

With the exception of the quite peculiar prohibition against operating on stones, in cases of lithiasis, all the prescriptions formulated in this ancient medical code remain current, if not in their letter, then at least in their spirit. The roots of modern medical ethics, embodied in law, are to be found in the *Oath*, whether it is a matter of technical secrets or of respect for human life. The absolute prohibitions of the Hippocratic code are qualified by contemporary law only in the case of abortion, which is now permitted under certain conditions.

The key word of this ethic, in the *Oath* as in the maxim of *Epidemics I*, is the "interest" of the patient. All—or almost all—the other rules flow from it. The first is the rule against administering lethal drugs. This prohibition implies that abuses were not rare in Hippocrates' time. To be sure, the law provided for punishment in the case of death by poisoning. A rich Athenian, responsible for supervising a choir of young people, was hauled before the courts because one of his choristers, in order to clear his throat, had drunk a medicine that killed him.[72] Plato, in the ideal legislation proposed in the *Laws*, takes a very severe line against a doctor who would administer even a nonlethal poison: this was to be punishable by death.[73] His harshness in this instance is probably explained by the de facto immunity from prosecution enjoyed by certain unscrupulous physicians who did not hesitate, in exchange for a good deal of money, to administer poison personally to an unwanted patient under the guise of treatment, or to supply poison discreetly to a third party who did not himself have the hereditary privilege of possessing "a poison from the Gorgon's snakes,"[74] indicating which doses were fatal and which not, so that revenge could be both flexible and measured. In addition, these evil doctors faced competition from pharmacopoles, or drug sellers, who may be thought of as the forerunners of modern pharmacists. But since the Greek term for medicine (*pharmakon*—from which both of the words "pharmacopole" and "pharmacist" are formed, by the way) also referred to poison, pharmacopoles in Hippocrates' time were able to sell both poison and medicine under the ambiguous name of *pharmakon*. Well attested in the fifth century in the plays of Aristophanes,[75] these pharmacopoles included some reputable experts who trained pupils exactly as physicians did. According to Theophrastus, one of them, Thrasyas of Mantinea, discovered a very potent poison, having a base of hemlock and poppy, that killed quickly and without suffering. His disciple Alexias was no less talented, but, Theophrastus adds, he was also knowledgable about medicine in general.[76] This is to say that the boundary between medicine and pharmacy, as between medicine and poison, was vague—so vague, in fact, that in the absence of any legislation regulating the sale of drugs, a commerce had developed by Hippocrates' time in more or less toxic products that were used for more or less honest purposes. It was against such a background that the absolute prohibition of the oath against giving poison to a patient or a third party acquired its full force and point.

We can therefore more easily grasp the moral need for a medical code that advocated respect for the patient and, more broadly, respect for life. Similarly, the prohibition against giving medicine to a woman to induce abortion is to be interpreted in a context in which such a prohibition was not assumed as a matter of course. We have seen that midwives, according to Plato, also knew how to induce abortion.[77] The moral grandeur of the Hippocratic oath consisted in its clear refusal to tolerate such practices, from which midwives did not shrink. And if one recalls, again on Plato's testimony, that these women acted also as procuresses, the contrast becomes still more pronounced between the conduct of midwives and the ethic of the *Oath*, which forebade a person from profiting from his or her profession in order to seduce any other person, even a slave.

All this, it may be objected, represented only an ideal code. What did it amount to in reality? How were these prescriptions put into effect in the daily practice of the art?

The cardinal rule of acting in the interest of the patient was not only the theoretical purpose of the physician's activity but also a practical guide with respect to the terms of his intervention. This concern for the patient is apt to appear suddenly in the middle of a passage when one least expects it. The author of *On Joints*, for example, describing a spectacular therapeutic procedure for setting a dislocated thigh, which we have already encountered in connection with the physician's assistants,[78] begins by carefully indicating the way in which the patient is to be suspended from a crossbeam, upside down:

One should suspend the patient by his feet from a cross-beam with a band, strong, but soft, and of good breadth. The feet should be about four fingers apart, or even less. He should also be bound round above the knee-caps with a broad, soft band stretching up to the beam; and the injured leg should be extended about two fingers' breadth further than the other. Let the head be about two cubits, more or less, from the ground. The patient should have his arms extended along the sides and fastened with something soft.[79]

What a lot of technical details to be observed in preparing for an operation! But then, abruptly, he adds an instruction that is irrelevant to the success of the treatment, but important from the point of view of the patient: "Let all these preparations be made while he is lying on his back, that the period of suspension may be as short as possible."

At the very heart of the physician's technique lies the human dimension of his art, suddenly coming into view, like a subliminal image that unexpectedly presents itself to consciousness. In everyday practice, this dimension generally assumed three forms: gentleness in treatment, courtesy toward the patient, and conversation with the patient.

Gentleness in Treatment

Gentleness in treatment was taken to be one of the characteristics of Greek medicine that distinguished it from Egyptian medicine. It will be recalled that the Greek physician Democedes, in treating King Darius, who had dislocated his foot jumping down from a horse, substituted softness for the roughness of the Egyptian physicians: "Darius submitted to his care, and then Democedes, using Greek remedies and gentle rather than forcible means, after the latter had been tried by others, succeeded in getting Darius his share of sleep and, in a while, healed him completely."[80]

Gentleness therefore amounted in the first place to a refusal to employ violent methods. Hippocratic surgery was to confirm Herodotus's account of the treatment administered by Democedes. Recounting a similar case having to do with treatment of a club foot, the author of *On Joints* stresses that it is necessary to put the deviated parts back into their natural position "by gentle means, and not violently."[81] The Hippocratic contrast between the use of force and gentleness in treatment is thus comparable to that of Herodotus.

The rejection of violent methods was manifested by smooth, gradual therapeutic procedures, some of which testify to real technical ingenuity on the part of Hippocratic medicine. Take, for example, the quite original method for gently squeezing out the chorion—the membrane enclosing the embryo—in the event that it was not expelled from the womb normally in the course of childbirth. The mother was placed in a standing position, either on a commode, or, if she was too weak, by leaving her in bed and raising it on an angle, having first softly strapped her to the bed so that she would not slip off; next two goatskins filled with water were placed on the floor, tied together, and, on top of them, newly carded wool to serve as a cushion, which was both soft and voluminous. On this cushion was placed the baby, and with the aid of a stilleto, a small hole was made in each of the goatskins: "The water running out, the goatskins shrink; shrinking with them, the infant pulls on the umbilical cord; and the cord pulls out the chorion."[82] Then the author concludes: "This is the best treatment in these cases and the least harmful." What better illustration could one find of the physician's astuteness in seeking to act gently, so as to avoid mistreating nature, in keeping with the famous maxim "To do good, or at least do no harm"?

Gentleness might sometimes take the form of controlled violence. In reducing dislocations and fractures, it was necessary to make use of instruments that exercised powerful forces of extension and counterextension while, at the same time, taking care to control these forces. The best instrument in this regard was the winch, which permitted the application of force to be graduated: "This reduction apparatus is easy to regulate as regards greater or lesser force, and has such power that, if one wanted to use such forcible manoeuvers for harm and not for healing, it is able to act strongly in this way also. . . . Such forces, then, are good where it is possible for the operator to regulate their use as to weaker or stronger."[83]

Here one senses the physician's wonder in the face of forces tamed by human ingenuity, and at the same time his fascination with the awesome power of an instrument that, though it is used to do good, could be used to do evil. The famous Hippocratic bench, with no modification whatever, would make a marvelous instrument of torture—for interrogating slaves, for example. But the prohibition of the oath serves to prevent any such abuse. The physician shall not allow himself to be transformed into a torturer.

Gentleness consisted, finally, in seeking to make the patient comfortable.

Comfort, of course, was a question of degree. When a patient is suspended by his feet to reduce a dislocation, or tied upside down to a ladder and the ladder let fall to the ground several times in a row to straighten out his spine; or when a pregnant woman is strapped to her bed and the bed dropped vertically on the ground each time she has contractions to assist delivery—one may well wonder where the gentleness is. All such ancient Greek treatments are bound to seem quite barbaric to us today. Even in these cases, however, gentleness was not wholly absent. It resided in the detail of the attention shown the patient, in the constant concern to make sure that what came into contact with the body was soft. The Hippocratic author did not cease to remind his readers, in every description of surgical operations, that it was necessary to use smooth straps, soft blankets, and leather cushions to avoid hurting the patient. It even occurred to him to note that these cushions had no other reason for their use than to prevent the patient from experiencing pain unnecessarily.[84]

Courtesies Owed by the Physician to the Patient

One Hippocratic physician, the author of *Epidemics VI*, ranks this concern for providing soft things to be placed in contact with the patient's body under the head of what might be called "courtesies," to use a somewhat old-fashioned word; that is to say, the particular kindnesses shown by the physician to the patient in order to be agreeable to him or her. The list of these small gestures comes as a surprise. Here it is: "Kindnesses to those who are ill. For example to do in a clean way his food or drink or whatever he sees, softly what he touches. Things that do no great harm and are easily got, such as cool drink where it is needed. Entrance, conversation. Position and clothing for the sick person, hair, nails, scents."[85]

What is surprising first of all is that here we have a chance to read the physician's actual working notes. They do not appear to be ready yet for publication, constituting instead a sort of memorandum for personal reference in which concise remarks are strung together in no particular order. But what is still more surprising is that the author places on the same level certain forms of attention that we would no longer today classify as courtesies. For us, the cleanliness of a patient's room or food is a matter of hygiene, not something attended to out of a desire to please the patient. By contrast, a slight departure from the prescribed diet, permitted in order to satisfy the wishes of a patient who asks for a cool drink, for example, is something that still today we would number among the small gestures of kindness a physician might make to a patient. Note, however, that this sort of graciousness runs counter to the sacrosanct principle "To do good, or at least to do no harm." The Hippocratic physician was aware of this. But he makes it clear that one may bend the rules only if the harmful consequences of doing so are either reversible or minimal. The author of the *Aphorisms* endorses a similar "courtesy," even though he does not use the word, when he makes this recommendation: "Food or drink which, though slightly inferior, is more palatable, is preferable to that which is superior but less palatable."[86]

Such a desire to please the patient testifies to a real humanitarian concern on the part of the physician. No doubt he was also motivated by a desire to satisfy the patient's whims in order to win his confidence—but perhaps, too, by a firm conviction that the patient's morale was not unrelated to his chances of recovery. It was probably this belief that justified another rather unusual practice, likewise mentioned by the author of *Epidemics VI*. This time it consisted not in pleasing the patient but in fooling him: "If the ear aches, wrap wool around your fingers, pour on warm oil, then put the wool in the palm of the hand and put it over the ear so that something will seem to him to come out. Then throw it in the fire. A deception."[87]

This feat of prestidigitation, which bordered on charlatanism, is exceptional in the annals of Hippocratic medicine. If the text of the manuscript is correct, it was in fact a "good lie" aimed at comforting the patient. The patient's imagination was therefore sometimes enlisted in the service of healing.

The Dialogue between Physician and Patient

Among the courtesies to be shown by the physician to the patient, the author of *Epidemics VI* lists, in addition to the physician's bearing—which extends as far as using perfume—his conversation.

The art of speaking was a necessary part of a physician's education, as we have seen, because he was liable to have to speak before an audience, whether a statutory assembly or some other assembled crowd, at one or more points in his career.[88] In addition, it needs again to be emphasized, the physician had to demonstrate his rhetorical ability in his visits with patients. If the coming of a physician to a patient's home was apt to arouse the curiosity of neighbors, who would then rush over on hearing of his arrival, it must also have been, for the patient, both a source of anxiety and relief. The prospect of a bitter potion, a scalpel, or a branding iron could not have improved his spirits. The physician needed to have a great talent for persuasion, or else be accompanied by a specialist in this art. The physician Herodicus of Leontini, in Sicily, was fortunate to have the celebrated Sophist Gorgias for a brother. Gorgias recalled joining Herodicus and other physicians of his acquaintance on their rounds: "Many a time I've gone with my brother or with other doctors to call on some sick person who refuses to take his medicine or allow the doctor to perform surgery or cauterization on him. And when the doctor failed to persuade him, I succeeded, by means of no other craft than oratory."[89]

Persuasive rhetoric of this sort was, in effect, a form of professional courtesy. But the originality of the Hippocratic manner of speaking lay elsewhere. It consisted in initiating a dialogue with the patient for the purpose of collecting information about the diagnosis or prognosis of the illness, or possibly about the course of treatment. For example, in the treatise *Prognostic*, the questioning of the patient serves to complete the information obtained through visual or tactile inspection in order to determine the precise significance of the signs observed.[90] A handbook on how to question patients seems not yet to have existed in Hippocrates' time. And while posterity did not always preserve this aspect of Hippocratic practice, it is significant that Rufus of Ephesus (first to second century A.D.) felt himself obliged at the end of his treatise *Medical Questions* to reply to the objection that his teaching was contrary to that of Hippocrates when he recommended questioning people about the nature of the waters where they lived or about endemic diseases in their localities: "I admire Hippocrates without reservation for his ingenious art; it has often led to fine discoveries; nonetheless I recommend to the physician who wishes to be instructed in all things not to neglect questioning either."[91]

To know how to question a patient was indispensable. But it was also necessary to know how to listen. Some notes made by the author of *Epidemics VI* suggest that the Hippocratic physician was indeed attached to this dual aspect of the dialogue initiated with the patient: "Arrangements for the sick person and inquiry about the disease: what is explained [by the patient], what kind of things, how it must be accepted; the reasoning."[92]

The manner in which the patient's responses were to be interpreted was an art on the same level as questioning. In the context of therapy it was particularly important. Applying a bandage in the case of a fracture, for example, was a delicate matter, for it could not be too tight, nor too loose. By questioning the patient, the physician could determine whether the wrapping was properly done: "These are the indications of . . . correct bandaging:—if you ask the patient whether the part is compressed and he says it is, but moderately and that chiefly at the fracture. A properly bandaged patient should always give a similar report of the operation throughout."[93]

The patient's response therefore served as a guide for the physician in the course of treatment—but only on the condition that the physician knew how to interpret it. Where he did, an attentive dialogue came to be established that marked the beginning of an authentic partnership between physician and patient in fighting illness. The most famous, and also the most unusual, formula for describing this collaborative effort is found in the first book of the *Epidemics*: "The art has three factors, the disease, the patient, the physician. The physician is the servant of the art. The patient must co-operate with the physician in combating the disease."[94] The role assigned to the patient in this passage is such that his relationship to the physician is now almost reversed. It is no longer the physician who stands at the center of the medical process, but rather the patient, to the extent that it is the patient's responsibility to fight the illness with the help of the physician.

The Duties of the Patient

Making the patient the primary agent of his own recovery appears to border on paradox. On the one hand, it is a sign of modesty on the part of the physician, who thus puts himself at the patient's service. But it also suggests that the sick person is to be considered not only as a patient, but as a responsible person who is obliged to work on his own behalf if he is to regain health. The patient is therefore conceived as having duties as well. Just as the physician is subject to a certain code of behavior, so a standard of conduct applies to the patient and the people surrounding him. Thus the physician is advised as follows at the beginning of the *Aphorisms*: "The physician must be ready, not only to do his duty himself, but also to secure the co-operation of the patient, of the attendants and of externals."[95]

There exists no formal statement of the duties of the patient. This is natural enough, given that the Hippocratic literature is addressed primarily to the physician. Nonetheless, hints can be found here and there as to what these duties were. They occasionally take the form of positive precepts, but more often have to be inferred from the author's complaints of lapses from good behavior on the part of the patient. This suggests that the relationship between physician and patient was sometimes less than perfectly harmonious.

From the precepts that assume a positive form, we know that the patient was expected to help work toward making the operation a success. This was at least the case with the most common operations, incision and cauterization. After having given all the necessary instructions concerning the position of the surgeon as he readied himself to incise or cauterize, the author of *In the Surgery* takes up more briefly the obligations of the person being operated upon: "Let the patient assist the surgeon with the other (free) part of his body standing, sitting, or lying so as to maintain most easily the proper posture, on his guard against slipping, collapse, displacement, pendency, so that the position and form of the part treated may be properly preserved during presentation, operation, and the attitude afterwards."[96]

A more active form of collaboration was sometimes demanded of the patient in other operations. Consider, for example, the admirable description of the putting back in place of a dislocated jaw—the procedure is no different than the one used today—where the assistance of the patient is explicitly required:

Someone should hold the patient's head, while the operator grasping the jaw with his fingers inside and out near the chin—the patient keeping it open as wide as he conveniently can—should move the jaw this way and that with his hand, and bid the patient keep it relaxed and assist the movement by yielding to it as far as possible. Then suddenly do a side-slip, having in mind three positions in the manoeuvre. For the deviation must be reduced to the natural direction, the jaw must be pressed backwards, and, following this, the patient must close his jaws and not gape.[97]

On two occasions during this operation, the patient needed to synchronize his movements with those of the physician. Success was not possible without the patient's cooperation.

This cooperation was required even in the case of operations that were the most frightening for the patient, such as cauterization of hemorrhoids.[98] We have some idea what this must have been like from the detailed description of the preparations that needed to be made. The patient was laid on his back with a pillow under his kidneys. The physician, for his part, prepared seven or eight white-hot irons. During the operation, aides held the patient by the hand and arms so that he would not move. Given this much, one might expect the author to caution the patient not to cry out in the course of the operation, which after all was as delicate for the physician as it was terrifying for the patient. Not at all. "[L]et him shout during the cautery," states the author of *Haemmorrhoids*, "for that makes the anus stick out more." The cooperation required of the patient in this instance is all the more remarkable since he had not only to overcome great fear during a painful operation, but also to cry out at just the right moment.

Failings of Patients

While it seems that cooperation on the part of the patient could be obtained immediately when the physician was present, it was apt to be only intermittent in his absence, when the patient was expected to comply with the physician's orders, above all in a treatment of long duration.

If we are to believe the physicians, patients are lacking in seriousness, and forget everything once the pain goes away. The condition appears to be a mild one? Then the patient disregards it—and the doctor's instructions. It is imperative, for example, that a patient who has suffered a dislocation of the foot remain immobile for twenty days. But the author of *On Fractures* declares in a cynical tone: "It is good to lie up during this period, but patients, despising the injury, do not bring themselves to this, but go about before they are well. This is the reason why most of them do not make a complete recovery, and the pain often returns."[99]

The condition appears more serious? The patient is worried at first, but then forgets about it altogether:"[W]hen the fracture [of the collarbone] is recent, patients take it seriously, thinking the damage is worse than it is . . . ; but as time goes on the patients, since they feel no pain and are not hindered either in getting about or eating, neglect the matter . . . and meanwhile the callus formation quickly develops."[100] Negligence, lack of steadfastness—such were the misdeeds of patients; they are reasonable only when in pain, or fearful for their lives.[101]

Still more serious was the fact that, in order to conceal their disobedience, patients were apt to take refuge in lying: "Keep a watch also on the faults of the patients, which often make them lie about the taking of things prescribed. For through not taking disagreeable drinks, purgative or other, they sometimes die."[102]

Monitoring the failings of patients was therefore very much a part of the Hippocratic approach to medicine. One quite specialized branch of prognosis consisted in identifying, during the course of a series of follow-up visits, unauthorized departures from the prescribed regimen. The author of *Prorrhetic II* devotes a long section to this subject.[103] No doubt he did not worry very much about detecting small lapses—these he was content to leave to the sensationalist devices of charlatans. But in order to detect major lapses, either in diet or in exercise, the method he recommended called for as much knowledge and perspicacity as that for determining the nature of the illness and forecasting its development. Above all, it meant taking into account the psychology of the patient, for "different patients carry out different instructions either easily or with difficulty."[104] Monitoring the patient's behavior properly was a time-consuming business from the physician's point of view: it assumed daily visits, at the same hour, preferably in the morning, for this was the time of day when the patient who had correctly followed the regimen would have uniform facial coloring—and the physician's eyesight would be at its keenest, his wits at their sharpest.

Thus the very patient who was supposed to be the person primarily responsible for his own recovery was nonetheless treated as a suspect under close watch, whose faults were to be brought to light by the physician using methods similar to those employed in tracking the disease.

The Physician as Victim of the Faults of the Patient

If the physician attached so much importance to the failings of his patients, it was of course in the patients' own interest that he did so: their survival was at stake. But the reputation of the physician was at issue as well. The author of *Decorum*, after having noted that patients sometimes died as a result of disobeying and lying, adds: "What they have done never results in a confession, but the blame is thrown upon the physician."[105]

Because physicians paid for the faults of their patients before the court of public opinion, in the last analysis it was the life of medicine itself that was at stake. It therefore should not come as a surprise that the author of the principal Hippocratic apology, the treatise *The Art*, makes a vigorous plea on its behalf, opposing the attitude of the competent physician, sound of mind and body, to the behavior of the patient, ignorant, anxious, and incapable of resisting disease, in order to excuse the failure of certain treatments:

As to those who would demolish the art by fatal cases of sickness, I wonder what adequate reason induces them to hold innocent the ill-luck of the victims, and to put all the blame upon the intelligence of those who practised the art of medicine. It amounts to this: while physicians may give wrong instructions, patients can never disobey orders. And yet it is much more likely that the sick cannot follow out the orders than that the physicians give wrong instructions. The physician sets about his task with healthy mind and healthy body, having considered the case and past cases of like characteristics to the present, so as to say how they were treated and cured. The patient knows neither what he is suffering from, nor the cause thereof; neither what will be the outcome of his present state, nor the usual results of like conditions. In this state he receives orders, suffering in the present and fearful of the future; full of the disease, and empty of food; wishful of treatment rather to enjoy immediate alleviation of his sickness than to recover his health; not in love with death, but powerless to endure. . . . Surely it is much more likely that the physician gives proper orders, which the patient not unnaturally is unable to follow; and not following them he meets with death, the cause of which illogical reasoners attribute to the innocent, allowing the guilty to go free.[106]

The metaphor of a trial crops up at the beginning and the end of this passage. The physician finds himself in the dock, accused of having killed his patient—unjustly, since it is the patient who, by disobeying the physician's orders, brought about his own death. Clearly this was nothing more than a metaphor: physicians in classical Greece were not responsible in the eyes of the law for the death of their patients. The idea of suing physicians in the courts for professional malpractice had not yet developed. But physicians were nonetheless directly affected by the misdeeds of patients, which threatened irreparable damage to their reputations.

The Hippocratic physicians were not alone in condemning their patients. One finds the following remark in Democritus: "[L]acking self-control, [men] perform contrary actions and betray health to their desires."[107]

The Faults of Physicians

One should not make too much of the accusations brought by physicians against patients. The offenses of patients are, after all, inherent in human nature. And physicians themselves are not exempt from its frailties.

The author of *On Joints*, while denouncing patients' lack of steadfastness, draws attention to a parallel and culpable indifference on the part of physicians. Let us go back to the passage we looked at earlier about patients suffering from a fracture of the collarbone. If this time the passage is reproduced in its entirety, it may be seen that the author's reproaches are not confined to patients alone:

Thus, when the fracture is recent, patients take it seriously, thinking the damage is worse than it is, and practitioners on their side are careful in applying proper treatment; but as time goes on the patients, since they feel no pain and are not hindered either in getting about or eating, neglect the matter, and physicians too, since they cannot make the parts look well, withdraw gradually, and are not displeased by the patients' carelessness, and meanwhile the callus formation quickly develops.[108]

These are harsh words so far as the patient is concerned, as we have seen; but the physician does not get off lightly. He, too, displays inconsistency and inattentiveness. But in his case the failing is much more serious because he does not have the excuse of ignorance to fall back upon. He evades his responsibilities in full knowledge of the facts of the case. Moreover, the term that the author uses to say that the physician shirks his duty, in withdrawing, is extremely strong in Greek: it is the same term that is used to describe soldiers who desert their post. If the patient is negligent, the physician is a deserter. In his absence, disease progresses, silently, swiftly. Thus the irreparable occurs.

SEVEN

The Physician and the Disease

Certain metaphors tell us more, implicitly or explicitly, than theories about the way in which the Hippocratic physician conceived the practice of his art. This was a drama with three characters, not only the physician and the patient, but the disease as well.

An Agonistic Conception of Disease

The metaphors that recur most often are those of struggle and combat. The disease, whether more or less powerful, or more or less rapid, attacks a patient, who in his turn is more or less resistant to it; and the treatment prescribed by the physician must do battle with the disease in order that the patient may escape the onslaught of illness. A race takes place between the disease, from the moment it attacks the patient, and the physician, who from the moment he intervenes plays the role of savior: "For if disease and treatment start together, the disease will not win the race, but it will if it start with an advantage," declares the author of *The Art*.[1] To treat is to oppose the disease. Thus an adversarial therapeutics, based on the clash of opposites, was fundamental to Hippocratic medicine. "[T]he physician must set himself against the established character of illness," says the author of *Nature of Man*;[2] and the author of the treatise *Breaths*, in his prologue, utters the formula that was to become the most famous of all: "opposites are cures for opposites."[3]

Hippocratic Nosology

Which diseases did the Hippocratic physician find himself confronted with in the practice of his art? What means did he have at his disposal in attempting to combat them?

This is not the place to discuss Hippocratic pathology and the basic principles of therapy that flowed from this theory—we will take up these matters
later, in connection with the discussion of rationalism. First we need to sketch
the major types of disease that the physician met with in the course of his
practice and the main forms of treatment that were available to him.

Hippocratic nosology is striking both for the richness and subtlety of the
physician's knowledge of disease and for the effort he made to organize this
material in broad categories. By Hippocrates' time, the majority of the diseases that constitute the nosology of Greek medicine were known. The
names of these diseases, whether already attested in the literature prior to
Hippocrates or appearing for the first time in the *Corpus Hippocraticum*, were
to serve as the foundation of Western medicine for centuries. But even in the
case of those that appeared for the first time in the corpus, one does not have
the impression that they were newly coined. The Hippocratic physicians
always spoke of them as if they were things that were known—another proof,
among many, that medicine did not begin with Hippocrates.

As an example of a disease whose name was attested before the time of
Hippocrates, consider the malady that affected the most famous mythical
patient of antiquity, Philoctetes. Homeric epic tells of the unfortunate pre-
dicament of this Thessalian chief, "who lay apart in the island, suffering
strong pains, in Lemnos the sacrosanct, where the sons of the Achaians had
left him in agony from the sore bite of the wicked water snake."[4] The pitiable
fate of Philoctetes, abandoned on account of his illness by the Achaeans in the
course of their expedition to Troy, then reclaimed by them ten years later
because his bow, inherited from Heracles, was indispensable to final victory
over the Trojans, was a special source of inspiration to the great tragic authors:
Aeschylus, Sophocles, and Euripides each composed a *Philoctetes*. In the *Iliad*,
Philoctetes' illness did not yet have a name, or at least the name is not
mentioned. By contrast, from Aeschylus on, it has the name *phagedaina*—
phagedaena, which means "the devouring [disease]."[5] The etymology of the
name plainly refers to the action of the malady: an ulcer, produced by the
snakebite, devoured Philoctetes' foot. This particular term is explained by
the archaic belief that diseases were monsters of a sort, endowed with peculiar
forces that ate into the patient from the outside and devoured him like wild
beasts.[6] The term reappears several times in the Hippocratic Collection,
where it denotes, as in the case of Philoctetes, a gnawing ulcer.[7] Modern
medical vocabulary preserves the legacy of this disease. Jean Hamburger's
dictionary of medicine lists the adjective "phagedenic" and gives the following definition: "Describes an ulceration having an extensive and unusually

destructive appearance, resistant and lacking histological specificity."[8] The modern definition nicely preserves what was essential about it from the beginning; namely, the destructive action of the ulcer. But how many doctors are still aware today that the first patient known to have had an phagedenic ulcer was Philoctetes?

It would be tedious to list all the names of diseases mentioned in the Hippocratic Collection. We will restrict ourselves here to citing a few names of diseases and afflictions that continue to figure in the most recent dictionaries of medicine: amblyopia, aphonia, aphtha, apoplexy, arthritis, asthma, cancer, coma, coryza, cholera, dropsy, dysuria, edema, emphysema, empyema, erysipelas, exanthema, tertian fever, quartan fever, hemeralopia, hemorrhoid, hepatitis, herpes, ileus, jaundice, leprosy, lethargy, lichen, lientery, lipothymia, lithiasis, mania, melancholy, meteorism, nephritis, ophthalmia, paraplegia, phagedenic (ulcer), phthisis, pleurisy, pneumonia, polypus, spasm, tenesmus, tetanus (along with its variant, opisthotonos), typhus. Even as long a list as this gives only a very partial idea of the variety of names for diseases contained in the Hippocratic Collection.

A comparison with older dictionaries—Littré's dictionary from last century, for instance—shows that other terms designating illnesses in the collection were preserved until comparatively recently, though they have since fallen out of use and no longer appear in current dictionaries: cardialgia, causus, cephalagy (replaced now by headache), epial fever, frenesia, leukophlegmasia, lipuria, peripneumonia, phlegmasia, podagra, strangury (replaced now by pollakiuria, a compound term formed from the Greek but unknown to Greek physicians of the ancient period).

Finally, other terms for illness familiar to Hippocratic physicians are not even listed in the dictionary compiled by Littré, who nonetheless was aware of them as the editor of the standard French edition of the collection. Some of these terms seem as foreign to the modern reader as the names of prehistoric animals: alphus, for example; also carus, and catochus.

Hippocratic Nosology and Modern Nosology

Even where the names of diseases commonly used in Hippocrates' time are still used in our own, one must be careful not to assume too much from the fact that a word has survived unchanged. In its modern use it may not always correspond to the same reality.

Of course, certain afflictions that have preserved the same name do in fact refer to the same thing. In particular, the situation with regard to surgical conditions, wounds, fractures, dislocations, and the like has not fundamentally changed. The same is true for certain other macroscopic external conditions; thus, for example, the nasal "polypus," or "polyp" (which is only the Greek name for "octopus"; that is to say, a marine animal having "many feet") is no different in Hippocrates than it is today. Even the description of certain internal conditions roughly corresponds to our present understanding of them. This is the case, for example, with tetanus, whose external symptoms are so characteristic, and dropsy, even though this older term has now been replaced by ascites and anasarca, as well as with cancer.

But other diseases, while keeping the same name, have changed partially or radically in meaning as a result of continuing medical progress. An example of a disease whose meaning has partially changed is pleurisy (Greek *pleuritis*). Pleurisy is defined today by the inflammation of the two serous membranes that form the pleurae. Pleurae were not known in Hippocrates' time, when pleurisy referred simply to a pain in the side. Leprosy may be cited as an example of a whole class of diseases that, despite the permanence of their name, has radically changed in meaning: in Hippocrates, leprosy (literally, desquamation) is only a mild skin condition, and not the disfiguring disease due to Hansen's bacillus.[9]

The gap between Hippocratic and modern nosology is due to the fact that systems of reference have changed, as contemporary historians of medicine are well aware. One of them judiciously remarks that "the carving up of nosological reality with the help of clinical symptomatology and a doctrine that attributed a preponderant role to the fluid parts of the organism has been replaced today by anatomical and etiological diagnosis, indeed by a molecular definition of lesions, that is to say by precisely those criteria which, leaving aside certain surgical conditions, were unavailable to the practitioners of antiquity."[10] Thus it is a tricky business, even for physicians, to make retrospective diagnoses of Hippocratic diseases or patients. One has only to consider the various retrospective diagnoses that have been proposed for the famous "plague" of Athens that arose at the end of the fifth century, immortalized in the account of the historian Thucydides.[11] Certain retrospective diagnoses have, of course, won unanimous approval among historians of science. For example, what Hippocratic physicians referred to as the "sacred disease," or the "disease called sacred," corresponds roughly to epilepsy.[12] Certain other diseases are well described and indisputably recognizable: mumps with orchitis, paludal fevers (known as tertian and quartan fevers), typhoid fevers, pneumonia, phthisis (or consumption), tetanus. But owing to the difficulty of converting ancient nosology into modern terms, we will restrict ourselves here for the most part to the picture of disease presented by the Hippocratic physicians themselves.

Principles of Classification of Diseases

In order to make sense of all these diseases, physicians had to find a way to order them. Alphabetical ordering, which seems such a familiar method to us, was never adopted by the physicians of Hippocrates' time.

One classification device, which was quite ancient, having been already employed in Egyptian medicine, consisted in treating every disease as being comparable with any other, beginning with diseases of the head and working on down to diseases of the feet—an ordering that scholars later were to call *a capite ad calcem* (from head to foot)—and in adopting for the presentation of each disease a standard framework that nonetheless allowed for subtle variations: first, identification of the disease and description of symptoms, then therapy and prognosis. This principle of composition, which amounts to placing accounts of each disease side by side in a continuous series, each account being similarly organized, was without doubt an archaic one in which juxtaposition prevailed over hierarchy. The same principle was applied earlier in Homer's *Iliad*, for example, in book 2, with its famous catalog of the Achaean contingents that took part in the Trojan War. The same principle may still be detected in certain works of the Hippocratic Collection, particularly in the two nosological treatises of Cnidian origin, *Diseases II* and *Internal Affections*, which are constituted solely by the juxtaposition of statements about particular diseases. They begin with diseases of the head, moving on to diseases of the throat and nose; next come the diseases of the breast and back. This juxtapositional style of thought is seen also in the multiplication of different varieties of a single disease, all once again presented as being on the same level. Thus the treatise *Internal Affections* presents three consumptions, three tetanuses, four jaundices, four kinds of kidney ailment.[13] Now we know from Galen that this manner of subdividing diseases into a fixed number of varieties was characteristic of Cnidian physicians, who distinguished not only (as *Internal Affections* attests) three consumptions, three tetanuses, four jaundices, and four diseases of the kidney, but also four stranguries, seven bilious diseases, and twelve diseases of the bladder.[14] Is this method of classifying diseases and dividing them up to be regarded merely as a sign of archaism or of the existence of a technical literature? It is, perhaps, a sign of both.

The fact nonetheless remains that this way of proceeding, according to which one disease follows another, was not adopted in the treatises that traditionally have been identified with the school of Cos. Nosological entities do not constitute the organizing principle of these works: even treatises that can be considered as encyclopedias of a sort, such as the *Aphorisms* and *Prenotions of Cos*, are not constructed in this manner. Diseases are typically discussed not on an individual basis, one by one, but instead are grouped together into categories that differ according to the various points of view from which they are discussed. Certain of these categories, or principles of classification, are already attested in Greek literature prior to Hippocrates.

Classification of Diseases: From Pindar to Hippocrates

The most ancient catalog of diseases that we have for Greece is found in a poem by Pindar, the third *Pythian Ode*, in which the poet evokes the medical feats of Asclepius, "the healer hero of all diseases":

> And those who came to him with flesh-devouring sores,
> with limbs gored by gray bronze or crushed beneath flung stones,
> all those with bodies broken, sun-struck or frost-bitten,
> he freed of their misery, each from his ailment.[15]

From this passage emerges a tripartite division of diseases: diseases that come into existence by themselves within the body; wounds; and finally illnesses due to the seasons. Such a division is not precisely reproduced in the Hippocratic treatises. Thanks to their greater concern for logical order, they tend to adopt a binary schema, opposing diseases due to some internal cause to diseases provoked by some external cause, as a result of which wounds and diseases caused by the seasons are put under the latter rubric. The treatise *Diseases I*, for example, states this principle of classification as follows: "Now all our diseases arise either from things inside the body, bile and phlegm, or from things outside it: from exertions and wounds, and from heat that makes it too hot, and cold that makes it too cold."[16]

Diseases and Seasons

If the great categories of diseases were now simplified, the subcategories were to become more refined. While Pindar divided the diseases caused by the seasons in two, diseases of summer and diseases of winter, the Hippocratic authors divided them in four. There were not only diseases of summer and winter, but also diseases of the intermediate seasons, spring and autumn. Thus the treatise of *Aphorisms*, in a quite celebrated passage that was to inspire the

Latin encyclopedist Celsus, groups diseases together according to the season in which they most readily appear:

In spring occur melancholia, madness, epilepsy, bloody flux, angina, colds, sore throats, coughs, skin eruptions and diseases, eruptions turning generally to ulcers, tumours and affections of the joints.

In summer occur some of the diseases just mentioned, and also continued fevers, ardent fevers, tertians, vomiting, diarrhoea, eye diseases, pains of the ears, ulcerations of the mouth, mortification of the genitals, sweats.

In autumn occur most summer diseases, with quartans, irregular fevers, enlarged spleen, dropsy, consumption, strangury, lientery, dysentery, sciatica, angina, asthma, ileus, epilepsy, madness, melancholia.

In winter occur pleurisy, pneumonia, lethargus, colds, sore throat, coughs, pains in the sides, chest and loins, headache, dizziness, apoplexy.[17]

These seasonal diseases are born and die with the rhythm of the seasons. Thus the author of *Nature of Man* declares:

[S]uch diseases as increase in the winter ought to cease in the summer, and such as increase in the summer ought to cease in the winter. . . . When diseases arise in spring, expect their departure in autumn. Such diseases as arise in autumn must have their departure in spring. Whenever a disease passes these limits, you may know that it will last a year. The physician too must treat diseases with the conviction that each of them is powerful in the body according to the season which is most conformable to it.[18]

Diseases and Places

To these principles of classification for diseases, which we find already in embryonic form in Pindar, Hippocratic physicians added others involving new factors.

Among the diseases that arose from the surrounding environment, there were not only general diseases due to the seasons but also local diseases dependent upon the orientation of cities. This distinction is made particularly by the author of *Airs, Waters, Places*, who, in the first part of his treatise, draws up four nosological categories corresponding to the four main orientations that cities can have. In cities exposed to hot and humid winds from the south, moist and phlegmatic diseases prevail, such as dysentery and diarrhea, and wet ophthalmia.[19] By contrast, in cities that are oppositely situated, that is to say toward the cold and dry winds of the north, the predominant diseases are dry and bilious, such as pleurisy, peripneumonia, causus, and dry ophthalmia.[20] Cities facing toward the west are the most insalubrious.[21] But this new classification of diseases as a function of the orientation of places was not totally independent of the classification of diseases according to seasons. The author of *Airs, Waters, Places* compares the orientation of places with the seasons: a city facing east resembles the spring by its settled climate; a city facing west recalls autumn because of its contrasts of temperature. An analogy is therefore established, more or less explicitly, between local diseases and seasonal diseases.

Diseases and Age of the Patient

Diseases did not vary only as a function of the surrounding environment, of seasons or places, but depended also upon the nature of the patient, on his or her sex and age. Thus the author of *Airs, Waters, Places* organizes its two nosological categories with reference to cities facing toward the south and toward the north while distinguishing between diseases of women and those of men, on the one hand, and between maladies of children and those of old persons on the other.[22] In the *Aphorisms*, the age of a person becomes a principle for classifying diseases comparable with that of seasons. Thus, having first been divided up according to the time of year in which they predominate, diseases are then classified according to the ages of the persons afflicted by them:

In the different ages the following complaints occur: to little children and babies, aphthae, vomiting, coughs, sleeplessness, terrors, inflammation of the navel, watery discharges from the ears.

At the approach of dentition, irritation of the gums, fevers, convulsions, diarrhoea, especially when cutting the canine teeth, and in the case of very fat children, and if the bowels are hard.

Among those who are older occur affections of the tonsils, curvature at the vertebra by the neck, asthma, stone, round worms, ascarides, warts, swellings by the ears, scrofula and tumours generally.

Older children and those approaching puberty suffer from most of the preceding maladies, from fevers of the more protracted type and from bleeding at the nose.

Most diseases of children reach a crisis in forty days, in seven months, in seven years, at the approach of puberty. But such as persist among boys without ceasing at puberty, or, in the case of girls, at the commencement of menstruation, are wont to become chronic.

Young men suffer from spitting of blood, phthisis, acute fevers, epilepsy and the other diseases, especially those mentioned above.

Those who are beyond this age suffer from asthma, pleurisy, pneumonia, lethargus, phrenitis, ardent fevers, chronic diarrhoea, cholera, dysentery, lientery, hemorrhoids.

Old men suffer from difficulty of breathing, catarrh accompanied by coughing, strangury, difficult micturition, pains at the joints, kidney disease, dizziness, apoplexy, cachexia, pruritus of the whole body, sleeplessness, watery discharges from the bowels, eyes, and nostrils, dullness of sight, cataract, hardness of hearing.[23]

Alternative Approaches to Classification

These various attempts to classify diseases using a series of criteria involving the nature of the affection, its causes and localization within the body, as well as the nature of the patient and the patient's sex and age had not yet managed by Hippocrates' time to produce a universally approved codification.

Beyond acknowledging the diversity of diseases, physicians sought to group them in more or less coherent ways. Some tried to reduce multiplicity to unity, on the model of certain pre-Socratic philosophers who endeavored to explain the multiplicity of the sensible world by reference to a single principle. Thus the author of the treatise *Breaths* considered that all diseases reduce to one and the same form, differing from each other only in respect of localization: "Now of all diseases the fashion is the same, but the seat varies. So while diseases are thought to be entirely unlike one another, owing to the difference in their seat, in reality all have one essence and one cause."[24]

This cause is air, which, according to the author, explained fevers as well as stomach aches, fluxes of humors, ruptures, dropsy, apoplexy, and the "sacred disease" (epilepsy). "If indeed I were to speak of all maladies," he concludes, "my discourse, while being longer, would not be in the least more true or more convincing."[25]

Such attempts at unification, while satisfying to those who looked for ways to organize the diversity of empirical data, were resisted by practitioners who felt they unacceptably simplified nosological reality. Thus the author of *Ancient Medicine* leads off his treatise with an attack on those who reduced the fundamental cause of diseases to one or two principles, such as hot, cold, dry, or wet.[26] As a practitioner himself, who was well aware of the complexity of the real world, he preferred to accumulate various categories that could be grouped together on the same level. The author of *Humours* provides a good example of this approach:

The fashions of diseases. Some are congenital and may be learned by inquiry, as also may those that are due to the district . . . Some are the result of the physical constitution, others of regimen, of the constitution of the [year],[27] of the seasons. Countries badly situated with respect to the seasons engender diseases analogous to the season. *E.g.* when it produces irregular heat or cold on the same day, diseases in the country are autumnal, and similarly in the case of the other seasons. Some spring from the smells of mud or marshes, others from waters, stone, for example, and diseases of the spleen; of this kind are waters because of winds good or bad.[28]

This list contains two categories of diseases we have already noted: local diseases and seasonal diseases. But it also introduces a new criterion that permitted a further category of diseases to be identified; namely, congenital maladies. All this proves that there was no fixed catalog. While some Hippocratic physicians tried to take in all of nosological reality by positing broad classes of disease, they did not quite succeed in wholly defining it. Again, what is striking about this enumeration from the treatise on *Humours* is that different categories are placed on the same level without any real attempt at organization. The very nature of the treatise itself is partially responsible: it consists, after all, of notes. But there is a deeper reason as well. The absence of hierarchy that we observe here was characteristic of a period that was prior to the invention of Aristotelian logic. Classification was still flexible and shifting, governed by interlocking principles. Thus while the author of *Humours* sets up places and seasons as the two criteria for classifying diseases, he talks at the same time of places being badly situated with respect to the seasons.

Classification of Fevers

Physicians felt more at ease when maladies could be organized in precise categories. This was especially the case with fevers, which they differentiated less by their intensity (the thermometer did not exist) than by the rhythm of their fluctuations. "Some fevers are continuous . . . ; there are semitertians, tertians, quartans, quintans, septans, nonans," declares the author of *Epidemics I* at the beginning of a long section on the classification of fevers, the most complex of those devised by Hippocratic physicians. Ordinarily they restricted themselves to four sorts of fevers: continuous, quotidian, tertian, and quartan. This, in any case, was the classification upheld by the author of *Nature of Man*.[29] Modern nomenclature has retained only three of its terms: continuous fever, on the one hand, and, on the other, tertian fever and quartan fever, the latter being characteristic of attacks of malaria due, respectively, to *Plasmodium vivax* or *Plasmodium ovale*, and *Plasmodium malariae*. Though ignorant of the exact cause of tertian and quartan fevers, the physicians of Hippocrates' time knew how to tell them apart and how to describe them correctly.

General Diseases and Individual Diseases

Though the classifications of diseases found in the Hippocratic Collection are apt to seem vague and variable, certain broad distinctions appear to have been universally accepted. This was true particularly in the case of the distinction between general diseases and individual diseases, clearly formulated in the treatise *Nature of Man*:

Whenever many men are attacked by one disease at the same time, the cause should be assigned to that which is most common, and which we all use most. This it is which we breathe in. For it is clear that the regimen of each of us is not the cause, since the disease attacks all in turn, both younger and older, men as much as women, those who drink wine as much as teetotallers, those who eat barley cake as much as those who live on bread, those who take much exercise as those who take little. For regimen could not be the cause, when no matter what regimen they have followed all men are attacked by the same disease. But when diseases of all sorts occur at one and the same time, it is clear that in each case the particular regimen is the cause.[30]

This distinction between individual diseases due to poor regimen and general diseases is also found, for example, in the treatise *Breaths*: "[T]here are two kinds of fevers; one is [common to all people], called pestilence [*loimos*], the other is [individual], attacking those who follow a bad regimen."[31] In the same way again, the author of *Regimen in Acute Diseases* contrasts common diseases of a pestilential nature (*loimodès*), which affect whole populations, with sporadic diseases.[32]

It goes without saying that such a distinction was not new in Hippocrates' time. Pestilence (*loimos*), a scourge falling upon an entire community, had haunted people's minds from the earliest times in Greece, in the same way as famine (*limos*). Well before the appearance of the first medical writings, it occupied a large place in Greek literature, not only among the epic and tragic poets but also among the historians. To cite only the most important examples, let us consider two mythical allusions and one historical description: the pestilence that decimates the Achaean expeditionary force before the gates of Troy at the beginning of the *Iliad*, the pestilence that ravages the city of Thebes at the beginning of Sophocles' *Oedipus Tyrannus*, and finally the pestilence described by Thucydides, which came to weaken the city of Athens during its long struggle against Sparta at the end of the fifth century.[33] Pestilence occupies, in fact, a much larger place in the mythical and historical literature of ancient Greece than in its medical literature. The technical writings of the Hippocratic Collection mention it only twice[34]—less often in fact than in the biographical writings of the collection, where reference is made to three waves of pestilence: the first, prior to Hippocrates, struck the army besieging Crisa during the First Sacred War,[35] just as the disease described by Homer diminished the army of the Achaeans laying siege to Troy; of the two others, both occurring during Hippocrates' lifetime, one afflicted Artaxerxes' army[36] and motivated his invitation to Hippocrates, and the other swept over Greece from the north, causing Hippocrates, who had refused to help the barbarians, to travel throughout the country with his disciples to give aid to his fellow Greeks.[37]

The concept of general disease that is opposed to individual disease appears on closer examination not always to apply to the same phenomena in all the Hippocratic treatises. In addition to plague, it can refer to local maladies that are peculiar to the inhabitants of a particular city. This dual meaning arises from a refinement of the analysis that one finds in the treatise *Airs, Waters, Places*. As against particular diseases caused by the regimen of individuals, its author distinguishes local diseases that affect the inhabitants of a city who are jointly subject to the same permanent local factors (geographic orientation with respect to prevailing winds, the nature of the soil, the nature of the waters), on the one hand, and, on the other, common diseases that arise at a given moment in a city and result from factors whose influence extends beyond municipal boundaries (seasons). In place of the traditional notion of general pestilential disease, therefore, a distinction was made that corresponded roughly to the modern distinction between endemic disease and epidemic disease. It needs to be kept in mind that this terminology did not yet exist in Hippocrates' time. The expression "endemic disease" does not occur until the time of Galen, the great physician of the imperial period.[38] In Hippocrates' time, only the term "epidemic" was applied to diseases. It designated, by contrast with individual diseases, a general disease or diseases that affected a large number of inhabitants. At no place in the writings of the Hippocratic authors is an epidemic connected with the idea of contagion. On their view, the general character of an epidemic was not due to the transmission of disease from one affected person to another by contact, but to the influence of the same general factors on each one of the persons affected by the disease (miasmas in the air they breathed, seasons, the exposure of places to the winds, and so on). Thus the term "epidemics" was given as a title to a series of seven books in the Hippocratic Collection examining those diseases that are predominant in a given place, in the course of a given year, having a given climatic constitution.[39]

Acute Diseases

Among individual diseases, one category seems to have been recognized by all the physicians of Hippocrates' time: "acute diseases." Some writers refer to them as such without further comment;[40] others qualify them as "diseases considered acute."[41] These were the most dangerous diseases, the ones that caused the most deaths in the absence of a pestilential epidemic. For this reason, physicians paid quite special attention to them. Two treatises are entirely devoted to them: on the one hand, the *Prognostic*, which, although its title gives no such indication, concerns prognosis in acute diseases;[42] and, on the other, as its title does indicate, the *Regimen in Acute Diseases*. The latter is our most detailed source of information about what physicians in Hippocrates' time intended by the term "acute diseases":

> I should most commend a physician who in acute diseases, which kill the great majority of patients, shows some superiority. Now the acute diseases are those to which the ancients have given the names of pleurisy, pneumonia, phrenitis, and ardent fever, and such as are akin to these, the fever of which is on the whole continuous. For whenever there is no general type of pestilence prevalent, but diseases are sporadic, acute diseases cause many times more deaths than all others put together.[43]

This passage, apart from the fact that it precisely defines what is meant by acute diseases, clearly shows the attempt at synthesis that has been made by the "moderns," at the time of Hippocrates, to reorganize under categories the various diseases that the "ancients" presented in juxtaposed fashion. These categories were, however, still in the process of being worked out. For just as Hippocratic physicians had only the term "epidemic disease" for general diseases, failing to grasp the distinction that was to become classic beginning in the Roman period between "epidemic" and "endemic" disease, so for particular diseases they had only the term "acute diseases," having not yet formulated the distinction between acute and chronic disease, though it already existed in embryonic form.[44] The latter distinction was to become fundamental to Western medicine as well—from before Galen's time, in fact, since it served as the organizing principle of the treatise composed in the first century A.D. by Aretaeus of Cappadocia, the first author to divide all diseases into two great classes, acute and chronic, for purposes both of pathology and of treatment.

Assessment of Hippocratic Nosology

The first thing one notes in studying "the voiceless people of the diseases that visit men day and night" (to recall Hesiod's phrase) is the extreme wealth of nosological terminology in the Hippocratic Collection. On the whole, this terminology was not a creation of Hippocratic physicians but rather a legacy of the ancients, and sometimes regarded as such. In the Cnidian writings, moreover, the various diseases were subdivided into meticulously codified types. One notes next an attempt at synthesis, at going beyond the multiplicity of these diseases by organizing them into broad categories. To be sure, this effort at synthesis was not an innovation of the Hippocratic period, either. We have already mentioned an earlier attempt by Pindar in the first half of the fifth century. But within the Hippocratic Collection itself, the consolidation of diseases was apt to be seen as something new by comparison with the nomenclature of the ancients. A conscious effort therefore was made prior to the great era of classification inaugurated by Aristotle and his school to organize diseases along different lines, some of which were to be adopted, refined, and codified by physicians who came after Hippocrates.

Classification of Remedies: From Pindar to Hippocrates

In addition to the classification of diseases, physicians made a parallel attempt to classify remedies. Here again the poet Pindar supplied an earlier and interesting example. In his ode praising Asclepius, he presented not only a classification of the diseases that the son of Apollo treated, but also a classification of the remedies that he employed to cure them:

> And those who came to him . . .
> he freed of their misery, each from his ailment,
>   and led them forth—
> some to the lull of soft spells, others by potions,
> still others with bandages steeped in medications
> culled from all quarters, and some he set right
> through surgery.[45]

The poet puts on the same level therapeutic methods that a modern historian of science would tend to categorize rather differently: incantations, or prayers sung to dispel evil, seem to us today to come under the head of magic, whereas the other methods—potions, unctions, and incisions—seem to have a more rational basis. By comparison with Pindar's list, the Hippocratic Collection marks both a rupture and a continuation. It marks a break with what went before to the extent that for the first time in the history of medicine rational methods came to be set apart from those of magic: incantations were not prescribed, but condemned.[46] It represents a continuation with the past to the extent that all the other therapeutic methods mentioned by Pindar—incisions, potions, and unctions—were used by Hippocratic physicians. Their elimination of magic in treatment was all the more remarkable since incantations continued to enjoy the same esteem as other methods of treatment in the popular medicine of Hippocrates' time. The attack by the author of *The Sacred Disease* upon charlatans who used incantations to treat epilepsy is evidence of this.[47] Further evidence is provided by Greek theater. Consider the famous lines that Sophocles gives Ajax, the hero from Salamis: "No good physician quavers incantations / When the malady he's treating needs the knife."[48] By this maxim, the dramatist intended to criticize not the therapeutic practice of incantation as such, only its improper application. Incantations and incisions both belonged among the paraphernalia of the physician in Sophocles as in Pindar.

A Therapeutic Triad: Medicines, Incisions, Cauterizations

What defined the physician in the popular mind of fifth-century Greece, however, was not efficacious speech but the lancet and the branding iron. In Greek literature, the expression "to cut and burn" (*temnein kai kaiein*) served as the identifying mark of medical activity, just as the cupping glass hung on the wall was its distinctive sign in the visual arts.

It was by means of a metaphor that plainly referred to the "burning and cutting" physician who sought to expel the scourge of disease that Aeschylus's Agamemnon, returned home victorious after long years away, expressed his determination to restore order to his kingdom.[49] Socrates, who led his disciples to reflect upon the activity of the professions, himself greatly contributed to the popularization of this image of the physician. Through his teaching, immortalized by Plato and Xenophon, the physician came to appear as the one who "cuts and burns." To cite just one example from among many others, in Plato's *Gorgias*, Socrates counsels a man who has committed a crime "to grit his teeth and present himself [to the judge] with grace and courage as to a doctor for cauterization and surgery."[50]

This, then, was the positive image of the physician, as one who acted vigorously by means of knife and fire on behalf of the patient. The same physician was also seen quite negatively, however, as one who by the same means tortured his patient and left him to suffer. Already in antiquity, well before Molière, physicians were ridiculed by comic authors, one of whom, the Athenian comic poet Plato, alluded to a patient who had been left covered with scabs by the Cnidian physician Euryphon.[51] At least one pre-Socratic philosopher helped spread this unfavorable image. Heraclitus spoke of doctors "who cut and cauterize and wretchedly torment the sick."[52]

Treatment by knife and fire remained the symbol of the physician's practice in the popular imagination because it represented what was most memorable and most painful from the point of view of the patient. Patients were sometimes also made to drink medicines (*pharmaka*). They balked at taking bitter potions, just as they refused treatment by knife and fire. The patients whom the Sophist Gorgias tried his best to convince refused "to take [their] medicine or allow the doctor to perform surgery or cauterization on [them]."[53]

This therapeutic triad of medicines, incisions, and cauterizations also figures in the Hippocratic Collection.[54] From the accounts found there, unlike the ones contained in the nonmedical literature, one learns that physicians ranked these three types of treatment according to their degree of effectiveness: "Those diseases that medicines do not cure," says the author of the *Aphorisms*, "are cured by the knife. Those that the knife does not cure are cured by fire. Those that fire does not cure must be considered incurable."[55]

There is not room here to go into these three categories of therapeutic method in great detail. We will therefore restrict ourselves to sketching the broad outlines of their use by Hippocratic physicians.

Evacuation

With regard to medicines, it is notable that most of them aimed at evacuating the "cavities" of the body. The Hippocratic physicians considered human beings to have two great cavities: the "upper cavity," which is to say the chest, and the "lower cavity," which is to say the stomach. Evacuation was therefore said to be either upwards or downwards. Vomiting and bowel evacuations were recommended either as preventive or curative measures. According to the author of *Nature of Man*, good hygiene required that vomiting be induced in winter and bowel evacuations in summer:

Emetics and clysters for the bowels should be used thus. Use emetics during the six winter months, for this period engenders more phlegm than does the summer, and in it occur the diseases that attack the head and the region above the diaphragm. But when the weather is hot use clysters, for the season is burning, the body bilious, heaviness is felt in the loins and the knees, feverishness comes on and colic in the belly. So the body must be cooled, and the humours that rise must be drawn downwards from these regions.[56]

It is above all in the case of diseases that these two types of evacuation were prescribed. Originally their purpose was to eliminate the disease, regarded as an impurity. We know that the same terms (belonging to the family *ka-*

thairein) were used in Greek to signify purgation and purification. The sick body was an impure body. There was therefore no difference in kind between medical treatment and rites of purification. In both cases it was necessary to remove an impurity. The language testifies here to a primitive identification of medicine and religion. But with the development of a more rational theory, of humors, evacuation was assigned a more specific role: to eliminate the humoral excess that was considered to be the cause of the disease. It was thus that Hippocratic physicians employed medicines that evacuated phlegm or bile. The author of *Nature of Man* thought it obvious that one could evacuate at will one of the four humors that, according to him, constituted the nature of man: "If you were to give a man a medicine which withdraws phlegm, he will vomit you phlegm; if you give him one which withdraws bile, he will vomit you bile. Similarly too black bile is purged away if you give a medicine which withdraws black bile. And if you wound a man's body so as to cause a wound, blood will flow from him."[57] The author does not say exactly how these selective evacuations were to be obtained.

Ordinarily, vomiting occurred following the absorption of food and drink. It was either spontaneous or facilitated by tickling the throat with a feather.[58] As for downward evacuations, they were provoked by clysters or, more drastically, by purgatives. One of the mildest purgatives was boiled ass's milk, or whey; the most powerful was hellebore. But physicians knew many other purgatives as well, as this passage from the *Regimen in Acute Diseases* suggests:

If the pain be under the diaphragm . . . , soften the bowels with black hellebore or peplium, mixing with the black hellebore daucus, seseli, cumin, anise or some other fragrant herb, and with the peplium juice of silphium. . . . Black hellebore causes evacuations that are better and more favourable to the crisis than does peplium; but peplium breaks flatulence better than black hellebore. Both, however, stop pain, as do many other evacuants; but these are the best I know of.[59]

Discovering the proper dosage of the most powerful purgatives was not a simple matter. Hellebore, for example, had only recently been mastered. Hippocrates' young relative Ctesias of Cnidus reported that neither his grandfather nor his father knew how to use it.[60] Even in Hippocrates' and Ctesias's time, accidents appear not to have been unusual. Xenophon noted in his *Anabasis* the case of the Lacedaemonian military strategist Chirisophus, who died from an evacuant taken to relieve fever.[61] But it was above all the Hippocratic physicians themselves who drew attention in their treatises to the harmful consequences of excessive evacuation, for which they had already coined the technical term "superpurgation."[62] The most careful of these physicians was the author of *Epidemics V*, who, despite taking great pains in these case studies objectively to describe the development of an affection and the treatment administered, did not refrain from commenting critically from time to time upon the outcome. In one such case, concerning treatment of a gangrenous hip, the author suggests at the end that the prescribed strength of the evacuant was poorly judged:

Scamandrus in Larissa had mortification in the hip; in time the bone came free. A large incision up to the bone was cut, and then cauterized. Then on the twelfth day after the incision, spasm began, and it increased. That leg was drawn up right to the ribs. And the contraction migrated to the other side. The leg was bent double and very tense and his other limbs trembled and his jaws were fixed. He died drawn up on the eighth day after the spasm came on. He was treated with fomentations made from leather bottles, and with heated vetch seeds over the whole body. He was given an enema and a little old excrement came out. He took the saturated (purgative) drug and repeated it. He did pass excrement. There was no help from what he drank. He slept a little. Having drunk the saturated drug [in its strong form] again at evening, he died at sunrise. It seemed that he would have survived longer if not for the strength of the medicine.[63]

This case study perfectly illustrates the different modes of therapeutic intervention that physicians had at their disposal in Hippocrates' time. In addition to the major triad (incision, cauterization, evacuation) there were fomentations and hot baths. But it is on the subject of evacuations that this passage is most instructive. A clyster was administered first. When it proved ineffective, stronger methods were employed: probably black hellebore. The dose must have been large, because the patient needed two tries to swallow all of it. But as this purgative did not produce the anticipated effect, it was prescribed again, only this time in still more concentrated form. The result was that the medicine in all likelihood killed the patient. The physician's final comment leaves no doubt about his opinion of the procedure.

The danger of evacuants was emphasized more generally by another Hippocratic physician: "But medications that clean bile or phlegm are a source of danger [for those who are treated], and of blame for the person treating."[64]

To complete the picture of upward and downward evacuations, it is necessary to mention two incidental methods. The class of lower evacuations also included diuretics.[65] Here is the recipe for one of them: "One administers the diuretic composed in this way: raisins and white chickpeas, two choenixes of peas [= 2.04 liters] and one of raisins [= 1.02 liters]; pour in three half-congiuses of water [= 4.8 liters]; after having decanted, expose to the evening dew and drink the next morning."[66] The dose is frighteningly large. Was the patient required to drink all of it? Probably so. Diuretics could prove to be as dangerous as purgatives. The author of *Epidemics V* cites the case of a patient in Larissa who died after having had his intestines "ulcerated by the excessive strength of the [acrid diuretic]."[67]

It was also thought possible to purge the head of its humors by means of evacuation from above. The method consisted of introducing irritant substances into the nostrils to provoke sneezing and discharges. In Hippocrates' time, however, the technical term for such substances had not yet been coined; only later would one speak of errhines (from the Greek *errinon*, meaning "that which is put in the nose"). Here is how a physician who came after Hippocrates described the procedure: "One employs errhines in the following way: one takes a thin tube, straight, six fingers long, and so disposed as to be able to fit in the nose. One fills the whole empty space of the tube with the medicine. One may choose a reed or a copper pipe. After having placed the tube in the nose, one breathes in to it from the end opposite to that by which the medicine is made to enter into the nose."[68] What was put up the patient's nose in this manner? One physician mentions peeled onion,[69] another pepper.[70] The poor patient!

Incision

Like the evacuant medicines, the knife served originally to expel illness through the elimination of impure liquids. The practice of bleeding, or venesection, which was employed almost as frequently as purgation, was known before Hippocrates' time. (It is exactly this operation, as we saw earlier, that is represented on the small perfume vase of the Louvre dating to about 470 B.C., or a decade or so prior to Hippocrates' birth.) Though the procedure was a common one, it nonetheless had to be learned. We have already mentioned the precise instructions that were given to the physician with regard to the proper position of his body and his hand in performing this operation.[71] The operation also assumed a knowledge of veins and arteries. Thus it is that the treatise *Nature of Man* presents a complete account of the blood vessels, with the express purpose of determining the points where bleeding can safely be done. The author concludes his presentation with the following words: "Bleeding then should be practised according to these principles. The habit should be cultivated of cutting as far as possible from the places where the pains are wont to occur and the blood to collect. In this way the change will be least sudden and violent, and you will change the habit so that the blood no longer collects in the same place."[72]

Bleeding could be done at many points of the body, chiefly the arms at the bend of the elbow and the legs behind the knee or at the ankle, but also the head and the area beneath the tongue.[73] Many diseases were thought to present suitable opportunities for bleeding. Some of the cases in which it was recommended seem surprising today. One physician went so far as to recommend bleeding at the ankle during a difficult childbirth: "If the pregnant woman goes a long time without being able to deliver and suffers for several days, and if she is young, in the prime of life and has much blood, it is necessary to incise the veins at the ankles and to draw blood, according to the strength of the subject."[74]

Unhelpful though this advice may be, the physician nonetheless exhibits a certain degree of circumspection. Knowing that surgical intervention weakens the patient, he advises resort to it only on the condition that the patient is robust. Another physician adds a similar note of caution in recommending venesection in the case of acute diseases: "The acute affections you treat with phlebotomy, if the disease seems to be severe, and patients are at the height of their youth and strength."[75]

This passage takes frank account of the dilemma faced by the physician. A strong disease called for a strong remedy, but it was necessary to make sure the remedy was not so strong that it weakened the patient to the point of death. One wonders how patients could have survived some of the purgations and phlebotomies to which they were subjected. Consider, for example, the strenuous course of treatment endured by a man in Oeniadae who sought relief for an upset stomach: "He drank various drugs to purge upward and downward, and was not benefited. But when he was bled in each arm in turn until he was bloodless, then he was benefited and freed from the trouble."[76] In the judgment of the physician, evacuants were inadequate to eliminate the cause of the illness; bleeding, a theoretically more forceful intervention, showed itself to be the more effective remedy.

Cauterization

We now come to the most powerful form of medication available to the physicians of antiquity, that which burns: "[O]f the caustics employed in medicine fire is the most powerful, though there are many others less powerful than it. Now affections that are too strong for the less powerful caustics plainly are not for this reason incurable; but those which are too strong for the most powerful plainly are incurable."[77]

Fire was regarded, therefore, as the treatment of last resort. Thus the author of *Diseases II*, confronted with a recurring disease of the head, recommends, in addition to three types of evacuants, no fewer than eight cauterizations of the skull, two beside the ears, two on the temples, two in back of the head, and two on the nose near the corners of the eyes. The physician ends on an optimistic note, declaring, "If a person [submits to] these things, he recovers."[78] The lucky patient who survived was left covered with scars, of course. One begins to understand why the comic playwrights of the period displayed such sarcasm toward practices of this kind.

Cauterization was supposed to block the advance of illness. The author of *Internal Affections*, considering a disease that he believes to be caused by the flow of bile and phlegm through the blood vessels, recommends that ten cauterizations be performed—four at the base of the right shoulder blade, two in the buttock, two in the middle of the thigh, one above the knee, one above the malleolus. This is surely a record! Then he adds triumphantly: "If a person is cauterized in this way, it will not allow the disease to migrate either upwards or downwards."[79]

But the strain of such treatments threatened to tax the unfortunate patient beyond his limits. Another physician, the author of *Epidemics V*, was well aware of this. He records the story of another inhabitant of Oeniadae, this one suffering from an abscess on the hip, who was heavily cauterized: "The scars were numerous, large, and close together. Much thick pus ran out. He died a few days after that, from the size and number of the wounds and from the weakness of his body."[80] The criticism implied here is shortly made explicit, as the author immediately goes on to note that if treatment had been restricted to one or two incisions to drain the pus, the patient would probably have been restored to health.

A Dietary Therapeutics

In addition to this first category of treatments relying on intervention in various forms—evacuative medicines, incisions, and cauterizations—the physician disposed of a second set of resources for fighting disease; these were associated with the diet and exercise habits of the patient.

While invasive methods of therapy had long been recognized as a fundamental part of traditional medicine, the art of regimen was considered in antiquity to have been a more recent achievement.[81] The most famous account in this connection is to be found in the *Republic*. To the pharmacological medicine of the Homeric epoch, Plato opposed the dietary medicine of his contemporaries. Plato did not regard this development as evidence of progress. The new medicine, which forced patients to observe a protracted course of treatment, diverted them in his view from fulfilling their duties as citizens.[82] But it seemed to represent progress from the point of view of physicians. The Hippocratic author who describes the regimen to be followed in acute diseases criticizes the pharmacological character of the therapeutics promoted by the authors of the *Cnidian Sentences*, and reproaches the ancients in general for having said nothing worthwhile about regimen.[83] A therapeutics that did not restrict itself to evacuation, incision, and cauterization in seeking to eliminate illness, but that adapted the regimen of the patient to the disease and its evolution, was indeed something new in the medicine of the late fifth century and early fourth century, as the reaction of Plato and other contemporaries confirms.

By "regimen" it is necessary to understand not only the patient's alimentary regime but also his habits of exercise. Other secondary elements entered into the art of regimen as well: baths, sometimes sleep, even the patient's sexual habits.

Alimentary Catalogs

To prescribe an alimentary regime for the patient, the physician had to know the "power of various foods and drinks, both what they are by nature and what by art."[84] The power of food and drink due to art is to be interpreted as referring to the results of the culinary art. This is why in the Hippocratic Collection, prior to the encyclopedic categorizations of the Aristotelian school, one meets with the first catalogs in Greek literature giving the properties of various diets. The longest and most complete of these catalogs is found in the treatise whose very title incorporates the word *regimen*—*Regimen*.[85] A briefer catalog occupies the last part of the treatise *Affections*.[86] Additional information is scattered throughout a good number of other treatises, particularly in *Regimen in Acute Diseases*.

The catalog of the *Regimen* is a mine of information about the diet and cuisine of the Greeks of the classical era. It reveals the properties of cereals, meats, fish, vegetables, fruits, eggs, cheeses, and, in beverages, of waters, wines, and vinegars. Here, for example, is what it tells us about animal meats. The ancient Greeks ate, as we do today, veal and beef, suckling pig and pork, lamb and mutton, but they also ate horse, donkey, and dog. As for game, in addition to hare, venison, and wild boar, they ate fox and porcupine. One learns, too, of the various methods for preserving meats, not only in salt, but also in wine and vinegar. More generally, what is striking about this catalog is the extraordinary variety of foods mentioned. For example, under the head of vegetables—a category that is broader than ours to the extent that it also takes in aromatic plants—the catalog of the *Regimen* cites some forty different names. But what is still more astonishing is the meticulous care with which the author specifies in each case the various properties of the foods that he cites; that is to say, the effects produced by each of them upon the body. Foods are said to heat or cool, moisten or dry out; they relax the bowels or tighten them; they are nourishing or slimming; they cause burps or wind. Certain of these properties may be combined in the same food. And the same food can change properties depending on its origin, its degree of freshness, and above all its preparation. To illustrate the subtlety of the distinctions made by physicians with regard to the various properties of foods, consider what the author of the *Regimen* has to say about barley and barley cakes:

Barley in its own nature is cold, moist and drying, but it has something purgative from the juice of the husks. This is proved by boiling unwinnowed barley, the decoction of which is very purgative; but if it be winnowed, it is more cooling and astringent. When it is parched, the moist and purgative quality is removed by the fire, and that which is left is cool and dry. When, therefore, it is necessary to cool and dry, barley meal thus used will do it, no matter how the cake is prepared; such, in fact, is the power of the barley cake. The meal together with the bran has less nourishment, but passes better by stool. That which is cleaned from the bran is more nourishing, but does not pass so well by stool. Barley cake made into a paste betimes, sprinkled with water but not well kneaded, is light, passes easily by stool, and cools. It cools because it is moistened with cold water; it passes by stool because that [*sic*] it is soon digested, and it is light because that [*sic*] a great part of the nourishment is secreted outside with the breath. For the passages, being too narrow for the nourishment, will not receive a new addition, and part of it is attenuated and secreted outside with the breath, while a part remains and causes flatulence; of this some is belched upwards, and some passes out downwards. A great part, therefore, of the nourishment passes out of the body. If you will give the barley cake as soon as it is mixed, it is drying, for the barley meal, being dry, and moist only by the water which is mixed with it, coming onto the belly attracts its moisture as being hot; for it is natural for the hot to attract the cold, and the cold the hot. The moisture of the belly thus being consumed it must necessarily grow dry, and when the water mixed with the barley cake has entered the belly it must grow cool. So when it is necessary to cool or dry a sufferer from diarrhoea or from any sort of inflammation, barley cake of this sort serves well. Barley cake that is dry and well kneaded does not dry so much, by reason that it is more tightly compressed, but it is very nourishing, because as it gently dissolves the passages admit the nourishment; so it passes slowly without occasioning wind either downwards or upwards. That which has been mixed beforehand and well kneaded nourishes less, but passes by stool and causes more wind.[87]

This text provides very precise information about the different ways for preparing barley cake, or *maza*, one of the most typical elements of the Greek diet. It was a cake of roasted barley flour, and could be made using flour of variable quality. The author distinguishes here between wholemeal flour and sifted flour. With regard to preparation, he distinguishes unkneaded cakes from kneaded cakes, and within these two categories he distinguishes cakes in which the flour has been mixed with some greater or smaller amount of water in advance from those in which the flour is mixed at the moment they are to be eaten. According to the nature of the ingredients or the manner of preparation, the effects of the cake on the body are subtly altered. One might have just as easily chosen as an example the many varieties of wheat bread. Hippocratic physicians also distinguished between those Greeks who were in the habit of eating barley cake and those who customarily ate wheat bread.[88]

Tisane and Ptisane

But if attention needs to be called particularly to barley, it is because this cereal served as the foundation for the regimen of patients in Hippocrates' time, and continued to play a large role in the regimen of patients in the centuries following. In modern French, an unsuspected legacy of this fact is preserved. Though the herbal decoction called *tisane* is well known (the same word is used in English), the etymology of the word is not. *Tisane* is a popular derivation from the Greek *ptisanè* via the Latin *ptisana*. Now, the Greek *ptisanè* (the learned equivalent of which in French is "ptisane") meant "winnowed barley," or "coarse-ground barley flour"—in French, *gruau*, the source of the English "gruel" (boiled meal). One finds glowing praise for this "ptisane" in the treatise devoted to the regimen of patients suffering acute illnesses:

Now I think that gruel made from barley has rightly been preferred over other cereal foods in acute diseases, and I commend those who preferred it; for the gluten of it is smooth, consistent, soothing, lubricant, moderately soft, thirst-quenching, easy of evacuation, should this property too be valuable, and it neither has astringency nor causes disturbance in the bowels or swells up in them. During the boiling, in fact, it has expanded to the utmost of its capacity.[89]

The end of this passage tells us that "ptisane" was boiled. It was therefore a decoction of winnowed barley. Physicians administered either the gruel obtained by boiling such barley, or the liquid extract of this gruel, strained through a fine linen cloth. This extract was called "juice of ptisane."

The alimentary regimen could therefore be graduated according to the strength of the disease and the resistance of the patient. Three sorts of regimen were distinguished.[90] Gruels and soups constituted an intermediate diet between a diet based on solid foods reserved for the strongest patients and one made up solely of liquids for the weakest. The intermediate category offered the doctor an option: he could prescribe the gruel itself, or simply the juice strained from it.

The Use of Beverages

Solid foods and soups were denied to the weakest patients. Their diet was restricted to beverages.[91] The physician therefore needed to know the properties of beverages as well as those of foods. The alimentary catalogs of the Hippocratic Collection do in fact lay out the advantages and disadvantages of various drinks, chiefly water and wine.[92] Here one finds the same subtle distinctions as in the case of foods, although water hardly inspires the author of the *Regimen*: he limits himself to contrasting water, cold and moist, with wine, dry and warm. The author of *Regimen in Acute Diseases* is somewhat more forthcoming with regard to the properties of water; but on balance he remains rather mistrustful, finding more inconveniences than benefits: water does not assuage thirst in fevers, and, he says, it is hard to digest![93] By contrast, many varieties of wine are mentioned: white and black (as the ancient Greeks called red wine), sometimes yellow, mild, light, or strong, sweet smelling or odorless, astringent, susceptible or not to being mixed with water. Many properties are identified in connection with these wines: they can be laxatives and diuretics or, conversely, constipatives and desiccants; others still are tonics. It is known that the Greek wines of antiquity were extremely strong, about 18 percent in alcoholic content, and so were generally prescribed to be mixed with water. But it would be a mistake to suppose they were never consumed in undiluted form. One Hippocratic physician, noting that certain Greeks were accustomed to drink pure wine, implies it would be dangerous to switch them abruptly to a diet of wine cut with water.[94] Others prescribed pure wine fairly frequently. "Strong drink dispels hunger," it is said in the *Aphorisms*.[95]

The praise of wine is clearest in the treatise *Affections*: "Wine and honey are held to be the best things for human beings, so long as they are administered appropriately and with moderation to both the well and the sick in accordance with their constitution; they are beneficial both alone and mixed, as indeed is anything else that has a value worth mentioning."[96]

Mead and Oxymel

Besides those drinks made from the grape (must, wine, vinegar), physicians relied above all, in planning the regimen of their patients, on beverages having a base of honey.

Mead, as the etymology of the word indicates, was honey mixed with a liquid. Mixed with milk, the honey formed a libation that in Homer was offered to the dead.[97] The mead used in medicine was honey mixed with water; it was therefore what we now call hydromel. But the Greek term *hydromeli* postdates Hippocrates' time. Mead could be drunk in its raw form or boiled. Boiling was recommended when the honey was of poor quality.[98] The author of *Regimen in Acute Diseases* makes a strenuous plea on behalf of this drink. He tells us that it had a reputation in the popular mind for weakening those who drank it. The explanation he gives for this false belief reveals an interesting detail about the life of the ancient Greeks. Certain people, probably out of despair, were known to starve themselves to death. Of these, some took hydromel—on account of which hydromel was supposed to hasten death. But according to the physician, hydromel was a fortifying drink, even more so than certain light wines, for pure honey is much more fortifying than pure wine, even when one takes two times less of it.

Oxymel was a mixture of honey and vinegar. Its dosage was variable, being either highly acidic or only lightly acidic. It was primarily used as an expectorant. Highly acidic oxymel was reserved for serious cases, and was to be used with caution. It was more a medicine than a drink. When one wished to give a patient oxymel regularly throughout the course of a long illness, only a small amount of vinegar was mixed in, just enough that its taste could be recognized.[99] That suggests therefore that the honey was diluted with water beforehand.

Exercise

After diet, exercise constituted the second major element of regimen, whether one was in good health or bad.

With the development of dietary medicine in the second half of the fifth century B.C. and the beginning of the fourth century, certain physicians favored a regime of exercise in treating their patients. Herodicus, who in the eyes of Plato symbolized this new therapeutic tendency, was its most famous representative. According to a reference made in the *Phaedrus*, his method consisted in prescribing long walks from Athens to Megara and back, a distance of some sixty kilometers (or almost forty miles).[100] This method was criticized in the Hippocratic Collection: "Herodicus killed fever patients with running, much wrestling, hot baths. A bad procedure. Fever is inimical to wrestling, walks, running, massage; that is trouble on trouble for them. Swelling of the blood vessels, redness, lividness, pallor, soft pains in the ribs."[101]

Although they condemned excesses, Hippocratic physicians recommended a balance between diet and exercise. The ideal was "to discover for the constitution of each individual a due proportion of food to exercise, with no inaccuracy either of excess or defect."[102]

There was therefore a catalog of exercises analogous to that of foods and drinks. The author of the *Regimen* distinguishes two kinds of exercises: on the one hand, natural exercises, mainly walks, though they had a vigorous aspect to them as well, and, on the other hand, more strenuous exercises such as swinging of the arms, running, and various sorts of wrestling. But the category of exercise also included activities that we would hardly think of classifying under this head today. This is particularly the case with the exercises that the author regards as properly called "natural":

Natural exercises are those of sight, hearing, voice and thought. The nature of sight is as follows. The soul, applying itself to what it can see, is moved and warmed. As it warms it dries, the moisture having been emptied out. Through hearing, when noise strikes the soul, the latter is shaken and exercised, and as it is exercised it is warmed and dried. By all the thoughts that come to a man the soul is warmed and dried; consuming the moisture it is exercised, it empties the flesh and it makes a man thin. Exercises of the voice, whether speech, reading or singing, all these move the soul. And as it moves it grows warm and dry, and consumes the moisture.[103]

Sight, hearing, voice, and thought therefore provide occasion for exercises of the soul that eventually have consequences for the condition of the body.

Also included among the activities that were considered by ancient physicians to be therapeutic was the purely passive exercise of balanced suspension. Very frequently encountered in the medicine of the Roman period, it was already known in Hippocrates' time.[104]

Although physicians generally contented themselves, when prescribing exercises, with distinguishing between walking and gymnastics (understood as including running and wrestling), the catalog given by the author of the *Regimen* showed much greater subtlety in dividing each kind of exercise into several varieties. Under walks, he distinguished morning promenades, walks taken after meals, and walks taken after gymnastic exercise. Similarly, he enumerated various sorts of running and wrestling, to which he attributed particular properties. So great, moreover, was the confidence of this author in the virtues of exercise, and of regimen in general, he held that proper regimen could actually make a person more intelligent.[105]

Baths

Less often mentioned than diet or exercise, baths nonetheless were part of the therapeutic arsenal of Hippocratic physicians. The use of baths in treating sickness was strongly affirmed by the author of *Regimen in Acute Diseases* in a passage of capital importance for reconstructing the way in which baths were administered: "The bath will be beneficial to many patients, sometimes when used continuously, sometimes at intervals."[106] But this is an ideal that was not always easy to achieve on account of the inadequate physical conditions that the physician was apt to encounter on visiting patients in their homes: "[F]ew houses have suitable apparatus and attendants to manage the bath properly."

It is true that the requirements listed by the physician in the rest of this passage are rather formidable. It was necessary that the room be free from smoke, which is to say that the water was not heated on a fire in the room where the bath was to take place. It was necessary that water be available in abundant supply. The patient should have to make only a short passage from his bed to the basin, which needed to be easy to get into and out of. It was necessary that the patient's servants take charge of pouring water on him and, depending on the case, of rubbing him with a cleansing paste. The patient, for his part, was to remain calm and quiet, doing nothing by himself. The bath did not involve immersion, as we are accustomed to experience it today, but was administered by affusions of water. Thus one bathed either the entire body or a part of it, depending on the case. There was a whole art to carrying out the affusions, which were to be frequent but not violent, unless the case required it. There was also a whole art to applying the soap, which was prepared in the form of a paste. It needed to be warm, abundant, and accompanied by a liberal affusion of water, followed immediately afterwards by another one. All this assumed that one had a large amount of water in reserve, cold and hot mixed together, and that it could be drawn rapidly. Finally, it was necessary to dry the patient using sponges rather than a strigil, or scraper. The head was to be perfectly dry, and the body was to be rubbed with oil before it had dried completely. It was necessary to avoid any chill. In short, all these requirements leave the impression of an almost ritual ceremony in which each gesture was to be carried out according to quite precise rules. For if there was a breach of any one or more of the rules, the result was that instead of doing good, the bath risked doing harm.

Several kinds of bath are prescribed in the Hippocratic Collection: hot baths, tepid or cold baths, baths taken on an empty stomach or after a meal. These were baths using soft water; saltwater baths were not unknown, however.[107] The general effect of a bath was to moisten the body. It was for this reason that baths were recommended more often in summer than in winter, and more often for the thin than the stout.[108] But each type had different effects.[109] And a single type could have opposite effects, depending on the way in which it was administered: "The hot bath, when employed in moderation, softens the body and increases it; when used to excess, it moistens the dry parts of the body, and dries out the moist ones; when the dry parts are moistened, it brings on weakness and fainting; when the moist parts are dried, they produce dryness and thirst."[110]

Similar to hot baths were steam baths, which caused perspiration.[111] Either a part or the whole of the body could be subjected to the vapor: the first case involved fumigations or fomentations, the latter something rather like a modern sauna. But physicians limited themselves to prescribing the procedure without going into detail about how it was physically to be carried out.

Along with these moist fumigations (*purian*), physicians occasionally prescribed fumigations using a dry medication that had been parched—aromatic plants (*thumian*), for example.[112]

Sleep and Sleeplessness

Alluding to the various elements that make up an individual's regimen, the author of *The Art* cites four: in addition to food, drink, and baths, he counts sleep.[113]

Sleep and insomnia were regarded by Hippocratic physicians primarily as an element of diagnosis and prognosis. Here is what the author of the *Prognosis* says of them: "As for sleep, the patient ought to follow the natural custom of being awake during the day and asleep during the night. Should this be changed it is rather a bad sign. Least harm will result if the patient sleep from early morning for a third part of the day. Sleep after this time is rather bad. The worst thing is not to sleep either during the day or during the night.

For either it will be pain and distress that cause the sleeplessness or delirium will follow this symptom."[114] More pithily, the *Aphorisms* twice enunciates the following maxim: "Sleep or sleeplessness, in undue measure, these are both bad symptoms."[115]

As for the other elements of regimen, physicians analyzed the different effects that sleep and sleeplessness could produce upon the body:

Sleep when fasting reduces and cools, if it be not prolonged, as it empties the body of the existing moisture; if, however, it be prolonged, it heats and melts the flesh, dissolves the body and enfeebles it. After a meal sleep warms and moistens, spreading the nourishment over the body. It is especially after early-morning walks that sleep is drying. Want of sleep, after a meal, is injurious, as it prevents the food from dissolving; to a fasting person it is less injurious, while it tends to reduce flesh.[116]

The author, noting that sleep aids digestion, seems to recommend a nap after meals. Although a patient's natural cycle may be normal, one physician suggests that sleep be prolonged in order to offset indigestion.[117] To re-establish a normal sleep / waking cycle, soporifics were already known.[118] But nothing is said about the details of their use.

All these elements of regimen (food, drink, baths, exercise, and in some cases sleep) usually figured in discussions of treatment in both a positive form (as prescriptions) and a negative form (as counterindications).

Sexual Life

Other elements of regimen were apt to be taken into account; for example, the patient's sexual life. Intercourse is mentioned by the author of the *Regimen* in his catalog of the various properties of the different elements of regimen: "Sexual intercourse reduces, moistens, and warms. It warms owing to the fatigue and the excretion of moisture; it reduces owing to the evacuation; it moistens because of the remnant in the body of the matters melted by the fatigue."[119]

Sexual relations were sometimes advised. "Venery helps diseases from phlegm," notes the author of *Epidemics VI*.[120] Sometimes they were prohibited. Thus, for example, it was necessary to abstain from sexual relations when one had suffered a contusion of the chest.[121] Some notes were addressed exclusively to women. A pregnant woman would deliver more easily if she abstained from sexual relations.[122] By contrast, one physician counseled young girls to marry as quickly as possible in case they suffered from delirium at the onset of menstruation, "for if they become pregnant, they get better."[123]

Diseases of Women and Their Treatment

We cannot close this chapter on the physician's relation to disease without mentioning the special place accorded to the diseases of women in the Hippocratic Collection. A vast set of treatises is exclusively devoted to the subject, as we have seen. Despite the difficulty that physicians were apt to experience in winning the confidence of women,[124] they could not fail to pay attention to them. The work that may be considered as distilling the essence of Hippocratic teaching, the *Aphorisms*, collects the information relating to the diseases of women in a special section.[125]

In addition to general diseases, women were liable to suffer from particular diseases that threatened to undermine their essential role in the survival of the race—their fertility. Barrenness was felt by women to be a sort of defect, on account of which their husbands might repudiate them. Greek theater, in both its tragic and comic branches, testifies to the ordeal that a sterile couple or an infertile wife often had to endure. They had recourse not only to doctors, but also to oracles. In Euripides' tragedy *Ion*, a couple that has long been sterile comes to consult the oracle at Delphi.[126] In a comic vein, Aristophanes recounts the story of a sterile woman who feigns labor for ten days and then presents her husband with a child, whom she has bought.[127]

Under these circumstances, it is not surprising to learn that the Hippocratic Collection contains tests for determining in principle whether or not a woman is sterile. Here is the test recorded in the *Aphorisms*: "If a woman does not conceive, and you wish to know if she will conceive, cover her round with wraps and burn perfumes underneath. If the smell seems to pass through the body to the mouth and nostrils, be assured that the woman is not barren through her own physical fault."[128]

To a modern sensibility, this test may seem absurd. But it did not seem at all absurd to Aristotle, who himself explains that one may determine whether women are fertile with the aid of pessaries inserted in the vagina, the odor of which ought to make its way into their breath.[129] In the same passage, Aristotle proposes a second, still more peculiar test. It is necessary to rub the eyes with a coloring substance. If this substance colors the woman's saliva, she is fertile. Now this test was previously to be found in a Hippocratic treatise: "If you wish to determine whether or not the woman is capable of having a child, rub the eyes with the red stone; if the medicine penetrates, the woman is capable of having a child; if not, she is not."[130] According to the philosopher, such tests made it possible to determine whether the passages through which the seed of the woman was secreted were obstructed. He expressly says that the eyes are the part of the body that furnish the most seed. Do such physiological explanations justify the tests proposed in the Hippocratic Collection? It is hard to say, for the tests themselves are unaccompanied by any attempt at justification. The claim that eyedrops pass from the eyes down into the mouth presumes in any case a fairly arcane knowledge of the structure of tear ducts.

Tests of fertility or sterility were much more varied than Aristotle implies, as the following passage from *Sterile Women* demonstrates. It lists five of them:

Exploratory methods for knowing if a woman will conceive: if you wish to know whether a woman will conceive, give [her] to drink on an empty stomach some butter and milk of a mother nursing a child; if the woman burps, she will conceive; if not, she will not conceive. Another: insert as a pessary in the vagina a bit of bitter almond oil wrapped in wool, and then in the morning check to see if the smell of the inserted material is exhaled through the mouth. If a smell is exhaled, she will conceive; if not, she will not conceive. Another exploratory method in the same vein: the woman in whom, following [insertion of] not overly strong pessaries, pains are felt in the joints and grinding of the teeth occurs, as well as dizzy spells with dimming of vision and yawning, can hope to conceive, more than one who does not experience any of this. Another: take a clove of garlic that you have cleaned and peeled, and insert into the womb as a pessary, and see if the next morning the odor is exhaled through the mouth; if it is exhaled, the woman will conceive; if not, she will not conceive. Does a woman wish to know if she will conceive? Have her drink dill crushed as finely as possible in some water and then go to sleep; if an itching seizes her around the navel, she will conceive; if not, she will not conceive.[131]

This strange science of tests must have been known to midwives as well. Plato alludes to such knowledge in the *Theaetetus* when he praises their art of "knowing about the kind of couples whose marriage will produce the best children."[132]

Let us suppose that the test is positive and that the woman is fertile. To favor the conception of a child, the physician does not hesitate to give the couple some advice. The woman is to go to her husband "at the end or at the beginning of her period; the best is when it is coming to an end; for these days are the most decisive."[133] Elsewhere, he says that she is to do this on an empty stomach.[134] Nor does the husband escape the physician's watchful eye. He is to choose a favorable season and follow an appropriate regimen: "The most efficacious season for conception is the spring. The man is not to be in a state of drunkenness; he is not to drink white wine, but wine as strong and pure as possible; he is to eat very strong foods and not to take hot baths; he is to be strong and in good health; he is to abstain from foods that are not suitable to the act."[135]

Quite specific instructions are given with regard to the decisive moment: "If the woman realizes that she has retained the seed, she must not go to her husband for a certain time, but remain quiet. She will know it from the fact that her husband says he ejaculated but she was not aware of it, having remained dry. If, by contrast, the womb gives back the seed the same day, she will be wet; and if she is wet, let her couple again with her husband until she retains the seed."[136]

If the couple has observed the physician's advice, and if the woman appears to have retained her husband's sperm, she can hope to become pregnant. While she waits to find out, the physician undertakes further tests. Here is an example of a test of pregnancy recorded in the *Aphorisms*: "If you wish to know whether a woman is with child, give her hydromel to drink [without supper] when she is going to sleep. If she has colic in the stomach she is with child, otherwise she is not."[137]

There even existed tests to determine whether a woman was pregnant with a girl or with a boy. Here is one of them: "Take some milk from the woman, mix some flour with this milk, make a little roll of bread and cook it over a low fire; if it is completely cooked, she is pregnant with a boy; if it is half-open, she is pregnant with a girl."[138] In the event this test was inconclusive, one could rely upon observation, which ultimately was a less arbitrary guide: "If you cannot tell that a woman is pregnant by another means, you will perceive it in this way: the eyes are drawn and more hollow, the white of the eyes does not have its natural whiteness, but seems more livid. All those who are pregnant have blemishes on the face and, at the beginning of pregnancy, lose their taste for wine, do not have a good appetite, are full of nausea and salivate."[139]

But observation was sometimes led astray by prejudices about the superiority of men over women, for immediately following these judicious remarks the physician adds: "Pregnant women who have blemishes on the face are pregnant with a girl; those who keep a clear complexion are pregnant most often with a boy. If the breasts are turned upwards, she is pregnant with a boy; if downwards, she is pregnant with a girl."[140] An analogous prejudice accounts for the belief that the "male embryo is usually on the right, the female on the left."[141]

Once it was confirmed that the woman was pregnant, she had to take special precautions. Several aphorisms are concerned with these. The woman was not to be given evacuants in the last months of pregancy, nor was she to be bled.[142] Her health was now more fragile; she was less likely to resist acute diseases.[143] The main risk was miscarriage. The physician needed to be trained to recognize the signs of this. The same prejudices that operated in the prognosis of pregnancy now reappear:

> Should the breasts of a woman with child suddenly become thin, she miscarries.
>
> When a woman is pregnant with twins, should either breast become thin, she loses one child. If the right breast become thin, she loses the male child; if the left, the female.[144]

Accidents that were liable to occur during childbirth and the maladies that were liable to occur afterwards also occupied the attention of physicians; they were to be summoned only in difficult cases, however, childbirth ordinarily being the responsibility of midwives.[145]

Let us for a moment come back to the test for fertility and sterility. If a woman who wished to have a child proved to be barren, it was the job of the physician to determine the causes of it and to propose a treatment. There is no question that Hippocratic physicians knew sterility could be due to the man, even if the man had not undergone an operation that might have rendered him sterile.[146] One aphorism clearly treats male sterility on a par with female sterility.[147] Contrary to an opinion that is too often repeated, the Greeks of the classical period did not systematically assign blame for sterility to women. From Aristotle, we know that a test existed for determining the fertility of the male comparable to those employed to decide if the female was fertile: "[T]he water-test is quite a fair one for infertility in the male semen, because the thin, cold semen quickly diffuses itself on the surface, whereas the fertile semen sinks to the bottom."[148]

Nonetheless, it was mainly female sterility that occupied the attention of the Hippocratic physicians. The principal cause of diseases in women was the condition of the womb. "The uterus is the cause of all these diseases," declares the author of *Places in Man*.[149] The modern term "hysteria," although it currently denotes a nonspecific neurosis in females, bears the trace of this ancient conception. The term derives in fact from *hystérè*, the Greek word for the womb. Originally, hysteria was supposed to be a specifically female complaint associated with the uterus. Given this general proposition, many particular causes of sterility could be imagined, having to do either with the condition of the womb itself, which might be either too cold, too moist, too hot, or too dry,[150] or the deviation, obstruction, or closure of the cervix, ulcerations or cancer of the uterus or of the cervix, inflammation or suppuration of the uterus, and so on. Female sterility was explained either by the fact that the womb could not receive or retain the male sperm, or by the fact that it prevented normal menstrual discharge, or that it did not provide a favorable environment for the coagulation of the seed and the development of the embryo.

To combat sterility and the diseases of women more generally, Hippocratic physicians employed a course of treatment that combined elements of the therapeutics of general diseases (notably evacuants, baths, fumigations, and diet) with remedies specific to women that involved the womb. It was possible to open and straighten out the cervix, for example, using probes made of pewter or lead.[151] To correct a prolapse of the uterus, the most spectacular treatment was succussion by ladder: the woman having been attached to a ladder by her feet, upside down, the shocks produced by raising and dropping the ladder onto the ground helped put the womb back into place, together with some manual adjustment; then the woman's legs were crossed and tied together, and she was left in this uncomfortable position for a day and a night, being given only some cold ptisane juice to drink.[152] A similar method was attributed to the Cnidian physician Euryphon.[153] In other cases, the patient was made to drink potions that were supposed to have the unique effect of evacuating the womb.[154] Evacuative clysters were injected into the uterus.[155] Pessaries, a kind of suppository, were inserted into the uterus. Moist or dry fumigations of the womb were carried out. Aromatic fumigations were used to pull the womb out, foul-smelling ones to push it back in. Treatment could be of long duration, lasting as much as four months or more.[156]

Certain preparations were intended to help beautify a woman's appearance: toothpastes for cleaning the teeth and perfuming the breath, creams for bringing a radiant glow to the face, and even a cream for getting rid of wrinkles.

It was in connection with the treatment of women that the art of the Hippocratic physician in his role as pharmacist was most lavishly—and sometimes disconcertingly—applied. The gynecological treatises preserve interminable lists of medicines combining the most familiar and the most unexpected animal, vegetable, and mineral substances. Among the ingredients that will seem extraordinary to the modern reader are human urine, Spanish fly, bull's bile and liver, dried donkey manure, snake fat, sea turtle's brain, beaver testicles, deer antlers, and the penis and marrow of the deer. In such a remarkably varied pharmacopeia, the legacy presumably of ages long obscured by time, the magical still crops up amid the rational.

Several of the products used came from distant lands. To take only one example, silphion, a plant that has since disappeared, grew in its wild state in Cyrenaica and was valued for medicinal purposes on account of its stalk, and above all for its juice. The medical school at Cyrene may have contributed to the diffusion of this medicine. Similarly it may be supposed that the Asclepiads of Cnidus helped establish the reputation of the "grain of Cnidus," frequently cited in the gynecological treatises. When it occurred to Hippocratic authors to indicate the geographical origin of the remedies they mention, or of their ingredients, as in the case of this grain from Cnidus, they named not only regions of the Greek world that they knew well[157] but also distant lands such as Egypt, renowned in Homer's time for its medicines,[158] Ethiopia, Media, and even India.[159] Greek medicine therefore did not have to wait for Alexander's famous expedition to the east in order to make use of exotic products.

PART III

Hippocrates and the Thought of His Time

The Hippocratic physician was first and foremost a practitioner. But he was also—and his obvious originality resided in just this—a thinker and a theoretician. In fact, it could hardly have been otherwise, as may be seen if the era and the environment in which he lived are taken into account.

The Age of Pericles was in every respect a time of intellectual ferment, extending and developing the infant tradition of scientific thought that had been born in Ionian Greece in the sixth century and inaugurated by thinkers from Miletus such as Thales, "who was the first to speak of nature,"[1] and his disciple Anaximander, who himself was the teacher of Anaximenes. But the curiosity of the first philosophers of the sixth century concerned the universe more than it did humanity. The anecdote related by Plato about Thales is symbolic of this state of affairs: "Thales was studying the stars, . . . and gazing aloft, when he fell into a well; and a witty and amusing Thracian servant-girl made fun of him because, she said, he was wild to know what was up in the sky but failed to see what was in front of him and under his feet."[2] In the fifth century, by contrast, reflection about the universe came to be enriched by reflection about humanity. "Many are the wonders," sings the chorus of Sophocles' *Antigone*, but "none is more wonderful than what is man."[3] In the sixth century, to be sure, Pythagoras, who was originally from the island of Samos, not far from Miletus, and who spread Ionian philosophy throughout Magna Graecia after his departure to Croton in southern Italy, had been interested not only in cosmology but also in the human soul and in the nature of the human body. Moreover, ties certainly existed between Pythagoras and the school of medicine at Croton.[4] But it was only from the middle of the fifth century that inquiry into the human condition, particularly under the influence of Sophists, historians, and ethnographers, but also of physicians, became the central preoccupation of philosophers. It was then, in the rather exceptional climate of intellectual excitement that prevailed at that time, that Greek man both discovered himself and questioned the nature of his being at the very moment of this self-discovery. Thus it was that the century of

1. Diogenes Laertius 1.24 (= Diels-Kranz 11A1).
2. Plato *Theaetetus* 174a.
3. Sophocles *Antigone* 332ff.
4. These ties were through the intermediary of Alcmaeon of Croton; see page 262.

Pericles saw the birth of rationalism, humanism, and science. With regard to each of these three events, Hippocratic medicine has things to tell us that are of the highest importance. The value and scope of this information has for too long been neglected by historians of Greek thought, who labored under a preconceived notion that the sciences were compartmentalized in Hippocrates' time in a way that they were not. Now, at last, Hippocratic thought is coming to be accepted as a rightful part of the study of classical Greece.

EIGHT

Hippocratic Rationalism
and the Divine

When one speaks of Greek rationalism in the Age of Pericles, one thinks immediately—and rightly so—of the historian Thucydides, who, unlike Herodotus, refused to explain the march of historical events by reference to divine intervention in human affairs. But less well appreciated is the fact that the Hippocratic Collection harbors a kindred spirit. There is no question that here and there in the language of these treatises traces can be found of an archaic view according to which disease was a demoniacal force that invaded the patient from outside in order to seize hold of him, with treatment consisting accordingly of an attempt to expel it from the body by means of a *pharmakon*, or medicinal evacuant, just as a *pharmakos*, or expiatory victim, was believed to bring about the expulsion of illness from the city. But Hippocratic thought either ignored or rejected any particular intervention on the part of a deity in the process of disease and any magical treatment through prayers, incantations, or purifications.

The Hippocratic physicians allied themselves with the enlightened minds of the Periclean Age who promoted the new rationalism, and criticized— sometimes strenuously—those who believed that a disease could be caused by the intervention of a particular divinity, contrasting the notion of divine causality with one of rational causality. They were prepared even to criticize soothsayers or interpreters of dreams when they encroached on the domain of medicine. The rational attitude of these physicians is all the more remarkable since belief in the efficacy of magical practices and in gods as healing agents is well attested in the popular mentality of the age, at the height of the fifth century. But it should not be deduced from this, as too often tends to be done, that the rationalism of the Hippocratic physicians was opposed to the notion of the divine or that it was incompatible with traditional religion. We will see, in fact, that things were more nuanced than this: the position of each of the

Hippocratic physicians regarding the divine was not necessarily the same, and even in those treatises where attacks against magico-religious medicine were the sharpest, this criticism was not intended to call into question the traditional religion of the temples and shrines.

Sacred Disease and Hippocratic Rationalism

The rationalist attitude of the Hippocratic physicians toward the sacred is particularly plain in connection with what the ancients called the "sacred disease" and what we call epilepsy.

Contrary to what one might suppose, the expression "sacred disease" was not in the fifth century the popular name of a disease for which a technical term was also used. It was in fact the term used by Hippocratic physicians. The author of one of the gynecological treatises, for example, describing the symptoms of an affection that caused a woman suddenly to lose the power of speech, indicates that the patient experienced "the same symptoms as people suffering from the sacred disease."[1] Since the sacred disease was taken as the frame of reference for describing another disease, it is clear that it was an affection that was well known to physicians and one whose symptoms were codified.[2]

However, in the majority of the passages of the *Corpus Hippocraticum* in which this disease is mentioned, it is referred to not as the "sacred disease" but as the "disease called sacred."[3] In employing this slightly variant phrase, the authors distanced themselves from a traditional name that did not correspond to the idea that they themselves had formed of the disease. None of them attributed a sacred character to it. The physiological explanations they proposed differed: according to some it was a disturbance in the motion of the blood, to others a disturbance in the motion of the air; according to some, the part of the body affected was the brain, to others the heart or the diaphragm.[4] Nonetheless, despite these differences of opinion, the rationalist spirit that guided their attempts at explanation was fundamentally the same. It was a matter, in their view, of physiological troubles due to natural causes.

Some of the Hippocratic physicians limited themselves to stating rational theories of the disease, as they would have done in the case of any other affection, without paying particular attention to its special name and the beliefs that this implied.[5] Others, by contrast, supplemented the exposition of their theories with polemics directed against those whose believed in the divine origin of the disease.

Soothsayers and Physicians

Let us begin by considering a little known but very significant example. Discussing the form of the sacred disease to which girls are susceptible at the moment of puberty, the author of the slender treatise *Diseases of Girls* describes the delirium to which it gives rise and offers a rational explanation for the attack, positing a flow of blood that spreads to the heart and the diaphragm instead of being discharged through the womb. Then he adds: "When the girl regains her reason, it is to Artemis that the women dedicate many offerings in general and, in particular, the most valuable feminine garments, on the recommendation of the soothsayers, but they are completely deceived. Deliverance from this disease occurs when the flow of blood is not blocked. For my part, I recommend to girls who suffer from such an affection to marry as soon as possible; for if they become pregnant, they get better."[6]

The opposition between physician and soothsayers hinted at here is radical. The seers believe in the divine origin of the disease and attribute it to the virginal Artemis. Furthermore, once the crisis is passed, they recommend that offerings be made to the goddess to thank her and to appease her, thereby preventing a recurrence of the attack. As against this advice, the Hippocratic author makes his own recommendation: unencumbered by taboos of morality or religion, he urges the girl to marry as soon as possible in order that the obstacle preventing the blood from draining out may be removed. The attack of the physician upon the soothsayers, whom he accuses of misleading the patient and her family, is brief but vehement, and gives us a sense of how bitter the rivalry between physicians and soothsayers at the patient's bedside must have been.

Such an attack is rare in the Hippocratic Collection, but it is not unique. The author of *Regimen in Acute Diseases*, warning his colleagues against inconsistencies in their treatment of acute diseases that might be seized upon to discredit the medical art as a whole, declares that "since among practitioners there will prove to be so much difference of opinion about acute diseases that the remedies which one physician gives in the belief that they are the best are considered by a second to be bad, laymen are likely to object to such that their art resembles divination; for diviners too think that the same bird, which they hold to be a happy omen on the left, is an unlucky one when on the right, while other diviners maintain the opposite."[7]

This document is exceptional for its content, since we have no other account attesting that the left side might be judged favorable by certain Greek diviners. But its spirit is very much in keeping with the rationalism of the Age of Pericles, and prefigures Cicero's critique in *De divinatione* opposing Greek divination, for which the right was the favorable side, to Roman divination, for which in general it was the left side.[8]

These two passages are the only ones in the Hippocratic Collection, however, in which soothsayers are singled out for attack.

Charlatans and Physicians

The best example of the sort of polemic mounted by the Hippocratic physicians against those who believed in the divine origin of the "disease called sacred," and of the sort of rationalist solution they advocated in place of such a belief, is to be found in the treatise *The Sacred Disease*. As its title suggests, the treatise is devoted entirely to this question. It is divided into two parts, the first polemical, the second analytical. In the first, it criticizes those who have sacralized the disease; in the second, it states the natural causes it maintains are responsible for the affection.

The polemical part contains an account of the highest importance for the history of ideas. For the first time, a rational medicine is posited in express opposition to a religious and magical medicine. With unequaled scope and vigor, the author lays into "those who first attributed a sacred character to this disease."[9] Here again we encounter the theme of the "first inventor," so dear to the century of discoveries that is identified with the name of Pericles. It bears comparison with the tragedy by a contemporary author, the Sophist Critias, entitled *Sisyphus*, which has to do with the man who "invented the belief in gods."[10] But whereas the mention of the "first inventor" is ordinarily accompanied by praise for his discovery—this is particularly the case with Critias, who praises the salutary fear inspired in men by belief in the gods—here it gives way to unusually harsh blame. The Hippocratic author compares these first inventors of the sacred disease to the "magicians, purifiers, charlatans, and quacks" of his own time.

To appreciate the violence of this attack fully, we may compare it to the scene in Sophocles' *Oedipus Tyrannus* where Oedipus, carried away by anger in his altercation with the soothsayer Tiresias, who has just revealed to him the truth about his origins that he did not wish to believe, calls Tiresias a "magus" and a "beggar."[11] The terms employed are analogous and the accusations comparable. By accusing Tiresias of being a magician and a mendicant, Oedipus brings two charges against him: first, that he has eyes only for his own gain; second, that he is blind with regard to his own art. These two accusations are repeated in the treatise *The Sacred Disease*. The Hippocratic author says that certain practitioners attribute the cause of each variety of the disease to a god because they are "in need of a livelihood."[12] However, this accusation is secondary in the Hippocratic treatise. The fundamental accusation is that they are incompetent: ignorance is said to be at the root of the sacralization of the disease. The author analyzes how his adversaries operate and denounces their deception in the following terms: "Being at a loss, and having no treatment which would help, they concealed and sheltered themselves behind superstition, and called this illness sacred, in order that their utter ignorance might not be manifest."[13] There is nothing subtle in this attack, any more than there is in that of Oedipus upon Tiresias.

That the words of a dramatic character who speaks in a fit of anger should so closely resemble the words of a man of science who defends a rational conception of medicine goes to show how fierce the attacks that Hippocratic physicians launched against the partisans of a magico-religious medicine could be. And if the attack in this case was launched with such passion, the reason is that the Hippocratic author's adversaries were not in fact as insignificant as he would have had his readers believe. At a time when the competence of physicians was not guaranteed by professional qualifications, and when the citizens of a democratic city, respectful of traditional religion and accustomed to hear reference made in the theater to divine healers, met in popular assembly to supervise the recruitment of public physicians, as in Athens,[14] the competition between enlightened physicians who had the interest of the patient at heart and charlatans who looked mainly to exploit the superstition and the ignorance of the people may well have been as heated as the rivalry between physicians and soothsayers.

An Account of Magico-Religious Medicine

The Hippocratic physician, though he denounced his adversaries' total ignorance of the medical art, nonetheless conceded that they had a certain talent both for disguising ignorance and for appearing knowledgable. To conceal their ignorance, they shifted responsibility onto the gods when the patient died but claimed all credit for themselves when the patient recovered. In order to give the impression of being masters of a higher science, they had recourse to a wide variety of tricks, in diagnosis as well as in treatment.

The best-known tricks concerned treatment. As a way of hedging their bets, these practitioners united magico-religious practices such as purifications and incantations, which rational medicine condemned, with various dietary restrictions that rational medicine was ready to admit were sound. The following passage gives a detailed account of these restrictions, which were comparable to the Orphico-Pythagorean interdicts without wholly co-inciding with them:

[T]hey forbade the use of baths, and of many foods that are unsuitable for sick folk—of sea fishes: red mullet, black-tail, hammer and the eel (these are the most harmful sorts); the flesh of goats, deer, pigs and dogs (meats that disturb most the digestive organs); the cock, pigeon and bustard, with all birds that are considered substantial foods; mint, leek and onion among the vegetables, as their pungent character is not at all suited to sick folk; the wearing of black (black is the sign of death); not to lie on or wear goat-skin, not to put foot on foot or hand on hand (all which conduct is inhibitive). These observances they impose because of the divine origin of the disease, claiming superior knowledge and alleging other causes, so that, should the patient recover, the reputation for cleverness may be theirs; but should he die, they may have a sure fund of excuses, with the defence that they are not at all to blame, but the gods. Having given nothing to eat or drink, and not having steeped their patients in baths, no blame can be laid, they say, upon them.[15]

Less well known, but perhaps more revealing of the skill of these therapists, were the subtle distinctions they made in diagnosing illness. Here is a very curious passage from *The Sacred Disease* in which the author describes the diagnostic method of his adversaries:

If the patient imitate a goat, if he roar, or suffer convulsions in the right side, they say that the Mother of the Gods is to blame. If he utter a piercing and loud cry, they liken him to a horse and blame Poseidon. Should he pass some excrement, as often happens under the stress of the disease, the surname Enodia is applied. If it be more frequent and thinner, like that of birds, it is Apollo Nomius. If he foam at the mouth and kick, Ares has the blame. When at night occur fears and terrors, delirium, jumpings from the bed and rushings out of doors, they say that Hecate is attacking or that heroes are assaulting.[16]

One must be grateful to the Hippocratic author for having preserved so detailed an account of the way in which his adversaries, as partisans of a religious medicine, introduced fine shades of difference among the symptoms of crisis in order to distinguish several varieties of the sacred disease and to attribute the cause of each to a different deity. Such an account gives us a better idea how this kind of medicine was able to compete with rational medicine. The diagnostic principle peculiar to magico-religious medicine recalls that of the nosological treatises of the Hippocratic Collection, where the subtle variations noted between symptoms license a distinction between types of diseases.[17] Of course, a fundamental difference remains between the two principles, to the extent that one assigns these varieties of disease to divine powers and the other to disturbances in the body. But their similarity nonetheless suggests that magico-religious medicine had been able to attain a rather high degree of sophistication at the very moment when rational medicine was beginning to blossom. We can thus better appreciate the paradox facing the Hippocratic polemicists: on the one hand, they felt justified in treating their adversaries as crude charlatans; on the other, they had to concede to them a certain sophistic talent—indeed, a certain positive knowledge of those aspects of regimen that were harmful to the patient.

Religious Medicine and the Popular Mind

By taking a close look at the representatives of religious medicine, then, we obtain a sense of the importance that the divine conception of disease must have enjoyed in the popular mind during the Periclean Age. The theater of Aeschylus, Sophocles, and Euripides, in which gods are seen to inflict diseases or to cure them, also testifies to its importance, although the evidence here is more indirect since the mythological nature of the subject matter of the classical tragedies may have led their authors to emphasize the religious aspect of the medicine they described. In any case, it is clear that the popular mentality reflected by the theater, in attributing the sacred disease to different deities as a function of the different symptoms presented, is consonant with the declarations of the charlatans. On learning of Phaedra's illness, the chorus of Euripides' *Hippolytus*, made up of the women of Troezen, wonders in a similar fashion about the various deities who may have provoked it:

> Is it Pan's frenzy that possesses you
> or is it Hecate's madness upon you, maid?
> Can it be the holy Corybantes,
> or the mighty Mother who rules the mountains?
> Are you wasted in suffering thus,
> for a sin against Dictynna, Queen of hunters?
> Are you perhaps unhallowed, having offered
> no sacrifice to her from taken victims?[18]

The catalog of deities invoked to explain the disease in this case is comparable to that attributed by the author of *The Sacred Disease* to his adversaries. Two deities, Hecate and Cybele, are mentioned in both works, Cybele being referred to as "Mother who rules the mountains" in Euripides, as "Mother of the Gods" in the Hippocratic account. In each case, the manner in which the deity takes possession of the patient—by attacking her—involves the same demoniacal conception of disease. The tragedy thus testifies to a popular credulity that charlatans could easily exploit, particularly when human remedies had shown themselves to be ineffective. Plato, in both the *Republic* and the *Laws*, was to be no less severe than Hippocrates in criticizing these neighborhood quacks, who, to make money, claimed to be able to compel the will of the gods through sacrifices, prayers, or incantations.[19]

A Rational Explanation of the Sacred Disease

Faced with competition from a popular medicine founded on a religious conception of disease, the Hippocratic author categorically denied any possible role in the production of disease for anthropomorphic deities and so rejected any form of therapy that aimed at appeasing the anger of the god or of purifying the patient. Instead, he advanced a natural cause—a flux of cold humors triggered by the change in winds—and proposed a natural treatment based on contraries, or opposites. Here is how he concludes his treatise: "For in this disease as in all others it is necessary, not to increase the illness, but to wear it down by applying to each what is most hostile to it, not that to which it is conformable. For what is conformity gives vigour and increase; what is hostile causes weakness and decay. Whoever knows how to cause in men by regimen moist and dry, hot or cold, he can cure this disease also, if he distinguish the seasons for useful treatment, without having recourse to purifications and magic."[20]

The Disease of the Scythians in Hippocrates and Herodotus

The "disease called sacred" is not the only affection mentioned in the Hippocratic Collection that occasioned criticism of a belief in the divine origin of disease. An entire chapter of the ethnographic section of the treatise *Airs, Waters, Places* comparing Europe and Asia is devoted to refuting the belief that the impotence of certain Scythians was caused by a deity.

The fate of these Scythians, called Anaries, who seemed similar to eunuchs, is well known. In the Hippocratic author's account, "when the Scythians approach a woman but cannot have intercourse, at first they take no notice and think no more about it. But when two, three or even more attempts are attended with no better success, thinking that they have sinned against Heaven they attribute thereto the cause, and put on women's clothes, holding that they have lost their manhood. So they play the woman, and with the women do the same work as women do."[21] The other men prostrate themselves before them, believing them to be holy and fearful lest the same malady affect them. To this religious explanation the author opposes his own rational explanation. Far from arising from a sin committed by man toward the gods, the affliction is to be explained mainly by the Scythians' way of life—the Scythians were great horsemen, and their constant riding impaired the pathways of the seminal fluid—but also by a treatment that was more harmful than helpful: at the onset of the illness, they cut the veins located behind the ears, which, in the author's opinion, by damaging the seminal pathways further, made the impotence permanent.

The refutation of religious belief found in this treatise is less markedly polemical than in *The Sacred Disease*. The reason for this is that the author is not dealing here with adversaries who were in a position to become competitors. It was not an opinion held by physicians or by people who claimed to be physicians, but the belief of a people who lived outside the area in which the Hippocratic physicians practiced medicine.

Just the same, even if the criticism is delivered without vehemence, the author clearly dismisses the explanation of the disease as being due to the personal intervention of a deity. The refutation consists in admitting the hypothesis of divine intervention in order to show that it entails consequences contrary to reality. If the disease were more divine than others, the author observes, it should mainly affect those who make the fewest sacrifices and offerings to the gods, which is to say the poor. But the disease affects mainly the rich. The rich are the only ones who own horses and ride. The hypothesis of personal intervention on the part of a deity therefore cannot be sustained.

The originality of the Hippocratic author's position can be seen to be still more pronounced when compared with that of Herodotus. The historian twice takes note of these Scythians, whom he calls Enaries rather than Anaries, in his *Histories*.[22] His account completes the one given by the Hippocratic author with regard to the identity of the deity who is supposed to be responsible for the disease. This deity is Aphrodite. She inflicted the malady upon the descendants of certain Scythians who were responsible for having pillaged her temple at Ascalon in Palestine. But while the Hippocratic author refutes this religious explanation at length, in order to propose a rational explanation in its place, Herodotus presents only the religious explanation, without any thought of calling it into question. The permanent character of the condition, and its disproportionate incidence in a part of the Scythian population, receive plainly discrepant explanations from the historian and the physician: the historian considers it to be due to the permanence of the religious sin, which is transmitted from generation to generation within the families whose ancestors committed the sin; the physician considers it to be due to the permanence of equitation as a way of life among the wealthy classes of Scythian society. Whereas the historian has not managed to get beyond the type of causality that operates in the myth of the great accursed family so widely disseminated by the Athenian tragic theater, the physician advances a natural explanation to account for this disease, as he does in the case of all other diseases. "Each of them has a nature of its own," he declares, "and none arises without its natural cause."[23]

The Divine and the Natural in Hippocratic Medicine

Nonetheless, even when Hippocratic physicians use rational arguments to oppose the notion that a deity might personally intervene in the sphere of human pathology, they are careful not to set science and religion against each other. It is significant that in the two treatises where a divine conception of disease is criticized at length, the notion of the divine per se, far from being rejected, is preserved by the Hippocratic author, who, however, gives it a new meaning.

Thus, the author of *Airs, Waters, Places* does not attack the divine explanation of the Scythians' illness head on. In fact, after having recalled that the Scythians attributed the impotence of the Anaries to a deity, the author gives his personal view of the matter: "I too think that these diseases are divine," he says. Translators have generally omitted to translate the Greek word *kai*, meaning "too," because unconsciously they are embarrassed that a rationalist physician should concede this much to a religious explanation. But in what immediately follows, the author actually dissociates himself from the religious explanation, while seeming to endorse it, by interpreting the notion of divinity in a different way. The passage as a whole reads: "I too think that these diseases are divine, and so are all others, no one being more divine or more human than any other: all are alike, and all divine. Each of them has a nature of its own, and none arises without its natural cause."[24] The Hippocratic physician therefore substitutes, in place of a more or less obscure divine justice that punishes the culpability of the individual by disease, a universe whose order is both divine and natural—one that, in explaining all diseases, frees the diseased person from all blame.

This is the same conception of the divine that we find in *The Sacred Disease*, expressed in terms so near to those of *Airs, Waters, Places* that the conclusion generally drawn—namely, that the two treatises are the work of the same author—seems highly probable. In particular, it is said in *The Sacred Disease*: "[T]here is no need to put the disease [called sacred] in a special class and to consider it more divine than the others; they are all divine and all human. Each has a nature and power of its own."[25]

This formula is precisely equivalent to that of *Airs, Waters, Places*. Here, too, the concept of the divine is emptied of all traditional anthropomorphic representation and defined instead by its accordance with the natural. Moreover, thanks to this latter treatise, it is possible to give specific examples of what the Hippocratic physician considered as divine. In the same chapter, in fact, he states: "The disease styled sacred comes from the same causes as others, from the things that come to and go from the body, from cold, sun, and from the changing restlessness of the winds. These things are divine."[26]

The divine embraces the permanent elements of the universe, independent of human beings, which have an influence upon human health and illness: the air that human beings inhale and exhale; the winds whose changes determine the modifications of the body, sun and cold. All these cosmological phenomena are thus capable of triggering or favoring pathological processes in the human body.

The Divine in Hippocrates and in Thucydides

In this respect, Hippocrates' rationalism differed from that of Thucydides. It may be useful to compare the historian's use of the notion of the "divine" with that of the Hippocratic physician. Thucydides did not limit himself to remarking the impotence of religion before the great malady brought by the "plague" of Athens,[27] but actually removed the notion of divine intercession from historical causality entirely, substituting for it a mechanism based on natural causes. For Thucydides, the "divine" was no longer anything more than a sort of allegation or belief of human beings, as for example in the dialogue of the Athenians and the Melians, where the weak Melians, besieged by the powerful Athenians, awaited rescue by the gods—a rescue that, in the event, did not occur.[28] In the work of the Hippocratic physician, by contrast, the notion of the "divine" was salvaged by incorporating it in an explanation of pathological phenomena that were judged to be both divine and human—divine to the extent that they had a cause and a nature independent of human beings, human to the extent that human beings could affect them through medical treatment. But the notion could be salvaged in this sense only on the condition that it had first been drained of all anthropomorphic content and that all possibility of intervention on the part of a particular deity had been denied, leaving only a rational conception of the divine and nothing else.

Traditional Religion and Medicine

Must we then conclude from the foregoing that if everything is divine, nothing is divine, and that by affirming as much the Hippocratic physician therefore called traditional religion into question? It turns out that matters are more complicated. In the two Hippocratic treatises in which the rational conception of the divine is asserted in identical terms, traditional religion plays a part as well.

In the treatise *Airs, Waters, Places*, traditional religion, with its gods who find it agreeable to receive offerings and sacrifices from human beings and to do them favors in return, is used as the premise of an argument designed to show that the disease of the Scythians cannot be attributed to a god, since the impotence disproportionately affects those who have the means to honor the gods by offerings and sacrifices. Thus the traditional belief in the gods, far from coming in for criticism, serves to denounce the falsity of a belief in the divine origin of a particular disease.

In the treatise *The Sacred Disease*, the position of the physician vis-à-vis religion is clearer still. He presents himself as the defender of traditional belief, accusing his adversaries of impiety and atheism: "[I]n my opinion their discussions show, not piety, as they think, but impiety rather, implying that the gods do not exist, and what they call piety and the divine is, as I shall prove, impious and unholy."[29] In particular, he implicates the impure and impious character of their method of treatment by purifications and incantations:

In making use, too, of purifications and incantations they do what I think is a very unholy and irreligious thing. For the sufferers from the disease they purify with blood and such like, as though they were polluted. . . . All such they ought to have treated in the opposite way; they should have brought them to the sanctuaries, with sacrifices and prayers, in supplication to the gods. As it is, however, they do nothing of the kind, but merely purify them. Of the purifying objects some they hide in the earth, others they throw into the sea, others they carry away to the mountains, where nobody can touch them or tread on them. Yet, if a god is indeed the cause, they ought to have taken them to the sanctuaries and offered them to him.[30]

This sort of criticism of the ritual practices of purification by blood recalls that made earlier by the philosopher Heraclitus: "They vainly purify themselves with blood when they are defiled."[31] And, as in the case of Heraclitus, who reproached such persons for "not knowing who the gods and who the heroes are," this criticism of the rites is made in the name of an elevated conception of divinity. Like Heraclitus, the Hippocratic physician contrasts his refined conception of divinity with that of his adversaries:

However, I hold that a man's body is not defiled by a god, the one being utterly corrupt the other perfectly holy. Nay, even should it have been defiled or in any way injured through some different agency, a god is more likely to purify and sanctify it than he is to cause defilement. At least it is godhead that purifies, sanctifies, and cleanses us from the greatest and most impious of our sins; and we ourselves fix boundaries to the sanctuaries and precincts of the gods, so that nobody may cross them unless he be pure; and when we enter we sprinkle ourselves, not as defiling ourselves thereby, but to wash away any pollution we may have already contracted. Such is my opinion about purifications.[32]

The conclusions the Hippocratic author draws are not as radical as the ones Heraclitus drew. While Heraclitus seemed to call into question religious rites in general—not only purifications but prayers to statues as well—in the name of reason, the Hippocratic physician makes a clear distinction between certain purificatory practices, on the one hand, and the rites of the religion of the sanctuaries on the other. He criticizes certain cathartic procedures employed by certain individuals, in the name of a quite pure conception of divinity, but he justifies the rites of the religion of the sanctuaries, ablutions, sacrifices, and prayers alike.

There coexisted then in the same physician two conceptions of the divine that seem to us quite different, but which to him did not seem in the least contradictory: on the one hand, in his capacity as physician, he believed in a unique causal order for all diseases, no matter which they might be—an order that was at once divine and natural; on the other hand, in his capacity as citizen, he took part in the traditional worship of the sanctuaries, even if he was inclined to question certain ritual practices that did not fit with the refined notion of the divine he had developed.

Ambiguity of the Notion of the Divine in the Treatise on Prognosis

Since the notion of the divine refers in the writings of the Hippocratic physicians both to divinity in the context of traditional polytheism and to atmospheric phenomena that cause illnesses, there is apt to be some ambiguity about the meaning of the word "divine." Thus the author of the *Prognostic*, after having remarked that the physician must know how to recognize diseases whose strength exceeds the patient's resistance, goes on to say: "It is necessary, therefore, to learn the natures of such diseases, how much they exceed the strength of men's bodies [and at the same time whether there is anything divine in the diseases], and to learn how to forecast them."[33]

From antiquity until the present day, interpreters have been divided over the sense of "divine" in this passage. Is it to be understood as implying that certain diseases resist treatment by the physician because they are caused by the gods? Or is one to suppose, by contrast, that "divine" refers to the atmospheric factors responsible for diseases? The range of responses that have been given may be explained in part by the fact the notion of the divine does not figure in the rest of the treatise. Accordingly, scholars are often led to justify a particular solution by comparing this text with other Hippocratic writings.

In favor of the first solution—namely, that there may be diseases (if only exceptionally) that are inflicted by the gods and that as a result do not fall within the competence of medicine[34]—one might cite the attitude of the Hippocratic author of the *Regimen* with regard to dreams. This physician distinguishes between two categories of dreams. "Divine" dreams, sent by the gods to cities or to individuals to notify them of impending happiness or misfortune, are matters for those who know the art of interpreting dreams. By contrast, dreams sent by the soul to foretell various states of the body fall within the competence of the physician.[35] One might suppose that, in a similar way, the author of the *Prognostic* admits the existence of a category of diseases sent by the gods that is beyond the physician's ability to treat. Using the *Regimen* in order to illuminate the *Prognostic* is risky, however, for the *Regimen*'s attitude toward the sacred gives it an altogether peculiar place in the Hippocratic Collection. Its author is in fact the only one of the Hippocratic writers who recommends combining rational treatment with prayers. He even goes so far as to indicate to which gods it is suitable to address prayers depending on the case to be treated. Thus he declares that "precautions must be taken, with change of regimen and prayers to the gods; in the case of good signs, to the Sun, to Heavenly Zeus, to Zeus, Protector of Home, to Athena, Protectress of Home, to Hermes and to Apollo; in the case of adverse signs, to the Averters of evil, to Earth and to the Heroes, that all dangers may be averted."[36]

Partisans of the second solution rely on treatises more representative of the school of Hippocrates; notably, on the two treatises in which there appears a "scientific" conception of the divine, *The Sacred Disease* and *Airs, Waters, Places*. On this view, rather than denoting instances of intervention by individual deities against which the physician finds himself powerless, the notion of the divine in the treatise *Prognostic* includes all those external factors—particularly climatic factors—that influence disease. Galen, a fervent supporter of this interpretation, rightly notes that at the end of the *Prognostic*, in a passing remark, the author stresses the need to take into account the constitution of the season in arriving at a prognosis.[37] It is quite possible that a concern for circular composition led him to link the divine of the beginning of the treatise with the constitution of the season mentioned at the end.

Whichever solution one adopts in order to account for the role of the divine in the *Prognostic*, two conclusions emerge from analysis of the various texts in which the question arises as to what the Hippocratic physicians understood by the sacred and the divine: first, that it is futile, despite a certain rationalist spirit common to these authors and characteristic of them, to hope to be able to reduce their various positions to a single view; second, that their rationalism, even when it was opposed to superstition and magic, did not amount to atheism. The rationalism of these physicians of the fifth century B.C. was more supple, more complex, and more malleable than that of nineteenth- and twentieth-century interpreters, who were sometimes inclined to force the opposition between the rational and the divine and, more generally, between reason and religion.

Miraculous Medicine of the Sanctuaries of Asclepius

Although the Hippocratic physicians came into conflict with certain diviners and charlatans who were in a position to compete with them in the practice of their art, they never openly challenged the religion of the great sanctuaries. This is all the more remarkable given the fact that at the very moment when the Hippocratic physicians were practicing, the religious medicine of the sanctuaries of Asclepius entered into a period of unprecedented popularity, thanks to miraculous healings in which the power of the god was manifested.

Asclepius had undergone a rather extraordinary transformation between the Homeric epoch and the classical era. Although already renowned for his medical knowledge in Homer, Asclepius was then only a human prince, from Tricca in Thessaly.[38] Later he became a healer-demigod, born of Apollo and a human mother, who was tragically struck down by Zeus for having abused his knowledge in bringing a mortal back to life out of a desire for gain.[39]

Finally he was transformed into a physician-god whose popularity following the Age of Pericles grew to such dimensions that his healing power eventually eclipsed even that of Apollo himself. Although the most ancient shrine of Asclepius was found in Tricca,[40] and although his sanctuary at Cos, the homeland of Hippocrates, was linked with that of Tricca,[41] it was the sanctuary of Epidaurus in the Peloponnesus that, more than any other, established the worship of Asclepius in the classical period. From Epidaurus his cult spread throughout the rest of continental Greece (its introduction at Athens dates from the last quarter of the fifth century), and into parts of insular Greece (at Lebena, on Crete) and Asia Minor (particularly at Pergamum), until finally it reached Rome, where he became known as Aesculapius. The miraculous healings of Asclepius in the classical era are well known through two accounts of the fourth century. One is a literary account, Aristophanes' comedy *Plutus*,[42] contemporary with the end of Hippocrates' life; the other is a slightly later epigraphic account, actually a series of accounts, of miraculous healings inscribed on steles found at Epidaurus.

In Aristophanes' play of the early fourth century, Plutus, the god of wealth, is portrayed as a blind old man. If he were not blind, wealth would be more justly distributed. A courageous peasant of Attica, who manages with the help of the Delphic oracle to meet Plutus and then to unmask him, offers to restore him his sight so that he may improve the lot of those who do not deserve their poverty. To this end, he brings Plutus "to lie down in the temple of Asclepius."[43] One night spent at the temple, in Asclepius's care, suffices for the blind man to regain his sight. Aristophanes' comic account of this recovery, related by the Athenian peasant's slave, is instructive. Many patients, suffering from all sorts of illness, came to sleep in the holy precinct of Asclepius. The god, aided by two goddesses of healing and health, Iaso and Panacea, was supposed to come during the night to make the rounds of all the patients who slept there and to treat them. Here is what happened when Asclepius came upon the god of wealth:

He sat down next to Plutus and began by palpating his head; next, taking a clean linen cloth, he wiped all around his eyelids. Panacea spread a purple veil over his head and over all his face. Then the god began to make a hissing sound. From inside the temple there rushed out two enormous snakes. . . . These two, gently sliding under the purple veil, licked all around the eyelids, or so it seemed to me. And in less time than it takes you to drink two cotyles of wine, Plutus was on his feet and could see. I began to clap my hands for joy and woke my master. The god slipped away inside the temple with his snakes.[44]

A recovery this miraculous could be dismissed as a case of exaggeration for comic effect. But the literary account is confirmed by the inscriptions preserved on the stelai at Epidaurus.

Before being partially recovered by archaeologists at the end of the last century, these stelai were known through Pausanias's *Periegesis*. Pausanias, the author of what was in effect the first *Blue Guide* to Greece, visited the sanctuary of Epidaurus in the second century B.C. He tells us: "Within the enclosure stood slabs; in my time six remained, but of old there were more. On them are inscribed the names of both the men and the women who have been healed by Asclepius, the disease also from which each suffered, and the means of cure. The dialect is Doric."[45]

Of the six stelai known to Pausanias, archaeologists have recovered three and a fragment of a fourth. They provide us with a total of seventy brief accounts of miraculous healings, probably composed by the temple personnel on the basis of votive offerings and engraved in stone in the second half of the fourth century for publicity purposes on behalf of the sanctuary. The stelai stood in the temple precinct in plain view for the edification of new pilgrims. As Pausanias noted, these accounts follow a roughly constant schema. The patient, whose name, native city, and disease are mentioned first, comes to the sanctuary in supplication of the god, sleeps in the incubation porch, sees the god in a dream, and arises the following morning healed. Several healings of the blind recorded on the stelai confirm the account found in Aristophanes' *Plutus*. Particularly notable is the case of an Athenian woman, whose initial reaction to so many miraculous cures was disbelief:

Ambrosia of Athens was blind in one eye. This one came in supplication to the god. Going round the sanctuary, she mocked certain healings that she judged unbelievable and impossible, namely that the lame and and blind were healed by the sole fact of having a vision while sleeping. Having lain down [in the incubation porch], she had a vision. It seemed to her that the god, standing above, said that he would heal her, but that in payment she had to deposit in the sanctuary a silver sow to commemorate her foolishness; after these words, he incised the diseased eye and poured a medicine into it. When day broke, she went away healed.[46]

The personal intervention of the god in the course of a dream was therefore held to be responsible for the recovery. The power of the god was such that he could cause blindness as well as restore sight to the blind. Aristophanes' *Plutus* had earlier indicated as much: while Asclepius restored the sight of the god of wealth, he aggravated the blindness of the demogogue Neoclides.[47] In a similar manner, the stelai of Epidaurus relate two cases where the god (temporarily) strikes blind an ungrateful patient who fails to pay the standard fee after having been healed. Here is one of these cases: "Hermon of Thasos. While he was blind, the god healed him. After that, as he did not bring the fee for the treatment, the god rendered him blind again. But, when he came and slept again in [the incubation porch], the god healed him once and for all."[48]

The curing of blindness seems somewhat less miraculous in the version of the Epidaurus stelai than in Aristophanes' account. The god intercedes directly, in a dream, without calling upon sacred snakes. But healing by the holy animals of the sanctuary is also attested by the stelai. In one case, a temple dog licks the eyes of a blind child and cures him;[49] in another, a sacred snake heals a "wild" or "savage" ulcer on a toe;[50] in still another, a goose bites the foot of a patient and cures him of gout.[51]

If one looks beyond these examples to consider all the other diseases whose cure is reported on the stelai of Epidaurus, the miraculous character of this medicine is found to go uncontradicted. No matter what the disease, the power of the god is manifested in the same way. His appearance in a dream and his subsequent action suffice to bring about healing. The god is even capable of acting at a distance. Proof of this is found in the case of a woman of Laconia:

Arete of Laconia. Dropsy. For her, while she stayed in Lacedaemon, her mother came to sleep in [the incubation porch] and had a dream. It seemed to her that the god, having removed the head of her daughter, had suspended her body with the neck hanging down; and that after the draining out of an abundant liquid he had taken down her body and replaced the head on the neck. Having had this dream, she returns to Lacedaemon where she finds her daughter who was healed and had had the same dream she did.[52]

Looking at the group of diseases as a whole, however, we get further information about religious medicine at Epidaurus. This gives us an idea both of the variety of affections for which the ill came to seek the help of Asclepius and also of the diversity of cities from which these persons came. The god treated women as well as men, and children as well as adults. He healed all sorts of patients. Besides the blind, those who came to him in search of a cure included the lame and the paralyzed, the mute, and women who were unable to conceive or who had difficulty giving birth; there were also persons suffering from ulcers, abscesses, or empyemas, or who had intestinal worms; other diseases, such as headache, dropsy, consumption, epilepsy, lithiasis, and gout, are more rarely attested.[53] As for the geographical origin of the ill who came to Epidaurus, the number of different places mentioned testifies to the influence of the sanctuary. Of some thirty persons whose native city is indicated, only four were from Epidaurus. An important group of those who came to consult the god were from different parts of the Peloponnesus, not only from nearby cities in the area such as Argos, Troezen, Hermione, and Halieis, but from cities in more distant regions as well, among them Pellene in Achaea, Caphyae in Arcadia, Messene in Messenia, and Sparta in Laconia. But the reputation of Epidaurus went well beyond the boundaries of the Peloponnesus to take in much of continental and insular Greece as well. In continental Greece, mention is made of pilgrims coming not only from Athens but from Thebes in Boeotia and Kirrha in Phocis, as well as from northern Greece, from Epirus, from Pherae and Heraclea in Thessaly, from Torone in Chalcidice, and from Lampsacus in the Hellespont. Considering insular Greece, together with islands near to Epidaurus such as Aegina and Ceos there is mention of islands much further away, such as Lesbos (and its city of Mytilene) and Chios, along the Asiatic coast, and Thasos, along the Thracian coast. One pilgrim even came from Asia Minor, from Cnidus, a city itself renowned for its medical center.[54]

Thus the variety of diseases treated, no less than the size of the area from which people afflicted by them came for help, provides evidence that the religious medicine of the great sanctuaries flourished in the fourth century B.C., if not already by the last quarter of the fifth century.

The Medicine of Asclepius and the Medicine of the Asclepiads

The evident success of the medicine of the priests of Asclepius, in some cases in areas that overlapped the sphere in which Asclepiad physicians from Cos and Cnidus were active, raises the question whether the miraculous medicine practiced in the temples was in competition with the rational medicine of the Asclepiads. The question needs to be addressed from two points of view.

The first is that of the clergy of the Asclepieum. To judge from the cures recorded on the stelai of Epidaurus, the temple priests seem clearly to have felt a need to defend their miraculous brand of medicine against the disbelieving reactions of rationalistically minded visitors. The rather large number of references to the skepticism shown by certain pilgrims on arriving in the sanctuary is telling in this regard. We have already noted the half-blind woman from Athens who toured the sanctuary and made fun of certain cures that she judged unbelievable or impossible. One might also mention the case of a man who had come on account of his fingers, all but one of which were paralyzed: "Looking at the tablets that were in the sanctuary, he did not believe the cures and mocked the inscriptions."[55] The daring words of a heathen are reported as well. "The god lies," he said, "when he claims to heal the lame!"[56] But in every instance this skepticism was overcome by the power of the god. Not content simply to heal, the god also lectured the incredulous, who were made to understand that an inquiring mind was only a sign of ignorance.

In any case, the sick had no alternative but to apply to Asclepius when physicians could do no more for them by human means or, what came to the same thing, when physicians refused to treat them, judging their condition to be incurable. Consider this votive epigram, left at Epidaurus by the orator Aeschines as a memorial of his healing there: "Despairing of human art, and placing all my hope in the Divinity, I left Athens, mother of beautiful children, and was cured in three months, Asclepius, by coming to thy grove, of an ulcer on my head that had continued for a year."[57]

Another example is furnished by the woman from Troezen who suffered from a worm in her stomach. The stele says only that she arrived in Epidaurus, without specifying the circumstances of her coming.[58] But Aelian, who reports the same story, begins thus: "A woman suffered from an intestinal worm, and the cleverest doctors despaired of curing her. Accordingly she went to Epidaurus and prayed the god that she might be rid of the complaint that was lodged in her."[59] There can be no clearer proof than this that religious medicine constituted the final recourse for patients who had been turned away by doctors.

Given that the divine physician seemed so powerful, was it not therefore in the interest of the attendants of the temple of Asclepius themselves to advise the sick to seek help from the god directly rather than go to human physicians? A case of healing preserved on one of the Epidaurus stelai plainly implies as much: "Eratocles of Troezen. He was empyematic. While he was at Troezen, the god appeared to him during his sleep: standing above him, he ordered him not to be cauterized but to come sleep in the sanctuary of Epidaurus. And once the deadline set by the god had passed, the pus burst and the sick man went away cured."[60] In this case, where physicians had recommended an operation that would have been doubly unpleasant for the patient even in the event it was a success—for cauterization was painful and left unsightly marks—the god, appearing in a dream, intercedes to invite the patient to come for treatment in his sanctuary, where he then makes an exact prognosis and brings about a cure by gentle methods that have none of the aftereffects of surgery. To the extent that this amounted to saying the god's prognosis was infallible and that divine treatment was both gentler and more effective than human treatment, what we are dealing with here is probably evidence of a rivalry between lay medicine and the medicine of the sanctuaries.

If we now look at the matter from the point of view of lay medicine, it seems astonishing not to find corresponding evidence of such a conflict in the writings that have come down to us under the name of Hippocrates. Nonetheless, everything we find in these writings seems to suggest that the rational medicine of the Hippocratics and the miraculous medicine of Epidaurus were utterly opposed. Though they treated the same diseases, they treated them by radically different methods. Let us take the case of epilepsy, which the author of *The Sacred Disease* refused to explain by the personal intervention of a deity, proposing instead to treat it by natural methods. By contrast, here is how the god of Epidaurus treated an inhabitant of Argos who was afflicted with epilepsy: "An inhabitant of Argos. Epileptic. This one having gone to sleep in [the incubation porch] had a vision. It seemed to him that the god standing above him pressed his ring upon his mouth, nostrils, and ears, and he got better."[61] The healing depended on a magical device, the ring, to which popular belief in Hippocrates' time attributed preventive, if not also curative, powers.[62] A Hippocratic physician, however, could in no way adhere to such a belief or advocate such a course of treatment. Nor could he endorse the whole series of cures, each more stunning than the last, that the staff of the sanctuary of Epidaurus had selected to promote the god's image as a healer.

It is not as though the Hippocratic physician refrained from noting surprising cures. Some of the cases recounted in the works of Hippocrates can even be compared to the miraculous healings of Epidaurus. Here, for example, is the story of the sudden healing of a paralytic following a shock: "Eumelus of Larissa grew rigid in his legs, arms, and jaws. He could not extend them or bend them . . . nor open his jaws. . . . On the twentieth day he fell backwards while sitting and severely struck his head on a stone, and darkness poured over him. Shortly later he stood up and was better."[63] Here the doctor limits himself to relating the facts of the matter without expressing judgment. Elsewhere he emphasizes the extraordinary character of the cure: "The man hit by an arrow in the gland at the groin, whom we had seen, was preserved in a most unexpected manner. The point was not removed because it was in too deep, nor was there any notable hemorrhage, nor inflammation, nor was he lamed. He had carried the point for six years up to the time of our departure."[64]

An analogous case has been preserved on the Epidaurus stelai. One Euhippus came to the sanctuary of Epidaurus, having lived for six years with the point of an arrow stuck in his jaw—which the god, naturally, removes without difficulty and without pain during the pilgrim's incubation.[65]

Similarities such as these serve only to bring out the differences between the two medicines. The Hippocratic physician notes the exceptional character of certain cures while resisting the inference that they constitute evidence of divine intervention. In religious medicine, by contrast, the exceptional becomes the rule, the normal manifestation of an almighty deity. The notion that the rational medicine of the Hippocratics might have emerged from the temples of Asclepius is therefore unimaginable.[66]

Nonetheless, despite the gap that separated the two medicines, the Hippocratics did not feel the need to keep their distance. Ordinarily, they kept silent. The only reference to be found in the Hippocratic Collection to the medicine of the sanctuaries is not unfavorable. In the course of his polemic against the charlatans who believe in the divine origin of epilepsy, the author of *The Sacred Disease* rebukes them for purifying patients with blood as if they were criminals. Then he indicates what in his view should have been done: "All such they ought to have treated in the opposite way; they should have brought them to the sanctuaries, with sacrifices and prayers, in supplication to the gods."[67]

This opinion, that the patients should have been taken instead to the sanctuaries, refers to the medicine of the sanctuaries, and possibly to incubation in the sanctuaries of Asclepius, a practice attested from the last quarter of the fifth century B.C.[68] To be sure, the reference is very ambiguous. The Hippocratic author does not absolutely recommend that patients be brought to the sanctuaries in all cases. His suggestion is influenced instead by the logic of a religious conception of disease that was not his own. He does not himself believe in the divine origin of diseases, in the traditional sense of the term, which is to say in diseases caused by the personal intervention of a deity. But he recognizes that others hold such a belief and that for them the sole therapeutic solution that corresponds to their elevated sense of the divine is to be found in the religious medicine of the great sanctuaries.

The respect shown by Hippocratic physicians toward religious medicine derived in part from the fact that, as Asclepiads, they claimed descent from Asclepius. For them, there was no incompatibility between rational medicine and the worship of their prestigious ancestor. Asclepius came after Apollo in the series of deities invoked as guarantors in the Hippocratic oath.[69] Those physicians who were actually members of the family of the Asclepiads, being tied to Asclepius not only by art but also by blood, presumably maintained a private cult in honor of the family's founder. This is all the more plausible in view of the fact, which admittedly is known to us from a slightly later period, that Nicias of Miletus, a physician who was a friend of the poet Theocritus, worshipped the god though he was tied to Asclepius only by art and not by blood.[70] Asclepius therefore constituted a link between the rational medicine of the Asclepiads and the religious medicine of the priests of Asclepius. More generally, the relations of Hippocrates and his family with the sanctuary of Apollo at Delphi[71] show that the practice of religion was not incompatible with the practice of rational medicine. Moreover, the religious privileges enjoyed by physicians who belonged, as Hippocrates did, to the aristocratic family of Asclepiads could have served only to reinforce their social prestige, and even to confer advantages in their medical career at a time when professional qualifications did not yet exist.

By putting Hippocrates and the Asclepiads in the context of the age in which they lived and practiced, we can better understand the position of the Hippocratic physicians vis-à-vis the sacred, even while allowing for the fact that not all Hippocratic physicians belonged to the Asclepiad family. Although they were capable of mounting a direct attack upon soothsayers and charlatans, to the extent that these were their competitors in a still unregulated profession, they were never opposed to the traditional religion of the great sanctuaries. Their rationalism enabled them to reconcile two distinct conceptions of the divine, one of which provided a foundation for medical science and the other for sanctified religion.

Decline of the Divine in the Explanation of Diseases: Pestilence in Sophocles, Hippocrates, and Thucydides

Despite the flexibility of Hippocratic rationalism in relation to the divine, the fact remains that the rational explanations proposed by physicians were often at odds with beliefs commonly held at the time. But given that physicians did not feel any need to insist on the difference between their views and received opinion, only by considering their views in relation to those expressed in contemporary literature, and particularly in tragedy, can we get a sense of how far the divine had receded as an explanatory factor in the thought of the Hippocratics as compared with traditional thinking.

The example that best illustrates this diminished emphasis is that of a disease that fell upon an entire community. Such a disease, which the Greeks called *loimos*, is usually referred to today as plague. But historians of medicine prefer to call it by the name *pestilence*, since plague, strictly speaking, is caused by Yersin's bacillus, which was unknown in Greece during the archaic and classical periods.[72]

Pestilence is mentioned several times in Greek tragedy. Aeschylus alludes to it as one of the two main reasons for the depopulation of cities—the other being war.[73] But only Sophocles places it at the center of one of his plays, *Oedipus Tyrannus*, which opens with the citizens of Thebes having fallen prey to a scourge ravaging the entire city. Here is the way in which the priest of Zeus describes the situation to Oedipus, the king of the city:

> King, you yourself
> have seen our city reeling like a wreck
> already; it can scarcely lift its prow
> out of the depths, out of the bloody surf.
> A blight is on the fruitful plants of the earth,
> a blight is on the cattle in the fields,
> a blight is on our women that no children
> are born to them; a God that carries fire,
> a deadly pestilence, is on our town,
> strikes us and spares not, and the house of Cadmus
> is emptied of its people while black Death
> grows rich in groaning and in lamentation.[74]

This theme of desolation is taken up again a bit later by the chorus of old people:

> Our sorrows defy number;
> all the ship's timbers are rotten;
> taking of thought is no spear for the driving away of the plague.
> There are no growing children in this famous land;
> there are no women bearing the pangs of childbirth.
> You may see them one with another, like birds swift on the wing,
> quicker than fire unmastered,
> speeding away to the coast of the Western God.
> In the unnumbered deaths
> of its people the city dies;
> those children that are born lie dead on the naked earth
> unpitied, spreading contagion of death.[75]

This notion of a general scourge that afflicts a city in each of the three great domains of life—vegetable, animal, and human—was not new in Greek literature in Sophocles' time. It was the legacy of an archaic conception present already in epic literature. In Homer, for example, at the beginning of the *Iliad*, a pestilence falls upon the camp of the Achaeans outside the gates of Troy; it strikes the animals first, mules and dogs, and then the men.[76] In Hesiod, the city of the unjust king, victim of pest and famine, sees its men waste away, its women cease to give birth, and its lands diminished by the loss of harvests and herds.[77] What unites the evocation of pestilence in Sophocles with that of Homer and Hesiod is chiefly the explanation that is given for it: the scourge is a divine punishment visited upon a whole community to punish the sin of a single member.

In Hippocrates, by contrast, there is no example of a generalized disease that falls upon all three natural domains at once. When the author of the treatise *Breaths* writes about pestilence, he stresses that this common disease does not attack human beings and animals indiscriminately, but sometimes affects human beings in general, sometimes this or that species of animal.[78]

It is above all with regard to the cause of pestilence that the difference between Hippocrates and Sophocles is clearly seen. The same term is used by both the physician and the playwright to explain pestilence: *miasma*, which is the source of the same word in English. But this term is not used in at all the same sense by the two authors. In *Oedipus Tyrannus*, as in the Greek tragedies as a whole, *miasma* denotes religious defilement, especially the defilement that results from the spilling of blood. Indeed, the Delphic oracle, consulted by Creon at the order of Oedipus, replies that in order to put an end to the pestilence it is necessary drive out from the land the *miasma* that caused it.[79] In this case, the source of defilement was the blood spilled in the murder of Laius, Oedipus's father. The whole tragedy, of course, consists in the discovery by Oedipus that he himself is the author of this foul act. The cause of the pestilence therefore is conceived in Sophocles as a sin against religion and morality, notwithstanding the fact that the sin was involuntary. In Hippocrates, on the other hand, the term *miasma*, though it is also used to denote the cause of pestilence, has been rid of all moral and religious connotation. "So whenever the air has been infected with such pollutions [miasmas] as are hostile to the human race," says the author of the *Breaths*, "then men fall sick."[80] What are we to understand these "miasmas" as implying in a medical context? According to ancient commentators, they were sorts of emanations that arose either from the earth or from swamps, or even from cadavers.

For the Hippocratic author, *miasma* was therefore a natural, physical cause. All notion of individual blame or responsibility has now disappeared. It is no longer a question of individual behavior in relation to religious and moral values, but human nature in the context of the surrounding environment. In the works of the physician, pestilence is due to a morbid element borne by the air, and selectively affects human beings, or the different animal species, according to the laws of compatibility or incompatibility between the element that causes the disease and the nature of each species, animal or human; in the works of the playwright, on the other hand, pestilence falls indiscriminately on all forms of life in the community to which the culpable individual belongs, as it did in Homer and Hesiod. Accordingly, there is a difference between the ways in which pestilence propagates itself under these two conceptions. While the dramatist makes reference to the dangers of contagion, the Hippocratic physician does not believe in the propagation of epidemic disease by simple contact. On this particular point, concerning the mode of transmission of disease, the archaic conception of the dramatic author paradoxically appears closer to the thinking of the modern physician than the rational conception of the medical author.

Given these divergences of opinion with regard to the cause of pestilence, it is clear that the means employed to put an end to it in tragedy and in Hippocratic medicine cannot be at all similar. In Sophocles' *Oedipus Tyrannus* there is no thought of calling upon a physician to combat the scourge. It is the gods, the oracles, and the soothsayers who must be consulted. The anguished chorus of old people, as spokesman of the people as a whole, invokes no fewer than seven deities in the hope that they may put an end to the scourge. But popular feeling is not the only thing that is at issue in the play. Oedipus, the leader of the city, who by his own wit alone had been able to solve the riddle of the sphinx, has no other recourse in the face of such a calamity than to send Creon to consult the oracle at Delphi and to summon Tiresias, the Theban seer—precisely as Achilles, at the beginning of the *Iliad*, urges the Achaeans to inquire of "some holy man, some prophet, even an interpreter of dreams."[81] The memory of Homer is so much a part of the play, in fact, that Oedipus, leader of the Thebans, is angered by Tiresias's revelations in just the same way that Agamemnon, leader of the Achaeans, was angered by the revelations of the seer Calchas. Nonetheless, this recourse to oracles and soothsayers is not merely a literary memory in Sophocles; it is also what actually took place in the real world. The records of the Delphic oracle contain some forty examples of responses given in connection with a pestilence. Among them is the response given to the Athenians when they fell victim to a pestilence in the sixth century. On that occasion, the Pythia advised them to "purify the city," a task they confided to one of the Seven Sages, Epimenides of Crete:

[Epimenides] took sheep, some black and others white, and brought them to the Areopagus; and there he let them go whither they pleased, instructing those who followed them to mark the spot where each sheep lay down and offer a sacrifice to the local divinity. And thus, it is said, the plague was stayed. Hence even to this day altars may be found in different parts of Attica with no name inscribed upon them, which are memorials of this atonement. According to some writers he declared the plague to have been caused by the pollution which Cylon brought on the city and showed them how to remove it. In consequence two young men, Cratinus and Ctesibius, were put to death and the city was delivered from the scourge.[82]

Even when the great "plague" of Athens broke out in the middle of the fifth century, at the beginning of the Peloponnesian War, its inhabitants resorted to supplication in the sanctuaries and oracles.[83] From the religious perspective, the end of a pestilence could be brought about only by driving out the miasma or by its purification in accordance with a religious ritual.

From the rational perspective of the Hippocratics, by contrast, the means to be employed fell exclusively within the province of medicine. Treatment consisted of protecting oneself against the cause; namely, the miasmas contained in the air. Consider the advice given by Polybus, Hippocrates' disciple:

[T]hese are the recommendations that should be made to patients. They should not change their regimen, as it is not the cause of their disease, but rather take care that their body be as thin and as weak as possible, by diminishing their usual food and drink gradually. For if the change of regimen be sudden, there is a risk that from the change too some disturbance will take place in the body, but regimen should be used in this way when it manifestly does no harm to a patient. Then care should be taken that inspiration be of the lightest, and also from a source as far removed as possible; the place should be moved as far as possible from that in which the disease is epidemic, and the body should be reduced, for such reduction will minimize the need of deep and frequent breathing.[84]

Aiming to prevent airborne miasmas from penetrating the body, the physician advises two things: diminishing the respiratory capacity of the subject by reducing his weight, and removing him from infested areas. This treatment, which is more preventive than curative, may raise a smile. But it relies on natural and rational procedures alone. These prudential counsels turn out not to be as obsolete as they may seem, if one compares them with the following instructions given out by an official body not many years ago:

The Office of Air Quality for the region of Basel (Switzerland) issued a warning on 27 July [1989] that air in the region contained high concentrations of ozone. Three measuring stations registered levels exceeding the limit value of 120 micrograms of ozone per cubic meter of air. Inhabitants of the region are therefore advised to avoid prolonged, strenuous activity. Persons suffering respiratory problems, as well as children, are particularly requested not to go outside.[85]

The originality of the Hippocratic physician's attitude toward pestilence may also be appreciated by comparing it with that of Thucydides regarding the great "plague" of Athens in 429. While Sophocles limits himself to a general and traditional characterization of the scourge in his *Oedipus Tyrannus*,[86] Thucydides gives a masterful description in which he distances himself from the conventional conception in favor of something closer to the new medical model.[87] He departs from conventional thinking to the extent that he notes the ineffectiveness of divine methods, which is to say supplications to the gods and oracles and so on, implying that religious defilements, such as the presence of cadavers in the sacred places of the city, were not the cause of the illness but rather its consequence. Thucydides is in accord with the medical literature in two respects: he describes the symptoms of the illness precisely, with the aid of a technical vocabulary analogous to that of the doctors; and his analysis of the pathological facts is thoroughly rational, as in the Hippocratic authors. But his dependence on the Hippocratics must not be exaggerated. The historian insists at the very outset of his description of the scourge on personal experience: he has personally suffered the illness and has seen firsthand many others who have been affected by it. He is therefore capable of describing the malady as a privileged witness, from both the outside and the inside, as it were, without needing to rely on others for information. In any case, not a single detailed account of a pestilence is to be found in the Hippocratic Collection. There is nothing to prove that Hippocrates himself witnessed the "plague" of Athens. It was only afterwards that the pestilence mentioned in his biographical writings came to be confounded with the great "plague" of Athens, and that Hippocrates was credited with having brought relief to the populace by lighting great fires to dry out the air.[88] But more than anything else, what separates Thucydides from the physicians of the Hippocratic Collection is his refusal to assign a cause: "All speculation as to its origin and its causes, if causes can be found adequate to produce so great a disturbance, I leave to other writers, whether lay or professional."[89]

For a Hippocratic physician, however, it was essential to know the cause of the illness. Treatment depended on it. "For knowledge of the cause of a disease," says the author of *Breaths*, "will enable one to administer to the body what things are advantageous [using opposites to combat the disease]."[90] Thucydides, for his part, faults the proponents of a rational medicine and those of a religious medicine on the same grounds. He stresses the powerlessness of each camp, drawing an eloquent parallel between them: "Neither were the physicians at first of any service, ignorant as they were of the proper way to treat it, but they died themselves the most thickly, as they visited the sick the most often; nor did any [other] human art succeed any better. Supplications in the temples, divinations, and so forth were found equally futile, till the overwhelming nature of the diaster at last put a stop to them altogether."[91]

One unexpected consequence of this refusal to speculate about causes is that the historian saw things more clearly than the physicians of his time. Not being the captive of the preconceptions that prevented specialists from admitting the possibility that an epidemic might be transmitted by contact, Thucydides was able explicitly to note the fact of contagion[92] and to observe, rightly, that physicians, by virtue of their contact with the sick, were the most vulnerable to infection.

The different explanations given for the origin of pestilence by the dramatist, the physician, and the historian allow us to situate them in relation to each other. The rational and natural causality of the Hippocratic physician stands opposed to the religious and moral causality of the tragic playwright, while the historian, though implicitly he challenges religious causality, shows himself to be openly skeptical of the rational explanations advanced by the physician. Sophocles may therefore be seen as representing the traditional cultural heritage; Hippocrates as embodying the rising tide of rationalism; and Thucydides as marking the beginning of a tradition of skeptical positivism that limits itself to describing facts and refuses to draw conclusions about causes.

NINE

Hippocrates and the
Birth of the Human Sciences

The fifth century B.C. may be thought of as giving birth not only to rationalism but also to humanism, so long as this term is understood in its broad sense as signifying mankind's reflection upon itself. The fifth century was the decisive period when man became aware of his place in the universe—and so of his own power of invention, which enabled him to pass from a state of nature to one of culture—and when he discovered that he was himself an object of science.

New Place of Man in the Universe

The medical literature of the Hippocratics greatly contributed to this redefinition of humanity in the Age of Pericles.

In the interval since the time of the Homeric epics, during which the Greeks advanced from lyric poetry to tragic poetry, they defined themselves above all in relation to the gods. The values they cared most about were piety and justice. If there existed a common denominator by which human beings could be conceived as being one, it was indeed this opposition between gods and men. The traditional view of the poets, contrasting the power and the knowledge of the gods with the weakness and foolishness of human beings, was still current in the theater of the classical period. In the striking scene that opens Sophocles' *Ajax*, in which the hero is found to have been driven mad by the goddess Athena, his enemy Odysseus draws a wise lesson from the spectacle, stressing the weakness of the human condition before the gods:

> *Odysseus*: . . . For I see the true state of all us that live—
>   We are dim shapes, no more, and weightless shadow.
> *Athena*: . . . One short day
>   Inclines the balance of all human things

To sink or rise again. Know that the gods
Love men of steady sense and hate the proud.[1]

Hippocratic medicine, to the extent that it ruled out, as we have seen, all personal intervention by the gods in the development of diseases, proposed another vision of humanity. The opposition between the divine and the human was thus neutralized from the medical point of view. Diseases "are all divine and all human," in the words of *The Sacred Disease*[2]—"no one being more divine or more human than any other," in the echoing words of *Airs, Waters, Places*.[3] Consequently, man was no longer to be situated in relation to the gods, but in relation to the universe that surrounded him.

In the view of the Hippocratic physicians, humanity could not be envisaged in its totality without taking account of the influences of the external environment in which human beings live. According to the treatise *Nature of Man*, for example, despite the permanence of man's natural constitution, composed of the four humors (blood, phlegm, yellow bile, and black bile), these humors nonetheless increase and decrease inside him with the rhythm of the seasons: phlegm, cold and moist, predominates in winter; blood, warm and moist, in spring; yellow bile, warm and dry, in summer; and black bile, cold and dry, in fall. "All these elements then," this author emphasizes, "are always comprised in the body of a man, but as the year goes round they become now greater and now less, each in turn and according to its nature."[4] In the world as seen by the Hippocratic physician, the tide of human affairs no longer rose and fell according to the whims of the gods or divine justice, as was still the case with Sophocles; it was rather a matter of the bodily humors growing larger and smaller according to the rhythm of the seasons, in keeping with a natural law.

Man and His Environment

This new vision of man as subject to the permanent influences of the external world in which he lives is masterfully presented in *Airs, Waters, Places*, which, as it has been said, was the first treatise of medical climatology in world literature, as well as the first treatise of anthropology.[5]

Written for the itinerant physician who arrives in an unfamiliar city, this work brings out in its first part all the factors that the physician must observe in order to make prognoses and treat whatever diseases, general or particular, may occur in the course of a year. The beginning of the treatise clearly lays out these different factors:

Whoever wishes to pursue properly the science of medicine must proceed thus. First he ought to consider what effects each season of the year can produce; for the seasons are not at all alike, but differ widely both in themselves and at their changes. The next point is the hot winds and the cold, especially those that are universal, but also those that are peculiar to each particular region. He must also consider the properties of the waters; for as these differ in taste and in weight, so the property of each is far different from that of any other. Therefore, on arrival at a town with which he is unfamiliar, a physician should examine its position with respect to the winds and to the risings of the sun. For a northern, a southern, an eastern, and a western aspect has each its own individual property. He must consider with the greatest care both these things and how the natives are off for water, whether they use marshy, soft waters, or such as are hard and come from rocky heights, or brackish and harsh. The soil too, whether bare and dry or wooded and watered, hollow and hot or high and cold. The mode of life also of the inhabitants that is pleasing to them, whether they are heavy drinkers, taking lunch, and inactive, or athletic, industrious, eating much and drinking little.

Using this evidence he must examine the several problems that arise. For if a physician know these things well, by preference all of them, but at any rate most, he will not, on arrival at a town with which he is unfamiliar, be ignorant of the local diseases, or of the nature of those that commonly prevail; so that he will not be at a loss in the treatment of diseases, or make blunders, as is likely to be the case if he have not this knowledge before he consider his several problems.[6]

The health of human beings depends therefore not only on the manner in which they live but on a whole series of natural factors that impose themselves upon every individual, no matter what a person's particular way of life may be. In the first place there are local factors, specific to the cities where they are prevalent, such as the orientation of a city with respect to the winds and the risings of the sun, the quality of the waters used by the inhabitants, and the nature of the soil; next there is a general factor that obtains in any city where the physician may need to go, the climatic constitution of the year, which is to say the weather in the different seasons. All these things produce effects upon individuals, who register them and react to them as a function of their nature, their sex, and their age. Mankind is thus defined by a network of factors, multiple and complex, that the physician must take into account, taking in as many of them as possible in their totality.

Man and His Habitat

To unravel this tangled skein of influences, operating in time and space both, the author of *Airs, Waters, Places* is obliged to make an unprecedented attempt at synthesis. This is particularly the case in his discussion of the orientation of places.

Taking as his point of departure the divided world of the Greek cities in which the Hippocratic physicians practiced, the author tries to go beyond the diversity of particular situations to identify those that are constant. He distinguishes four categories of cities, corresponding to the four main directions in which cities can be positioned with respect to the sun and the winds. To each type of city corresponds a type of person. In cities exposed to warm and moist winds from the south, the inhabitants tend to have a phlegmatic constitution, while in cities oriented toward the cold and dry winds from the north, the inhabitants tend to have a bilious constitution; cities facing to the east are the healthiest; those facing to the west are the most unhealthy.[7] In the healthiest cities, the inhabitants "are of better complexion and more blooming . . . [and] clear-voiced."[8] By contrast, in the least-healthy cities "they are likely to be pale and sickly . . . [and] have deep, hoarse voices."[9] The author therefore posits a necessary relation between the orientation of places and the constitution of human beings.

This relation is not restricted to physical characteristics, but also embraces character and intelligence, as certain passing remarks indicate. The inhabitants of cities exposed to northerly winds have "characters [that] incline to fierceness, not to mildness,"[10] and the inhabitants of cities facing toward the east have "better temper and intelligence than those who are exposed to the north."[11] Estimating the influence of environment therefore depends on considering human beings in their totality.

Moreover, the physical environment does not affect human beings alone. It acts also on all the other productions of nature, including plants and animals. After having emphasized that the people of cities that face eastwards are, in respect of character and intelligence, superior to those of cities exposed to the elements of the north, the physician locates his observation in a wider context, noting that it is true "just as all things growing there are better."[12]

The Classification of Cities in Hesiod and Hippocrates

We can see how innovative this classification of cities and people actually was by comparing it with the oldest such classification known to us, formulated two or three centuries before Hippocrates by Hesiod in his poem *Works and Days*. There Hesiod contrasts two types of cities, one in which men prosper, the other in which they waste away.[13] This picture is not dissimilar to the one presented by the Hippocratic physician of salubrious and insalubrious cities. The question of childbirth figures importantly in both the poet's description of the prosperous city and the physician's description of the salubrious city: "[W]omen bear children that resemble their parents," says Hesiod; likewise, Hippocrates says, "The women there very readily conceive and have easy deliveries."[14] Moreover, in the picture of the opposite kind of city, the poet and physician both insist on diseases that affect people: pestilence in Hesiod's case; in the case of the Hippocratic physician, any and all diseases that may befall them.[15]

These similarities in the description of two cities of contrary destinies serve only to make the differences between the explanation proposed by the poet and the one proposed by the physician more noticeable. For the poet, it is a question of the relation in each case between men and gods. For the physician, it is the relation between men and their environment that must be taken into account: the winds and the sun have either a beneficial or a baleful influence on men according to whether the city is well or badly situated.

For the ancient divine and moral law, then, the physician substituted a rational and natural law. And in doing this, the Hippocratic author established the first principles of a science that was to regain favor only much later in modern times, under the name of ecology.

Man and Climate

Human beings, according to the author of *Airs, Waters, Places*, show the effects not only of the local conditions of their physical environment but also of the general conditions of its climate. "For with the seasons men's diseases, like their digestive organs, suffer change," he declares in the introduction to his treatise. Then he concludes his examination of the factors that have an effect upon the health of men and upon their diseases with a long discussion of the influence of the seasons.[16]

Just as there exists a salubrious type of city, so there exists a healthy type of climatic constitution. The healthiest year is described as follows: "If the signs prove normal when the stars set and rise; if there be rains in autumn, if the winter be moderate, neither too mild nor unseasonably cold, and if the rains be seasonable in spring and in summer, the year is likely to be very healthy."[17] What salubrious cities and healthy years have in common is a sense of proportion, or moderation (*métriotès*). The healthiest city is one where there is a balance between hot and cold, as in the most balanced season of the year, springtime.[18] The healthiest year is that in which each of the seasons is in balance, both internally and with respect to the others.

Human beings therefore enjoy the best health when the external influences that act upon them, whether these be local or general, are balanced and moderate. The notion of moderation, traditionally applied by the Greeks to human conduct, is transposed by the physician to the natural environment in which human beings reside. But this transposition did not come about without certain shifts in terminology. In the moral domain, the behavior opposed to moderation (*métriotès*) is excess (*hybris*). For this notion of excess, the new perspective of the physician substitutes the notion of change (*métabolè*). Bad conditions, whether local or climatic, arise through change. Speaking of the most unfavorable orientation for a city, the author asserts: "Such a situation for a city is precisely like autumn in respect of the changes [*métabolas*] of the day, seeing that the difference between sunrise and afternoon is great."[19] And with regard to climate, he recommends that one "should be especially on one's guard against the most violent changes [*métabolas*] of the seasons."[20]

Man and the Stars: Medicine and Astronomy

While local factors involve only the winds and the sun—the orientation of places being defined in relation to these things—climatic factors introduce a new field of observation: the stars. In his introduction to *Airs, Waters, Places*, the author places changes of seasons and the rising and setting of the stars on the same level: "For knowing the changes of the seasons, and the risings and settings of the stars, with the circumstances of each of these phenomena, he will know beforehand the nature of the year that is coming."[21] Then, in his discussion of climate, after having drawn attention to the dangers that come with changes of seasons, he continues: "One must also guard against the risings of the stars, especially of the Dog Star, then of Arcturus, and also of the setting of the Pleiades. For it is especially at these times that diseases come to a crisis. Some prove fatal, some come to an end, all others change to another form and another constitution."[22]

Man therefore lives according to the rhythm not only of the changing seasons but also of the motion of celestial bodies. This dimension of medicine is strongly insisted upon by the author. Moving at once to preempt an objection from those who would construe it as merely an idle digression about celestial phenomena, he forcefully declares: "[T]he contribution of astronomy [*astronomiè*] to medicine is not a very small one but a very great one indeed."[23] The physician must therefore also be an astronomer, which is to say he must know the science of the rising and setting of the constellations. This declaration has rather the air of a manifesto about it. It takes on an importance that is all the greater for the history of science in that the term "astronomy" occurs here for the first time in Greek literature.[24]

The belief in the influence of the stars upon the health and illness of human beings no doubt has deep roots in the most ancient Greek thought. Already, in the *Iliad*, it is clearly stated, on the occasion of a comparison of Achilles with a star, that the constellation of the Dog of Orion, when it rises in autumn, "brings on the great fever for unfortunate mortals."[25] When the Hippocratic physician instructs his readers to "guard against the risings of the stars, especially of the Dog Star," he is repeating a belief as old as Homer. But if he feels the need to reply to a possible objection, openly asserting the usefulness of astronomy in medicine, it is probably because in his time this science was as much contested as admired.

The science of the stars fascinated some scholars, for example the Sophist Hippias, a proponent of encyclopedic knowledge,[26] or the disciples of Socrates whom Aristophanes portrays in his comedy *The Clouds* (423 B.C.).[27] Others, more interested in the day-to-day problems of human life, were reluctant to join in. Thus the Sophist Protagoras judged this science to be useless in the education of young people.[28] It seems reasonable, then, to suppose that some physicians must also have been skeptical about the application of astronomy to medicine, and ready to dismiss the pretention to explain man in terms of the universe that surrounded him as futile.

The conviction of the author of *Airs, Waters, Places* is all the more remarkable for that. Man, he believes, is part of his environment. Medicine cannot ignore this fact, and so it must therefore be both ecological and meteorological in its approach to man.

On Certain Extensions of the Theory of the Influence of Places and Climate on Man

The idea that places and climate exercised an influence upon the physical and moral character of human beings was not to remain confined to medical circles.

In the event, the treatise *Airs, Waters, Places* did not have to wait for Montesquieu's statement in the eighteenth century of the theory of the influence of climate on human tissues in order to be appreciated. Plato, whose admiration for Hippocrates we have already noted several times, was probably an attentive reader of this treatise. In a passage in the *Laws*, he advises the lawmaker who must found a city to take into account several factors pointed out earlier by the Hippocratic physician: "And that's another point about the choice of sites . . . that we mustn't forget. Some localities are more likely than others to produce comparatively good (or bad) characters. . . . Some sites are suitable or unsuitable because of varying winds or periods of heat, others because of the quality of the water; in some cases the very food grown in the soil can nourish or poison not only the body but the soul as well."[29]

Such considerations were not only of concern to the lawmaker who must decide upon the siting of a city, but also to the architect who must build it. Thus, more than four centuries after Plato, the Roman architect Vitruvius was to affirm the necessity of knowing that part of medicine relating to climate, waters, and places. At the beginning of his treatise *On Architecture*, he says: "[The architect] must know the art of medicine in its relation to the regions of the earth (which the Greeks call *climata*); and to the characters of the atmosphere, of localities (wholesome or pestilential), of water-supply."[30]

From Medicine to Ethnography and Anthropology

If the treatise *Airs, Waters, Places* made a major contribution to the birth of the human sciences, it was not only by virtue of its medical part, but also on account of a rather unexpected extension of the work to support a comparison, which was to become famous, between the peoples of Europe and of Asia.[31] Thus it succeeded in passing from medicine to the realm of ethnography. The change of subject seemed so remarkable that subsequently many wondered whether the treatise was actually the work of a single author and not two distinct treatises written by two different authors, one a physician and the other an ethnographer. It is true that the framework within which man is viewed is not the same in the two parts: in the medical part, the city (*polis*) is the basis for the human typology; in the ethnographic part, it is the people (*ethnos*). However the anthropology that serves as the foundation of analysis in each of the two parts is identical: human beings owe their physical peculiarities mainly to the influence of climate; humanity considered in all its aspects, moral as well as physical, is shaped by climate; the notions of equilibrium (*métriotès*) and change (*métabolè*) of seasons are fundamental to the analysis of the effects of climate on human beings. Examination of the style of the treatise confirms that the author of its two parts is the same. A single author, a physician, therefore managed to extend the etiological method suggested to him by his medical experience to questions of ethnography. It can hardly be supposed that this enlargement of the work, which involved the study of many different peoples and thus presumed a broad knowledge of the inhabited world, acquired by consulting specialized works and perhaps through travel as well, was simply tacked on to the medical section afterwards.

The Description of Peoples

The first thing that strikes the reader about the ethnographic part of the treatise is the detail of the information it contains and the mastery with which it is described.

Thanks to the curiosity of this physician, peoples whom history would otherwise have condemned to oblivion for their lack of notable achievements now come back into plain view. This is particularly the case with the inhabitants of the valley of the Phasis in Colchis, the present-day Rioni River that passes through Georgia before emptying into the Black Sea. Here is the description of this people, which is unique in Greek literature and supplies one of the first two literary accounts of lacustrian villages:[32]

Now let me turn to the dwellers on the Phasis. Their land is marshy, hot, wet, and wooded; copious violent rains fall there during every season. The inhabitants live in the marshes, and their dwellings are of wood and reeds, built in the water. They make little use of walking in the city and the harbour, but sail up and down in dug-outs made from a single log, for canals are numerous. The waters which they drink are hot and stagnant, putrefied by the sun and swollen by the rains. The Phasis itself is the most stagnant and most sluggish of all rivers. The fruits that grow in this country are all stunted, flabby, and imperfect, owing to the excess of water, and for this reason they do not ripen. Much fog from the waters envelops the land. For these causes, therefore, the physique of the Phasians is different from that of other folk. They are tall in stature, and of a gross habit of body, while neither joint nor vein is visible. Their complexion is yellowish, as though they have suffered from jaundice. Of all men they have the deepest voice, because the air they breathe is not clear, but moist and turbid. They are by nature disinclined for physical fatigue. There are but slight changes of the seasons, either in respect of heat or of cold. The winds are mostly moist, except for one breeze peculiar to the country, called *cenchron*, which sometimes blows strong, violent and hot. The north wind rarely blows, and when it does it is weak and gentle.[33]

So evocative a description gives one the impression of reading a firsthand report composed by a traveling physician who seems to have observed the land, the climate, and the physique of the inhabitants and their way of life with his own eyes. His account does not appear to be borrowed from a book or any such secondary source. This impression is confirmed by the fact that certain details would have gone unperceived by an observer who did not have available to him the interpretive schema elaborated by the physician in the first part of the treatise. The description is, in fact, guided by the observation of all the factors that the author recommends be taken into consideration upon the physician's arrival in a city unknown to him: the climate, the winds, the waters, the soil, the way of life of its inhabitants. From an ethnographic perspective, all of these things explain the body and mind of peoples in the same way that, from a medical perspective, they explain the constitution of human beings and their diseases. What is remarkable about this description of the country of the Phasis and its inhabitants is that the people reflect their environment: they are wet, heavy, and slow, like the swamps on which they live, characterized by a hot and foggy atmosphere, and like the Phasis, which flows lazily to the sea, without there being any contrast between the seasons to draw the natives out of their indolence.

Nothing in all of this shows that the author of *Airs, Waters, Places* was actually Hippocrates himself; but equally nothing shows that he was not. Is it altogether unreasonable to suppose that Hippocrates might have traveled beyond the perimeter of the world in which the Hippocratic school practiced medicine and seen with his own eyes these people who lived in the region of the Phasis?

A Comparison between Europe and Asia

The next thing that strikes the reader about this second ethnographic part of the treatise is the entirely novel attempt at synthesis that is made in order to organize the differences between the body and mind of the peoples of Europe and of Asia, which the author explains by reference to general laws of nature.

But before turning to these general laws, one needs to be aware of what was involved in making a comparison of this sort between Europe and Asia. To treat of the peoples of Europe and Asia in Hippocrates' time meant treating of the peoples of the entire known world. From the beginnings of Greek ethnography—which may be traced back to the work of Hecataeus of Miletus, whose *Periegesis* was written at the end of the sixth century B.C. or the beginning of the fifth—the earth as a whole, represented by the Greeks as a bronze disk encircled by the river Oceanus, was divided into two continents, Europe and Asia. Europe extended from southern Spain as far as Lake Maeotis (the present-day Sea of Azov). Asia included not only the Persian Empire but also the known part of Africa, which is to say Egypt and Libya. The second part of *Airs, Waters, Places* is therefore a sort of treatise of world ethnography, and one that is all the more valuable since Hecataeus's foundational work has come down to us only in the form of scant fragments.

The ambition of the Hippocratic physician was not, however, to describe the peoples of the whole world in an exhaustive manner, but to explain the most important differences distinguishing them from one another. The originality of the project consists in just this, and derives from the fact that the author approached ethnography from the point of view of medicine. In expanding his method of analyzing people who are ill to cover people who are well, he gave ethnographic research a whole new dimension.

Peoples and Climate

The fundamental idea of this treatise—which was to enjoy a brilliant career in the history of ideas, finding its most celebrated expression in Montesquieu's *Spirit of the Laws* (1748)—was that the major physical and moral differences between the peoples of Asia and Europe were chiefly due to climate. This notion is highlighted at the outset of the physician's exposition:

I hold that Asia differs very widely from Europe in the nature of all its inhabitants and of all its vegetation. For everything in Asia grows to far greater beauty and size; the one region is less wild than the other, the character of the inhabitants is milder and more gentle. The cause of this is the temperate climate, because it lies towards the east midway between the risings of the sun, and farther away than is Europe from the cold. Growth and freedom from wildness are most fostered when nothing is forcibly predominant, but equality in every respect prevails.[34]

Even so, not all parts of Asia benefit from the same favorable climate. The median part, which coincides roughly with Ionia, has the best climate and produces the tallest and most handsome men:

[T]he region . . . situated midway between the heat and the cold is very fruitful, very wooded and very mild; it has splendid water, whether from rain or from springs. While it is not burnt up with the heat nor dried up by drought and want of water, it is not oppressed with cold, nor yet damp and wet with excessive rains and snow. Here the harvests are likely to be plentiful. . . . The cattle too reared there are likely to flourish. . . . The men will be well nourished, of very fine physique and very tall, differing from one another but little either in physique or stature.[35]

By contrast, the peoples of Europe live in a climate of sharp contrasts, with the exception of the Scythians, whose climate is dominated by the cold, just as that of the Egyptians in Asia is dominated by the heat. Now where the climate is one of sharp contrasts, the author maintains, people will differ physically from one another. The reason he gives is that the human seed suffers from the change of seasons. If this ethnographer were not a physician by training, such a physiological explanation probably would not have occurred to him.

But while the temperate climate of Asia has the advantage of producing taller and more handsome people than the more varied climate of Europe, it has the disadvantage of making the people there less courageous:

[T]he chief reason why Asiatics are less warlike and more gentle in character than the Europeans is the uniformity of the seasons, which show no violent changes either towards heat or towards cold, but are equable. For there occur no mental shocks nor violent physical change, which are more likely to steel the temper and impart to it a fierce passion than is a monotonous sameness. For it is changes of all things that rouse the temper of man and prevent its stagnation. For these reasons, I think, Asiatics are feeble.[36]

Climate is therefore held to be the essential cause of the physical and moral characteristics of a people. To this is added a secondary cause of a different kind, for it does not arise from the natural environment. This is a human factor that the Greeks called *nomoi*, a term that covers both customs and laws.

Laws and the Spirit of Peoples

Customs and laws (*nomoi*) are to peoples what regimen (*diaita*) is to individuals. Just as regimen influences the health of individuals, so habits and laws have an influence on peoples.

This is apparent most particularly in the moral domain. To explain why Asiatics are less courageous than Europeans, the author, having already noted the unduly equable climate of Asia, goes on to invoke the influence of laws on the people as well:

Their institutions are a contributory cause, the greater part of Asia being governed by kings. Now where men are not their own masters and independent, but are ruled by despots, they are not keen on military efficiency but on not appearing warlike. For the risks they run are not similar. Subjects are likely to be forced to undergo military service, fatigue and death, in order to benefit their masters, and to be parted from their wives, their children and their friends. All their worthy, brave deeds merely serve to aggrandize and raise up their lords, while the harvest they themselves reap is danger and death. Moreover, the land of men like these must be desert, owing to their enemies and to their laziness, so that even if a naturally brave and spirited man is born his temper is changed by their institutions.[37]

The conjunction of the influence of climate and that of laws also helps account for the courage of Europeans. For to the effects of the contrasting seasons that are felt particularly in Europe must now be added the motivations that Europeans draw from the political regime under which they live, which is one of liberty, and therefore opposed to the despotic regime of Asia:

Wherefore Europeans are more warlike, and also because of their institutions, not being under kings as are Asiatics. For, as I said above, where there are kings, there must be the greatest cowards. For men's souls are enslaved, and refuse to run risks readily and recklessly to increase the power of somebody else. But independent people, taking risks on their own behalf and not on behalf of others, are willing and eager to go into danger, for they themselves enjoy the prize of victory. So institutions contribute a great deal to the formation of courageousness.[38]

The influence of law on the spirit of peoples therefore tends to run in the same direction as climate. But it may happen that law offsets the effect of climate. This is the case in Asia where peoples enjoy a political regime analogous to that of Europe—the author has in mind mainly, but not exclusively, the Greek cities of Asia Minor—on which account they prove to be the most courageous of the Asiatics. The power of law to modify the natural character of men and to counteract the influence of climate reinforces the author's conviction that the form of government is a component of the psychology of peoples.

The Physique of Peoples and Their Customs

Although the influence of what the Greeks called *nomos* may have been perceptible most of all in the moral sphere, the author also notes cases where customs act upon physique.

The Scythians, a people of the north of Europe, were in the habit of cauterizing themselves in many parts of the body. According to the physician, this was a way of remedying the moistness and softness of their natural constitution due to a climate that was too uniformly damp and cold. For if they did not cauterize themselves, they did not have enough strength to bend back a bow or to throw a javelin: cauterizations had the effect of removing the humoral excess in their joints and giving them the energy they otherwise lacked. This, then, is an instance of a custom that acts upon the physical nature of man and combats the influence of climate.

The customs whose influence upon physique is most pronounced are those that operate on the body of the young child when it is still malleable. This is the reason why the author of *Airs, Waters, Places* meticulously notes whether or not peoples observe the custom of swaddling their babies. To revert to the example of the Scythians, he thinks that if they are knock-kneed and squat it is "firstly because, unlike the Egyptians, they do not use swaddling clothes."[39] But his attention is drawn above all to two spectacular customs involving children.

The first is specific to a Scythian people that inhabited the area of Lake

Maeotis (Sea of Azov) and were called the Sauromates. Their peculiarity consisted in the fact that the women went to war, like the Amazons, and underwent an operation for this purpose in infancy:

Their women, so long as they are virgins, ride, shoot, throw the javelin while mounted, and fight with their enemies. They do not lay aside their virginity until they have killed three of their enemies, and they do not marry before they have performed the traditional sacred rites. A woman who takes to herself a husband no longer rides, unless she is compelled to do so by a general expedition. They have no right breast; for while they are yet babies their mothers make red-hot a bronze instrument constructed for this very purpose and apply it to the right breast and cauterize it, so that its growth is arrested, and all its strength and bulk are diverted to the right shoulder and right arm.[40]

Here then is a custom practiced upon the bodies of women from infancy that modifies their natural capacities by increasing the strength of the right arm, as a result of which they can more easily handle the bow and throw the javelin. The explanation proposed by the author is the same as in the case of the cauterizations performed by the Scythians: the custom involves a deliberate operation intended to remedy innate inadequacies and to improve natural endowments for purposes of combat.

The second custom to which infants were subject concerns a people who actually owed their name to this practice: the Macrocephalics, or Longheads.[41] Unlike the foregoing custom, this one was not adopted with utilitarian aims in mind. In this case, an Asian people elongated the heads of its children because it considered the form to be a sign of nobility. The physician's description is entirely centered on this custom and on the effects that it produced upon nature:

The races that differ but little from one another I will omit, and describe the condition only of those which differ greatly, whether it be through nature (*physis*) or through custom (*nomos*). I will begin with the Longheads. There is no other race at all with heads like theirs. Originally custom was chiefly responsible for the length of the head, but now custom is reinforced by nature. Those that have the longest heads they consider the noblest, and their custom is as follows. As soon as a child is born they remodel its head with their hands, while it is still soft and the body tender, and force it to increase in length by applying bandages and suitable appliances, which spoil the roundness of the head and increase its length. Custom originally so acted that through force such a nature came into being; but as time went on the process became natural, so that custom no longer exercised compulsion. For the seed comes from all parts of the body, healthy seed from healthy parts, diseased seed from diseased parts. If, therefore, bald parents have for the most part bald children, grey-eyed parents grey-eyed

children, squinting parents squinting children, and so on with other physical peculiarities, what prevents a long-headed parent having a long-headed child? At the
present time long-headedness is less common than it was, for owing to intercourse
with other [peoples] the custom is less prevalent.[42]

The great originality of this passage, compared with the preceding ones,
comes from the fact that the physical modification imposed by custom has
become, in a secondary stage, a natural character that is hereditarily transmitted. The acquired has become innate. But the innateness of the acquired
character remains fragile if the custom disappears.

The ethnographic physician's commentary on the relation between custom (*nomos*) and nature (*physis*) proved to be of great importance for the
history of ideas. For it marked the first time that the pair *nomos/physis* appeared in Greek literature. In modern terms, it corresponds roughly to the
familiar opposition between culture and nature. Surely the Hippocratic physician was not the creator of this conceptual tool; he introduces it in his
discussion without feeling the need to justify it. But the use that he makes of it
is original. We know that certain Sophists, or disciples of Sophists, such as
Antiphon or the Callicles of Plato's *Gorgias*, used the antithesis *nomos/physis*
in a subversive way in politics and ethics to devalue law, seen as an arbitrary
and restrictive institution, in favor of nature, the true order that justified the
strongest law. Because he was a man of science, the author of *Airs, Waters,
Places* made much more nuanced use of it. While recognizing the power of
nature, he also emphasized the force of custom, and imagined a relation
between the two that involved not only opposition, as the Sophists did, but
also collaboration. The Hippocratic physician thus occupied a middle ground
between the old conception, which made of *nomos* the "king of all things
mortal and immortal,"[43] and the Sophistic conception, in which *nomos* had
become a mere social convention.

On the Threshold of a General Anthropology

Climate and custom: thus the two principal factors that, according to the
ethnographic physician, accounted for the differences between the peoples of
Europe and of Asia, whether they were Greek or barbarian.

It may seem surprising that he did not go beyond the traditional division of
the world into two continents arbitrarily separated by Lake Maeotis (the
modern Sea of Azov). The factors that he identified as explaining the physical
and moral differences between peoples might have led him to challenge this

division of the world, or at least to ignore it. By the end of the treatise, in fact, he seems to have gotten beyond it. In a final section treating of the influence of the soil on the minds and bodies of human beings, he seems to have extracted the rules of a general anthropology in which the differences between Europe and Asia begin to fade away. It may also seem surprising to find a certain inconsistency in the explanations given: sometimes the physician relies on climate to explain human beings and the world in which they live, sometimes on climate and the world to explain human beings.

But one must not require extreme rigor of an infant science. What needs to be emphasized instead is the unprecedented effort on the part of the Hippocratic physician to conceive of man, whether as an individual or as a race, in terms of the rational factors that apply indiscriminately to all human beings. In this sense, he stands as the first founder of a human science.

Ethnography in Herodotus and Hippocrates

The originality of the ethnographic method of the author of *Airs, Waters, Places* appears more clearly still if we compare it with that of his contemporary, Herodotus. Both wrote about the same peoples of Europe and Asia, and both reflected upon the greater courage of Europeans in relation to Asiatics in the light of the great clash between the two races during the Persian Wars.

Before developing the comparison between Herodotus and Hippocrates (as we may as well refer to the author of *Airs, Waters, Places* from now on, for the sake of convenience), it should be acknowledged that the ethnographic material they present is not the same, even though there are undeniable points of resemblance. For example, while Hippocrates divides the world into two continents, Europe and Asia, Herodotus divides it into three: Europe, Asia, and Libya; or again, while Herodotus places the boundary between Europe and Asia along the Phasis (today the Rioni River), Hippocrates locates it at Lake Maeotis (the Sea of Azov). Their accounts are apt to diverge even when they concern the same peoples: for Hippocrates, the Sauromates are a Scythian people, but for Herodotus they are a distinct race, neighbors of the Scythians;[44] and while Hippocrates and Herodotus agree on the whole in reporting the way of life of the Sauromate women, they differ with regard to a single detail, the number of enemies whom they must kill before marrying: one according to Herodotus, three according to Hippocrates.[45] From these discrepancies, it can clearly be seen that Hippocrates did not use Herodotus as a source of information, and that the *Periegesis* by Hecataeus of Miletus, who is usually regarded as the founder of geography and ethnography, was not the only work consulted by either the historian or the physician. The ethno-graphic sources available to them—oral sources, of course, but also written ones—must have been richer and more varied than the meager fragments of Hecataeus that have survived. In ethnography, as also in history and medicine, the works of Herodotus and of Hippocrates did not represent absolute begin-nings. If we are sometimes inclined to suppose they did, it is only because the loss of the technical literature that came before has distorted our perspective of them.

Nonetheless we have no choice but to stick to what has survived. The comparison between Herodotus and Hippocrates, in cases where the eth-nographic material is comparable, shows that the physician had a knack for synthesis and a sense of coherence that the historian lacked. Let us turn once again to one of the European peoples, the Scythians, to whom both men devoted a detailed discussion.

The lengthy presentation that Herodotus gives of this people on the occa-sion of the expedition of the Persian king Darius against them[46] is the best example of what Herodotus brought to the field of ethnography that was new. It is justly renowned for the richness of its information, particularly regarding the customs of the Scythians, a people whom he himself had vis-ited. He describes, often in a very picturesque way, their religion, their gods, their sacrifices, their seers, their funerals, and their practices in war—things that were all to go unmentioned later by Hippocrates. But one will search in vain in Herodotus for any clear overview of the discussion of the Scythians as a whole, or of the leading ideas that structure it: the material is indeed rich, but it can hardly be regarded as having been mastered, even if one disregards the adventitious sections, often quite long, which Herodotus inserts at will throughout his account.

In Hippocrates, by contrast, everything is clearly ordered: first comes the way of life of the Scythians; then their physical constitution as determined by a cold and damp climate; then the unprolific character of the Scythians—this as a consequence of their physical constitution, and also of their way of life—some of whom are actually afflicted with impotence.[47] This mastery in the exposition of the argument as a whole is displayed also within each of the sections. Thus the author sketches a precise picture, dense and evocative of the way of life of these nomads, and exhibits a talent for uniting the pictur-esque detail with a vision of the whole the like of which is not to be found in any of the other Greek authors who wrote of the Scythians, not in Hero-dotus, nor even in the geographer Strabo:

What is called the Scythian desert is level grassland, without trees, and fairly well-watered. For there are large rivers which drain the water from the plains. There too live the Scythians who are called Nomads because they have no houses but live in wagons. The smallest have four wheels, others six wheels. They are covered over with felt and are constructed, like houses, sometimes in two compartments and sometimes in three, which are proof against rain, snow, and wind. The wagons are drawn by two or by three yoke of hornless oxen. They have no horns because of the cold. Now in these wagons live the women, while the men ride alone on horseback, followed by the sheep they have, their cattle, and their horses. They remain in the same place just as long as there is sufficient fodder for their animals; when it gives out they migrate. They themselves eat boiled meats and drink mares' milk. They have a sweetmeat called *hippace*, which is a cheese from the milk of mares (*hippoi*).[48]

Herodotus also speaks of these Scythian nomads, whom he nicely calls "house-carriers" (the word in Greek for snails), describing a people who "shoot with bows from horseback; they live off herds of cattle, not from tillage, and their dwellings are on their wagons";[49] in another place he mentions the "hornless breed of cattle" found in Scythia, for which he proposes the same explanation as Hippocrates—the cold Scythian climate.[50] But these remain scattered remarks: the historian does not know how to insert picturesque details, as the physician does, within a framework for analyzing the world.

The same ethnographic datum may also receive markedly different explanations from the historian and the physician. Such is the case with the nomadism of the Scythians. While the physician accounts for it by the need to find food for their animals,[51] Herodotus sees in it one of the cleverest human inventions for surprising the enemy, or fleeing from him, in time of war.[52] Where the historian admires what he regards as an unusual creative facet of human genius, the physician sees only one example among others of the necessary relation between living beings and their environment. Where the one expresses his astonishment before the exceptional, the other places the exceptional within a rational framework of explanation.

Similarities between Herodotus and Hippocrates

It should not be supposed that Herodotus ignored the influence of environment on man altogether. Indeed, there exist certain rather striking points of resemblance between the accounts of the historian and the physician in this regard.

First of all, it likewise occurs to Herodotus to appeal to climate in order to explain the health or illness of human beings. Thus he declares in connection with the Egyptians: "Indeed, in general the Egyptians are the healthiest of all men (after the Libyans), and it is because, I think, of their climate; for their seasons do not change much, one from the other. It is in changes that diseases grow most among men, and in no matter does change make such difference as in changes of seasons."[53]

It is a pity that a large accidental gap in the treatise *Airs, Waters, Places* prevents us from knowing what the physician had to say about the Egyptians and the Libyans, and so deprives us of the opportunity to compare his thinking with that of Herodotus on this point. But the idea that the major changes in the seasons are the principal cause of diseases is fundamental in this treatise, as indeed in other Hippocratic treatises as well—particularly in the *Aphorisms*, where it is said, in terms very near to those of Herodotus: "It is chiefly the changes of the seasons which produce diseases."[54]

Next, Herodotus, like Hippocrates, uses the theory of the influence of the soil on both physique and personality to explain differences among peoples. The quite famous passage referring to this constitutes the final anecdote of the *Histories*, rather carelessly tacked onto the account at the end. Whereas the narrative of the clashes between the Greeks and barbarians closes with the return of the Greeks after the naval battle of Cape Mycale, which marked the end of the Persian Wars (479 B.C.), the final anecdote takes the reader back to the beginning of the *Histories*, to the time of Cyrus the Great and the roots of Persian dominance. When Cyrus had succeeded in subjecting Asia to his rule, one of his counsellors proposed that he move on. Herodotus reports in a direct style the proposition made by the counsellor, a certain Artembares, and the wise response that Cyrus gave him:

"[L]et us move from this land of ours [said Artembares]—for it is little and rocky, too— and take something better than it." . . . When Cyrus heard that, he was not amazed at their argument but said that they should do as they said; but in that case they should prepare to be no longer those who rule but those who would be ruled. "From soft countries come soft men. It is not possible that from the same land stems a growth of wondrous fruit and men who are good soldiers." So the Persians took this to heart and went away; their judgment had been overcome by that of Cyrus, and they chose to rule, living in a wretched land, rather than to sow the level plains and be slaves to others.[55]

Implicit in Cyrus's reply is a sort of law that asserts a relation of identity to obtain between man and the land ("From soft countries come soft men"), a more general formulation of which is to be found in Hippocrates: "For in general you will find assimilated to the nature of the land both the physique and the characteristics of the inhabitants."[56]

Hippocrates illustrates his law by two brief and opposed examples, the first corresponding to the soft countries that produce soft men and the second to the rough countries that produce rough men: "For where the land is rich, soft, and well-watered . . . , there the inhabitants are fleshy, ill-articulated, moist, lazy, and generally cowardly in character. . . . But where the land is bare, waterless, rough . . . , there you will see men who are hard, lean, well-articulated, well-braced, and hairy; such natures will be found energetic, vigilant, stubborn and independent in character and temper . . . , and in war of more than average courage."[57]

Two of the great explanatory factors of Hippocratic anthropology and ethnography, climate and land, were therefore also formulated by Herodotus. Since Herodotus and Hippocrates composed their works independently of each other, it is probable that such ideas were already current in Ionian science prior to both the Father of History and the Father of Medicine.

A further resemblance may be noted in connection with a secondary series of factors that operate in Hippocratic ethnography; namely, the influence of laws and customs on the behavior of peoples. We have seen how, in Hippocrates, the political regime is held to have an effect upon the mind of a people, a government based on liberty tending to promote courage, a despotic one, cowardice. Now Herodotus, remarking the progress of the Athenians after exchanging a tyrannical regime for one of equality, notes the influence of this change of political regime in terms that are very close to those used by Hippocrates: "It is not only in respect of one thing but of everything that equality and free speech are clearly a good; take the case of Athens, which under the rule of princes proved no better in war than any of her neighbors but, once rid of those princes, was far the first of all. What this makes clear is that when held in subjection they would not do their best, for they were working for a taskmaster, but, when freed, they sought to win, because each was trying to achieve for his very self."[58]

The Originality of Hippocrates in Relation to Herodotus

But despite the resemblance between the texts of Hippocrates and Herodotus, there remain great differences that serve to bring out the originality of the Hippocratic method.

The first difference bears upon the role assigned to arguments from environmental influence. In Hippocrates, throughout his comparison of Europe with Asia, the climatic factor constitutes the framework within which the most significant physical and moral differences between peoples are to be accounted for. In Herodotus, by contrast, it is mentioned only in passing, on the occasion of a particular example, and does not play the role of a recurrent etiological system in the rest of the *Histories*. Thus, after having stated, with regard to a people of the south, that climate is an important factor in health and illness, Herodotus no longer makes any reference to it when he speaks of the disease affecting a people of the north—the Scythians' impotence—but at this juncture adopts instead the religious explanation that was common among the Scythians themselves, having to do with the curse of the goddess Artemis. We have already had an opportunity, in the preceding chapter on the divine, to compare this religious explanation with the rational explanation of the Hippocratic physician.[59] It needs to be added here that the physician's explanation of this particular case fits logically into a larger explanatory scheme, in which climate plays an essential role. One must not be misled by the fact that one detail in particular, relating to the way of life of the Scythians—the constant horse riding of its wealthiest class—is insisted upon in connection with the disease. The analysis of this disease is to be understood as part of a more general argument about the nature of the Scythians, whom the author has described as being the least fertile in the world. The disease therefore emerges under conditions favorable to its development. Now, the author says, if the Scythians are by nature unprolific, this is because their nature is cold and wet; and if their nature is cold and wet, this is because the climate itself is cold and wet. In working back through the causal chain, one uncovers the preponderant explanatory factor; namely, climate.

The coherence of the Hippocratic position becomes clearer still when it is compared to the incoherence, or at least the inconsistency, of Herodotus, who gives explanations as he needs them, on an ad hoc basis, at one moment attributing diseases to climate, at another to the gods.

The second difference, which follows from the first, is that Herodotus, to the extent that he cannot draw upon a coherent etiological system of human data, is obliged to invoke several sets of causes at once in order to account for such a fact, causes that the Hippocratic physician would consider internally inconsistent. The explanation that Herodotus gives for the outcome of the conflict between Europe and Asia in the Persian Wars provides an example. Against all expectation, Greece was saved from the menace of Persian despotism at the battle of Salamis in 480, though a substantial imbalance of forces in favor of the barbarian seemed to predict the opposite. How to explain the unexplainable? Herodotus does not make a clear choice between a divine explanation and a human explanation. On the one hand, he makes Themistocles say that the gods were the architects of the victory, thus adopting the chief reason given earlier by Aeschylus in his *Persians*,[60] and on the other he has Demaratus, a Spartan exiled to the court of the great king, say that the courage of the Greeks, acquired thanks to their political regime, was superior to that of the barbarians.[61] Herodotus seems not to see the contradiction between these two kinds of causes. For Hippocrates, by contrast, all personal intervention on the part of the gods having been ruled out, the only possible explanation is the personal courage of human beings. And to account for the courage of the Europeans, as opposed to the cowardice of the Asiatics, Hippocrates gives a new explanation that is consistent with an etiological system characterized by the preeminence of the climatic factor. While courage for Herodotus is an acquired trait, the product of law, for Hippocrates it becomes an innate quality, the product of climate, favored by law.

Climate and Peoples in Hippocrates and Aristotle

This new explanation of the nature of peoples by climate, formulated for the first time by Hippocrates, was to prove immediately popular. Aristotle, the son of a physician and an attentive reader of Hippocrates, later took up the idea in his *Politics*, declaring:

The nations inhabiting the cold places and those of Europe are full of spirit but somewhat deficient in intelligence and skill, so that they continue comparatively free, but lacking in political organization and capacity to rule their neighbours. The peoples of Asia on the other hand are intelligent and skilful in temperament, but lack spirit, so that they are in continuous subjection and slavery. But the Greek race participates in both characters, just as it occupies the middle position geographically, for it is both spirited and intelligent; hence it continues to be free and to have very good political institutions, and to be capable of ruling all mankind if it attains constitutional unity.[62]

For Aristotle, as for Hippocrates, climate determined the presence of courage in Europeans and its absence in Asiatics, though the climatic determinism is simplified in Aristotle, by comparison with Hippocrates, since now either cold or heat intervenes, and no longer the contrast, or lack of contrast, among seasons. But Aristotle introduced an important modification in replacing Hippocrates' bipartite Europe-Asia scheme by a tripartite Europe-Greece-Asia scheme. Situated between the two extreme poles represented on the one side by the European peoples, inhabitants of cold lands, courageous but unintelligent, and on the other by the Asiatic peoples, inhabitants of warm lands, and for this reason intelligent but pusillanimous, the Greek race occupied a doubly fortunate middle position. The temperate climate meant that it enjoyed both the qualities of courage and intelligence, and so possessed the characteristics needed to dominate the rest of the world if it were politically unified.

The climatic determinism that served in Hippocrates to implicitly justify the Greeks in putting a halt to Persian imperialism became in Aristotle a justification for the hope of a Panhellenic imperialism that his own student, Alexander, was to bring about in his own way. Aristotle thus reestablished a tradition of Hellenocentrism that Ionian ethnography had tried to gloss over.

The History of Man and the Archaeology of Medicine

The Hippocratic physicians not only placed human beings within the context of their environment in reflecting upon the causes of diseases. They also retraced the history of mankind in reflecting upon the art of medicine. To see how they did this it will be necessary to take our leave of *Airs, Waters, Places* and take up the treatise *Ancient Medicine*.

This work presents a reconstruction of the birth of medicine. In so doing, it helps to illuminate a decisive moment in the history of humanity, the point at which man passed from a state of savagery to a state of civilization. This reconstruction was part of a "first *Querelle des anciens et des modernes*" that took place in the fifth century B.C., echoes of which can be found in several passages of the Hippocratic Collection.[63] Was medicine obliged to follow the lead of tradition, or did it need to be reestablished on the basis of new principles? The Hippocratic author occupies an ambiguous position in this quarrel. He unquestionably sides with the ancients to the extent that he defends traditional medicine against innovators who desired to provide the art with new foundations.[64] But, at the same time, when he retraces the history of medicine as far back as its origins, he adopts the conception of historical development shared by the most modern minds of his own time—a conception founded on the idea of progress.

In Hesiod's time, the Greeks held a pessimistic view of the human condition. The history of humanity, seen through the myth of races, appeared then as a progressive decline from a golden age to an iron age, as it were. In the fifth century, by contrast, the human chronicle was seen as a progression from a state of savagery—the opposite of a golden age—toward a state of progressive civilization, thanks to the discovery of various arts (*technai*). This theme of progress, whose source may be found in the thought of the Sophists and pre-Socratic philosophers of the fifth century, such as Protagoras and Democritus, was sufficiently fashionable that it was used by the three great tragic authors, by Aeschylus in *Prometheus Bound*, by Sophocles in a celebrated chorus of *Antigone*, and by Euripides in a tirade delivered by the Athenian king Theseus in the *Suppliant Women*. This picture of human progress is also found in the work of Thucydides, at the very beginning, where he recounts the advance of civilization in ancient Greece. Prominent among the arts that made progress possible in Thucydides' account, along with agriculture and navigation, is the saving art of medicine, which delivered men from diseases and from death. Aeschylus's Prometheus boasts of having shown to men the "blendings of mild simples [soothing medicines] with which they drive away all kinds of sickness."[65] Sophocles, for his part, ranks medicine among the marvelous inventions of man—though man has no means of escape from death, "escape from hopeless diseases he has found in the depths of his mind."[66]

Under these circumstances, one better appreciates why a physician should have attempted to reconstruct the birth and development of the medical art in a historical setting. Considering that the author of *Ancient Medicine* had a dietetic conception of medicine, it is perhaps not surprising that he held the birth of medicine to coincide with the discovery of dietary principles. On this view, it was the discovery of an alimentary regime adapted to the needs of the ill that marked the beginning of medicine proper; but it had been preceded by the discovery of a parallel regime suited to the healthy. These twin discoveries allowed human beings to pass from a brutish and unhappy life, in which they ate as beasts, to a civilized one.

The Discovery of Cooking

The first of these discoveries was none other than that of cooking. But the author of *Ancient Medicine* refrained from calling it by this name, for he saw in it the first stage of medicine, or at least a preliminary step in the direction of medicine. Here is how he characterizes this initial discovery:

To trace the matter yet further back, I hold that not even the mode of living and nourishment enjoyed at the present time by men in health would have been discovered, had a man been satisfied with the same food and drink as satisfy an ox, a horse, and every animal save man, for example the products of the earth—fruits, wood and grass. For on these they are nourished, grow, and live without pain, having no need at all of any other kind of living. Yet I am of [the] opinion that to begin with man also used this sort of nourishment. Our present ways of living have, I think, been discovered and elaborated during a long period of time. For many and terrible were the sufferings of men from strong and brutish living when they partook of crude foods, uncompounded and possessing [strong qualities]. . . . For this reason the ancients too seem to me to have sought for nourishment that harmonized with their constitution, and to have discovered that which we use now. So from wheat, after steeping it, winnowing, grinding and sifting, kneading, baking, they produced bread, and from barley they produced cake. Experimenting with food they boiled or baked, after mixing, many other things, combining the strong and uncompounded with the weaker components so as to adapt all to the constitution and power of man, thinking that from foods which, being too strong, the human constitution cannot assimilate when eating, will come pain, disease, and death, while from such as can be assimilated will come nourishment, growth, and health. To this discovery and research what juster or more appropriate name could be given than medicine, seeing that it has been discovered with a view to the health, saving and nourishment of man, in the place of that mode of living from which came the pain, disease and death?[67]

The first discovery consisted in adapting diet to human nature by various culinary operations, the main ones being cooking and mixing. It had major consequences for the course of human history, snatching man from animality and so delivering him from an unfortunate fate. Paradoxically, it was the weakness of man that in the end proved to be the cause of his greatness. Endowed with too frail a constitution to partake of the same diet as animals without suffering harm, man was forced to discover an art for modifying natural foods in order to adapt them to his nature. Humanism, it may therefore be said, was born with cooking.

The Discovery of Medicine

To this discovery relating to the diet of persons in good health a second one came to be added that extended and perfected the first: the discovery of the diet best suited to sick persons. Here is how the author of *Ancient Medicine* envisages this second stage, which marked the birth of medicine proper:

Let us consider also whether the acknowledged art of medicine, that was discovered for the treatment of the sick and has both a name and artists, has the same object as the other art, and what its origin was. In my opinion, as I said at the beginning, nobody would have even sought for medicine, if the same ways of life had suited both the sick and those in health. At any rate even at the present day such as do not use medical science, foreigners and some Greeks, live as do those in health, just as they please, and would neither forgo nor restrict the satisfaction of any of their desires. But those who sought for and discovered medicine, having the same intention as the men I discussed above [i.e., those who discovered the diet appropriate to healthy persons], in the first place, I think, lessened the bulk of the foods, and, without altering their character, greatly diminished their quantity. But they found that this treatment was sufficient only occasionally, and though clearly beneficial with some patients, it was not so in all cases, as some were in such a condition that they could not assimilate even small quantities of food. As such patients were thought to need weaker nutriment, slops were invented by mixing with much water small quantities of strong foods, and by taking away from their strength by compounding and boiling. Those who were not able to assimilate them were refused even these slops, and were reduced to taking liquids, these moreover being so regulated in composition and quantity as to be moderate, and nothing was administered that was either more or less, or less compounded, than it ought to be.[68]

The author is strict in insisting on the continuity of the two discoveries. They rested on the same reasoning and had the same purpose: to adapt diet to the needs of human beings, whether they were healthy or sick. But the second discovery was more complex than the first, for the degree of weakness in patients varied according to the strength of the disease. And so, whereas a single diet sufficed for persons in good health, it was necessary to devise several diets for sick persons: a solid diet for those who were least ill, a liquid diet for those who were weakest, and a diet of "slops," or soups, for the class of patients who fell in between. Medicine was therefore a sort of customized cuisine. More than this, it was the sign of a superior degree of humanism in which not all men shared. Incidentally, but significantly, the author of *Ancient Medicine* mentions in his description of the second discovery that medicine was unknown to barbarians. Consequently, if cooking represented the highest degree of a humanism that included foreigners as well as Greeks, medicine corresponded to the most evolved form of humanism—Hellenism. Despite his attempt to conceive of humanity in general terms, the Hippocratic physician was unable wholly to free himself from a characteristic kind of Hellenocentrism.

The History of Man and the Discovery of the Arts

The significance of this reconstruction of human history, marked by the passage from a state of nature to a state of culture owing to the discovery of a single art, can be fully appreciated only if it is restored to its historical context as part of a series of classic texts composed in the fifth century that related the birth of civilization to the discovery of the arts in general. The best known of these take the form of speeches that the three great tragic authors, Aeschylus, Sophocles, and Euripides, put into the mouths of their characters for the edification of their audiences. They have several themes in common.

The evolution of humanity is characterized in all these works not as a continuous form of progress but as a rupture between two periods, one negative, in which men were deprived of all things, the other positive, in which men enjoyed the benefits brought by the arts. Before the discovery of cooking, men led a life that the author of *Ancient Medicine* describes as "savage." Now it is this same term—"savage"—that is used to describe the life of the first men in Euripides' *Suppliant Women*, where the king of Athens, Theseus, retraces the evolution of humanity.[69] According to the Hippocratic physician, the diet of those savage times entailed terrible suffering and mortal illnesses; similarly, in Aeschylus's *Prometheus Bound*, men who had fallen ill are said to have wasted away, without any hope of relief, before the appearance of medicine.[70]

But the human condition utterly changed from the moment that men came into possession of the civilizing arts. In *Ancient Medicine*, the strong and bestial nourishment that brought on suffering, illness, and death is replaced by a diet that brings recovery from sickness and health. The life of men in Aeschylus's *Prometheus* and Euripides' *Suppliants* undergoes a comparable change. There a confused and brutish existence gives way to conscious and organized life.[71] The difference between these accounts is that whereas the physician attributes this change to a single art, cooking and medicine, the tragic authors appeal to a whole series of arts necessary to the survival and happiness of human beings. Medicine, which is not even mentioned in the play by Euripides, is only one art among others in the play by Aeschylus. Nonetheless, it is a very important art, and one that introduces a radical change into the life of men, just as in *Ancient Medicine*. Here is how Prometheus presents the discovery of medicine to the chorus: "If you hear the rest, you will marvel even more at what crafts and what resources I contrived. Greatest was this: when one of mankind was sick, there was no defense for him—neither healing food nor drink nor unguent; for lack of drugs they wasted, until I showed them blendings of mild simples with which they drive away all kinds of sickness."[72]

Naturally the conception of medicine is not exactly the same in Aeschylus's *Prometheus* and *Ancient Medicine*; for the tragic author treatment is pharmacological, while for the Hippocratic physician it is dietetic. But this difference is overshadowed by the fact that both authors attach importance to the notion of "mixing" in the discovery of therapeutics,[73] and that both underscore the decisive contribution made by medicine to the advancement of humanity.

Medicine: Gift of the Gods or Discovery of Men?

Despite these similarities, the medical treatise and the tragic drama disagree about what caused the appearance of medicine. In Aeschylus, this beneficent art is the gift of a deity; in Hippocrates, it is a discovery made by man.

This difference marks a dividing line in the explanation of human progress among thinkers of the fifth century. For some—particularly Aeschylus in the *Prometheus*, but also Euripides in the *Suppliant Women*—the gods sponsored human progress through their gift of the arts; for others, man invented the arts through the application of his own intelligence. In Sophocles' *Antigone*, for example, the chorus admires the ingenuity of man for having "taught himself" the arts, among which it counts medicine.[74] The author of *Ancient Medicine* likewise belongs to this second group. True to the rationalist spirit of the Hippocratic Collection, he attributes the twin discoveries concerning diet to human agency—sometimes to men, sometimes to one man.

To be sure, he does not ignore the traditional belief that the discovery of medicine was due originally to a god. But instead of arguing against it, he skillfully makes use of it in order to praise the actual discovery of medicine by men: "[T]he first discoverers," he says, ". . . thought the art worthy to be ascribed to a god, as in fact is the usual belief."[75] The reference here to divinity is simply a matter of customary reverence; it takes away nothing from the realism of the analysis. The author of *Ancient Medicine* forcefully insists on the role of necessity and need in supplying motivation for research and discovery. The harsh conditions of primitive life provided science with its initial impetus: because a bestial diet, so far from being useful to the first human beings, actually caused suffering, illness, and death, the diet of people in good health came to be studied and discovered; and because the diet of people in good health did not suit people who were sick, men were forced to seek and find the various diets appropriate to various sorts of illness. This relation of cause and effect, asserted to obtain between necessity and need, on the one hand, and research and discovery on the other, is affirmed by no other text of the fifth century with such clarity. Among the rare direct remarks made by a dramatic author in this connection, there is this maxim taken from one of Euripides' tragedies: "Need commands intelligence, even in a dolt."[76]

Was the Art of Medicine Discovered in Its Entirety?

A final difference between *Ancient Medicine* and Aeschylus's *Prometheus* brings out what is original about the Hippocratic physician's conception of progress in medicine.

The dramatic author uses Prometheus to express an unfailingly optimistic view of the power of medicine, whose remedies dispel "all kinds of sickness."[77] Promethean medicine appears therefore as a total science, utterly complete from the moment it was first revealed to human beings. The medical author expresses a more qualified optimism. There is no question that he shares Aeschylus's enthusiastic admiration for the discoveries of medicine. In one of the passages that best illustrates the fifth-century Greek faith in rationalism, the Hippocratic physician urges admiration for the manner in which men, after having emerged from a condition of profound ignorance, managed to achieve by means of reason, rather than by chance, splendid and correct discoveries.[78] Although the first discoveries were decisive in enabling medicine to attain the highest exactitude in several areas, the evolution of medical science was nonetheless not yet complete. Discoveries continued to be made in his own time, the author notes, and would go on being made in the future, whether in connection with the regimen of healthy persons, as a result of research by athletic trainers, or with the regimen of sick persons, as a result of the practice of actual physicians. Such a conception of open-ended progress seems obvious to a modern mind—but it deserves to be emphasized here, for it was new in the fifth century.

In fact, other authors in the Hippocratic Collection held a rather similar view to that of Prometheus in Aeschylus's play, in the sense that they too were persuaded that medicine was wholly known. Thus the author of *Places in Man* declares: "Medicine in its present state is, it seems to me, by now completely discovered"; and, a bit further on: "For the whole of medicine has been established, and the excellent principles discovered in it clearly have very little need of good luck."[79] Similarly, according to the author of *The Art*, medicine is a totally discovered art whose limits are not a result of its being unfinished, but of the very nature of therapeutic methods.[80]

By comparison with such overconfident practitioners, the author of *Ancient Medicine* is remarkable for his gradualist and open view of the evolution of the art; just the same, he remains an optimist. One sentence from this treatise clearly sums up his admiration for past discoveries and his hope for discoveries yet to come: "But medicine has long had all its means to hand, and has discovered both a principle and a method, through which the discoveries made during a long period are many and excellent, while full discovery will be made, if the inquirer be competent, conduct his researches with knowledge of the discoveries already made, and make them his starting-point."[81]

The Method for Reconstructing the Past

To reconstruct the "archaeology" of medicine, the author of *Ancient Medicine* employs a method comparable to that which the historian Thucydides uses at the beginning of his work to sketch the development of Greece from the earliest times. What unites the physician and the historian is their common recourse to the notion of "probability,"[82] and above all to analogy with the present in order to ground their reconstruction of the past. In the work of both authors, the contemporary barbarian world—and even parts of the Greek world that had not yet been touched by civilization—are taken to provide some probable indication of what the way of life of the ancients was like. In Thucydides, appeal is made to local customs in a part of continental Greece for insight into the way in which the ancients considered and practiced pillage; and the world beyond continental Greece is cited in connection with the ancients' habit of wearing a belt in sporting competitions.[83] In Hippocrates, a part of the Greek world, and the whole of the barbarian world, are consulted as sources of information about the way of life of the ancients before the discovery of medicine—on the assumption that since they are ignorant of medicine, they therefore behave when they are sick as the ancients must have behaved when medicine did not yet exist.[84]

These and other such similarities make it clear that, despite their many obvious differences, the Hippocratic author of *Ancient Medicine* shares with the historian Thucydides and the three tragic playwrights, Aeschylus, Sophocles, and Euripides, an optimistic view of human history. For all of them, what enabled mankind to pass from a primitive state where all things were opposed to its survival to a state of civilization was the discovery of the arts.

The Sources of the Reconstruction of the Past

It has usually been supposed that the Sophists and the pre-Socratic philosophers of the fifth century were the chief sources for the history of humanity retraced by the author of *Ancient Medicine*.

The most senior of the Sophists, Protagoras of Abdera, has long been cited in this connection. None of his works has come down to us, but we know that one of them was in fact called *On the Original State of Humanity*; and indeed Plato, in the *Protagoras*,[85] has the Sophist cast the story of primitive humanity and the birth of civilization in the form of the Promethean myth. No doubt this is a reasonably faithful reflection of what one would have encountered in the original work. Let us briefly recall the main elements of the myth of Prometheus in the version given it by Protagoras. At the moment when the gods created living creatures, human beings and animals, by a mixture of earth and fire, they asked Prometheus and his brother Epimetheus to distribute the various qualities among all living things. Epimetheus wished to take charge of the task, and asked Prometheus to come back to inspect his work only when it was done. Epimetheus began by harmoniously distributing all the qualities among the various animal species so that they would all survive; but when he came to human beings, there was nothing left. Then his brother turned up unexpectedly to inspect the distribution. Seeing that the animals were well provided for and that man was totally impoverished, without shoes or clothing or arms, he took it upon himself to steal the art of fire possessed by Hephaestus and the other arts possessed by Athena. Men thus found themselves equipped with the necessities of life. But as they lived in isolation, they risked decimation by wild beasts, for they were lacking the art of politics. Zeus, fearing the complete disappearance of mankind, sent Hermes to deliver political virtue to each man, which is to say justice. In this way, cities came to be formed, and men survived.

Certain similarities can, of course, be detected between Protagoras's version of the Promethean myth and the account given in *Ancient Medicine*. According to Protagoras, men found their very existence threatened before the discovery of the arts and political virtue, just as they did, according to the Hippocratic physician, before the discovery of cooking and medicine. Moreover, the dual acquisition of the arts and political virtue, which according to the Sophist occurred over time, bears comparison with the dual discovery of cooking and medicine as described in the Hippocratic treatise. But as against these similarities, which frankly are rather loose, there is an important difference having to do with the place of the physician in human progress. Compared with the Hippocratic author's lengthy discussions of diet and medicine, the skimpy details about animal nourishment and the brief allusion to human medicine found in Protagoras's version of the myth of Prometheus do not carry much weight.[86] The little information we have relating indirectly to his theory is therefore not enough to allow us to conclude that Protagoras actually influenced the Hippocratic author.

Among the pre-Socratic philosophers who are commonly thought to have inspired the author of *Ancient Medicine*, mention is most often made of Democritus, who treated of the history of mankind in his (lost) *Little World-System*. Particular emphasis is given to the role assigned in *Ancient Medicine* to necessity and need as points of departure for the discovery of the art, which is supposed to be a Democritean idea. In support of this claim, parallels are frequently cited between the argument of the Hippocratic treatise and the account given by the historian Diodorus of Sicily (first century B.C.) in the beginning of his *Bibliotheca historica* of the life of the first human beings and the gradual birth of civilization. Here is what Diodorus says:

[T]he first men to be born, they say, led an undisciplined and bestial life, setting out one by one to secure their sustenance and taking for their food both the tenderest herbs and the fruits of wild trees. Then, since they were attacked by the wild beasts, they came to each other's aid, being instructed by expediency, and when gathered together in this way by reason of their fear, they gradually came to recognize their mutual characteristics. And though the sounds which they made were at first unintelligible and indistinct, yet gradually they came to give articulation to their speech. . . .

Now the first men, since none of the things useful for life had yet been discovered, led a wretched existence, having no clothing to cover them, knowing not the use of dwelling and fire, and also being totally ignorant of cultivated food. For since they also even neglected the harvesting of the wild food, they laid by no store of its fruits against their needs; consequently large numbers of them perished in the winters because of the cold and the lack of food. Little by little, however, experience taught them both to take to the caves in winter and to store such fruits as could be preserved. And when they had become acquainted with fire and other useful things, the arts also and whatever else is capable of furthering man's social life were gradually discovered. Indeed, speaking generally, in all things it was necessity itself that became man's teacher, supplying in appropriate fashion instruction in every matter to a creature which was well endowed by nature and had, as its assistants for every purpose, hands and speech and sagacity of mind.

And as regards the first origin of men and their earliest manner of life we shall be satisfied with what has been said, since we would keep due proportion in our account.[87]

Aspects of this very detailed picture do indeed converge with the account found in *Ancient Medicine*: at the root of the discovery of the arts was need; the discovery occurred over time; and, prior to this discovery, the first human beings led a brutish life. But in order to conclude that Democritus was responsible for these points of contact, we would have to be sure that Democritus was the source for Diodorus, which is impossible to prove—for the works of the philosopher of Abdera are all lost, and only one title is known to us. On other grounds we are certainly justified in assuming that Democritus explained the progressive emergence of the arts according to their degree of necessity. His judgment about music is revealing in this regard. Music he considered a young art; the reason for its relative youth, he says, is that "necessity did not foster it, but it was born of surplus."[88] Nonetheless, we cannot legitimately make broad inferences on the basis of so fragmentary a piece of evidence, about the way in which Democritus retraced human history. The influence of this pre-Socratic philosopher on *Ancient Medicine*, typically asserted as something obvious, is in fact a commonplace without any solid foundation.

A less tenuous link can be asserted with another pre-Socratic thinker, Archelaus of Athens. A disciple of Anaxagoras of Clazomenae, Archelaus seems to have played an important role in the history of ideas. He is supposed to have been the first to introduce Ionian philosophy to Athens and to have been Socrates' teacher. Like the author of *Ancient Medicine*, Archelaus considered that the first men had the same diet as animals and that at this stage of history their life was short; he distinguishes also, following this first difficult stage, a second stage where men became separated from other living creatures by virtue of the establishment of laws, the arts, and cities.[89] But despite these similarities, one must be wary of inferring a direct influence upon the physician by the Athenian philosopher. So far as we can judge from our very indirect knowledge of Archelaus's theories, there is less than perfect agreement at the level of detail: the first men, according to Archelaus, fed on mud. More than this, the author of *Ancient Medicine*, who in his polemic against innovative physicians denounces the importance accorded by some colleagues to heat and cold, could hardly subscribe to the doctrine of a philosopher who explained the genesis of all living things by the mixture of heat and cold.[90]

In summary, our knowledge of the pre-Socratic philosophers, as of the Sophists, is too indirect and too full of gaps to allow us to conclude with confidence that a particular thinker had a decisive influence upon *Ancient Medicine*. The various resemblances we have noted testify to the existence of a common fund of ideas that each thinker was able to draw upon and adapt to his subject. At all events, the altogether remarkable coherence of the theory advanced in *Ancient Medicine* rules out the chance that it may have been the work of an editor or compiler. It is more justly regarded as an original piece of work than as a reflection of the work of others. It stands, in any case, as the only theory of the fifth century B.C. about the evolution of humanity that has come down to us intact. As such, it constitutes an account of the highest importance for anyone writing a history of man's inquiry into his own origins.

TEN

Challenges to Medicine and the Birth of Epistemology

The Age of Pericles, while a period of genuine enthusiasm for what reason had managed to discover, was at the same time one in which the achievements of reason were challenged. On the one hand, the second half of the fifth century witnessed the appearance of works defining rules of art—called *technai*—in the most varied disciplines. The best known were manuals of oratorical art. Such manuals flourished in many other domains as well: besides medicine, dietetics, and cooking, there were manuals devoted to gymnastics, wrestling, riding, architecture, sculpture, painting, and music. But on the other hand, just as these arts were coming into existence, arguments—often quite passionate ones—arose over whether they really existed at all, or, at the least, over which methods were appropriate to them. The Hippocratic Collection gives the best picture of what these polemics were like, for it is the sole corpus of the fifth century to have preserved examples of these treatises on art, or *technai*, in their entirety.

Experts in Denigration

What comes as the greatest surprise is the fact that the very existence of such arts was being sharply challenged at the very moment when specialists were at work laying down the rules that governed them. The observations of the Hippocratic treatise *The Art* are highly illuminating in this regard. The author begins with a striking formula: "Some there are who have made an art [*technen*] of vilifying the arts [*technas*]." The whole object of his treatise is to show that an art of medicine did indeed exist, while replying to the various objections made by his detractors. *The Art* is, of course, not the earliest indication we have that criticisms were brought against physicians. We have seen in particular that their greed had been denounced by poets such as

Pindar, and by philosophers such as Heraclitus, in addition to comic play-wrights.[1] But it is the earliest evidence we have of an attack on medicine itself and of the way in which it was defended. One is astonished to discover how bitter the disputes were, how direct and how violent the assaults of those who challenged the art, and how caustic the irony of its defenders, who accused their adversaries of ignorance, innate wickedness, indeed of madness, and so transformed these denigrators of the art of medicine into sick persons in need of medical treatment.[2] While polemics are often to be found in the Hippo-cratic Collection, nowhere do they occupy as great a place as in the treatise *The Art*.

It would be interesting to know who these adversaries were, who dared to attack the existence of arts in general and that of medicine in particular. In keeping with the practice of scholarly disputation in the fifth century, they remain hopelessly anonymous. The Hippocratic physician refers to them frequently by some plural circumlocution such as "those who thus invade the art of medicine," "those who attribute recovery to chance and deny the existence of the art," and so on; or, more rarely, by a collective singular form such as "my opponent" or "he who upholds the contrary thesis." It is there-fore impossible to identify them with certainty. Nonetheless, one may count among these adversaries the disciples of the elder Sophist Protagoras. "Expert in disputation," as he was known, the Sophist of Abdera had written a work marshaling all the objections that a layman might bring against specialists of art in general and of each art in particular. This work, entitled *On Wrestling and the Other Arts*, was still very famous in Plato's time.[3] Since the work is known to have examined each art in particular, it must have included objec-tions against the art of medicine. It is not impossible that *The Art* was in fact a reply to attacks that ultimately derived from this work by Protagoras. Objec-tions to the existence of the art of medicine may therefore have come from Sophistic circles.

Medicine Does Not Exist

There remains in any case some doubt as to the actual identity of those who made a practice of denigrating medicine. But the essential thing is that we know the arguments they employed to demonstrate that medicine did not exist. Indeed, they appear quite clearly illuminated in the lucid discussion in *The Art*. The first argument was that the recovery of patients treated by physicians was a matter of chance and not of art, since some patients died despite the aid of physicians. Here is how the Hippocratic physician describes this objection: "It is conceded that of those treated by medicine some are healed. But because not all are healed the art is blamed, and those who malign it, because there are some who succumb to diseases, assert that those who escape do so through luck and not through the art."[4]

This kind of argument against the existence of medicine was to continue to fuel polemics against the art for quite some time. An echo of it can be found in Cicero's treatise *On the Nature of the Gods*: "Nor do all sick persons get well, but that does not prove that there is no art of medicine."[5] The second argument used by adversaries was that some who were ill got well without summoning doctors. The Hippocratic author does not contest the fact, but turns the argument around:

Now my opponent will object that in the past many, even without calling in a physician, have been cured of their sickness, and I agree that he is right. But I hold that it is possible to profit by the art of medicine even without calling in a physician, not indeed so as to know what is correct medical treatment and what is incorrect, but so as by chance to employ in self-treatment the same means as would have been employed had a physician actually been called in. And it is surely strong proof of the existence of the art, that it both exists and is powerful, if it is obvious that even those who do not believe in it recover through it.[6]

A third and final argument advanced by adversaries was aimed at physicians who refused to treat cases that they judged to be incurable.[7] We have already had the opportunity to examine this argument, as well as the scathing reply of the author of *The Art*, in connection with the prognosis of incurable cases and the problem of refusing treatment.[8] There is no need to take it up again here.

The Birth of Epistemology

The merit of the treatise *The Art* is not merely that it supplies us with extremely detailed information about the attacks to which physicians were exposed. It also shows us how this challenge turned out to have a positive effect by encouraging practitioners to reflect upon the basis of their art. Without these experts in denigration, the Hippocratic physician no doubt would not have found himself in a position to state his own conception of the art of medicine as forcefully as he did in this treatise.

Thanks to *The Art*, then, we are able to form some idea of what the first debates over science were like, coming as they did at a moment when science was consciously being brought into existence and this existence reaffirmed in the face of contrary claims made by those who were hostile to it. It would not be an exaggeration, in fact, to say of *The Art* that it contains the first recorded signs of interest in epistemological issues. What is remarkable about the author of this treatise is that he was fully aware of the fact that not only the existence of medicine as an art was at stake in this debate, but equally the existence of every other art and science. The general form given to the argument at the outset of the author's refutation is proof of this, for it undertakes to mount a defense on behalf of all the arts, not just of medicine. One is struck moreover by the difficulty of the argument itself, which assumes a thorough knowledge of philosophy. This physician knows, for example, how to juggle notions of being and nonbeing:

Now it seems to me that generally speaking there is no art which does not exist; in fact it is absurd to regard as non-existent one of the things that exist. Since what substance could there be of non-existents, and who could behold them and declare that they exist? For if really it be possible to see the non-existent, as it is to see the existent, I do not know how a man could regard as non-existent what he can both see with his eyes and with his mind think that it exists. Nay, it cannot be so; but the existent is always seen and known, and the non-existent is neither seen nor known. Now reality is known when the arts have been already [taught], and there is no art which is not seen as the result of some [form].[9]

Underlying this argument, which may be considered the first attempt at general epistemology bequeathed to us by antiquity, one first of all notices traces of the philosophy of Parmenides of Elea. The propositions of Parmenidean philosophy relating to being and nonbeing are applied here to the reality or nonreality of the sciences. Indeed, just as Parmenides affirms the impossibility of being's not being, and of nonbeing's being, so the Hippocratic physician affirms the impossibility of a science that does not exist and of a nonscience that does exist. But if he draws inspiration from the principles of Eleatic philosophy, he transposes them into a realistic perspective. For to the extent that he introduces as grounds for asserting the existence of being not only thought but also vision ("the existent is always seen and known"), he clearly distances himself from the doctrine of the Eleatics. According to this doctrine, only thought can grasp being; vision, like the other senses, perceives only becoming. The author's realism leads him therefore to combine the evidence of reason with that of the senses: each science is both seen and known. It is known, he says, because it is taught. It is therefore the fact that the teaching of a science exists that proves the very existence of this science. To be sure, the argument appears rather unusual to a modern mind, for teaching has lost its former prestige and no longer stands as a sign of infallibility. But for the ancients, a science existed only if it were taught. This idea was, at the least, generally accepted by the Hippocratic author's contemporaries, whether they were opponents or partisans of the Sophists.[10] What seems frankly puzzling to a modern mind is the author's claim that "science" (*technè*) is seen because it has a "form" (*eidos*). The strange character of this formulation arises in part from the fact that technical terms, at the dawn of scientific thought, still had quite broad extension and took in both the concrete and the abstract. The Greek word *technè* in the Periclean Age denoted both art and science; it was applied equally to the art of the blacksmith or the doctor as to the science of speaking. As for the Greek word *eidos*, which was to be the source of the English word "idea," its ancient etymology is well established: it originally referred to "that which is seen," the "visible form" of a thing. This concrete sense was still very much current in the fifth century. Even so, the author nowhere says exactly what he means by the "visible form" of "art" or of "science." The reason is that, for him, the meaning was altogether obvious. To take the example of medicine, this "visible form" probably indicated the different procedures that the physician carries out in a certain order and according to certain defined norms in order to realize his art,[11] which is to say in observing and treating the patient, whether in his office or at the patient's bedside. Once more one encounters, here on the theoretical level, that visual—indeed spectacular—aspect of the physician's trade whose importance we stressed earlier in our description of the actual practice of medicine.

Name and Reality of the Art

This exercise in general epistemology, in which the author of *The Art* attempts to demonstrate the existence of the sciences, concludes with a secondary argument that finds its source in the philosophy of language: "I for my part think that the names also of the arts have been given them because of their [forms] [*eidea*]; for it is absurd—nay impossible—to hold that [forms] spring from names. For names are [institutions of nature], but [forms] are not [institutions] but the offspring of nature."[12]

To properly appreciate the import of this argument, it needs to be put back in the context of the debates of the period over language. Owing to the impetus provided by the Sophists in particular, a lively interest had already developed in the nature of language as it related to the world. Among the Sophists, the leading specialist in these questions was Prodicos of Ceos. Prodicos was prepared to reveal the entire truth about how words applied to the world if one paid him the tidy sum of fifty drachmas; those who were willing only to pay one drachma, like Socrates, stood to learn very little. With regard to this problem, concerning the relation between names and the realities that they referred to, two extreme positions were contested: the realist theory and the nominalist theory.[13] According to the first, names correspond by nature to the realities they pick out; language, in other words, is natural. According to the second, names are attributed to objects in the real world by custom; on this view, language is conventional. The theory of language that serves as the basis for the demonstration given by the author of *The Art* is more subtle. It lies between the two extremes. Like the proponents of nominalism, the author believes that names are institutions; but like the proponents of realism, he holds that a relation obtains between language and the reality it names. In proposing the altogether original definition of language as an artifact of nature, he recognized the special character of language insisted upon by the nominalist theory while preserving an analogy between the series of names and the series of realities they refer to. Names are natural institutions modeled on realities that themselves are productions of nature. The force of this is to say that the very existence of names is a sign of the existence of the realities that they name. Accordingly, the secondary argument advanced by the Hippocratic author consists in asserting that the various sciences exist by virtue of the fact that they possess different names.

It may readily be seen that this first attempt at a general epistemology derives very largely from the philosophical problems that were being debated at the time—ontological problems in particular. But it came to assume great importance in the history of ideas, not only because it constitutes the most ancient evidence we have of epistemology in the sense of discourse about knowledge, but above all because this account was written by a scientist and not by a philosopher. We know that epistemology was long to remain the province of philosophers, and that philosophical epistemology is traditionally said to begin with Plato. But in fact this style of thought predates Plato, and derives from a time when it was the concern not only of Sophists and philosophers, but also of men of science.

Two Paths to Knowledge

If the author of *The Art* relies upon ontology in developing a general argument about epistemology, it is nonetheless the case that when he restricts his attention to medicine proper, he deals with problems that are nearer to what we expect an analysis of knowledge to be concerned with. He establishes in particular a distinction between two categories of illness to which correspond two modes of knowledge: apparent, or manifest, affections involve sight and touch; hidden diseases, which is to say diseases lodged in the cavities of the body, involve the intellect. It is in connection with this distinction that we meet with one of the finest phrases of the treatise: "[W]hat escapes the eyesight is mastered by the eye of the mind."[14] This formula is the first attestation of the metaphor of the "mind's eye," or the "eye of the soul," which was to become popular not only among the Greeks and the Romans but also in European literature much later. If the formulation appears new, at least to judge from the texts that have come down to us, the distinction between two paths to knowledge, one via the senses and the other via the mind, was not a new idea in Greek thought. Comparison has rightly been made with the following fragment of Democritus of Abdera, which distinguishes two types of knowledge, one due to the senses, the other to the intellect: "There are two forms of knowledge, one genuine and the other dark. To the dark belong all these: sight, hearing, smell, taste, touch. The dark [is] separated from [the genuine]. When the dark can no longer see more finely or hear or smell or taste or perceive by touch, but something finer [is to be examined, genuine knowledge takes over]."[15]

Nonetheless, there is a significant difference between the philosopher's view and that of the physician. Whereas Democritus devalues the knowledge of the senses, which is described as "obscure," in order to privilege knowledge gained by the intellect, which is called "authentic," the Hippocratic physician does not doubt for a moment the validity of visual evidence, for he knows full well the value of visual observation in the practice of his art. Moreover, according to the physician, knowledge obtained by means of the intellect does not possess the immediacy of visual information. In fact, investigation was slower in the case of hidden diseases, for the "attendant . . . , as he could neither see the trouble with his eyes nor learn it with his ears, tried to track it by reasoning."[16] Thus those who criticized medicine for its slowness in investigating the source of illness indicted it unjustly, for it is "not the art [that] is to blame, but the constitution of human bodies."[17] Finally, the Hippocratic physician, though he joined the philosopher in opposing the two modes of knowledge, envisaged a collaboration between intellect and vision for the diagnosis of hidden diseases. In a highly ingenious passage, he shows that medicine makes use of visible signs, whether natural or induced, such as exhalation of breath, evacuation of humors, or elimination of sweat, to inform the mind about the nature of invisible diseases.[18] Thus we can see that medical practice was capable of enriching and nuancing the philosophy of knowledge to a considerable degree.

Science or Luck?

The author of *The Art* provides a splendid example of the Hippocratic physician's aptitude for reflecting upon his own activity and upon the conditions that needed to be met if this activity were to be considered a *technè*—an art, a science.

The best way to define these necessary conditions is on the basis of a concept that was opposed to that of *technè*: the concept of *tuchè*. In the fifth century, this antithesis between science and chance structured discussions of the various activities that pretended to the status of art or of science. This antithesis appeared even in the theater. Euripides expresses it nicely, and vividly, in his *Alcestis*, when he says that "what is produced by chance is not captured by art."[19] But it was most frequently employed before Plato and Aristotle in the technical writings of the physicians. Already, in *Ancient Medicine*, the notion of chance is used to reject the absurd hypothesis that the art of medicine does not exist: "[I]f an art of medicine did not exist at all, . . . the treatment of the sick would be in all respects haphazard."[20] And when he praises the discoveries of medicine, he makes it clear that they are the result "not of chance, but of inquiry rightly and correctly conducted."[21] This antithesis occupies an important place in *The Art*, notably in the reply made to the first argument of the adversaries of medicine, which, as the reader will recall, claimed that patients who recover from illness "do so through luck and not through the art." His reply is based on this antithesis throughout:

Now I, too, do not rob luck of any of its prerogatives, but I am nevertheless of [the] opinion that when diseases are badly treated ill luck generally follows, and good luck when they are treated well. Again, how is it possible for patients to attribute their recoveries to anything else except the art, seeing that it was by using it and serving it that they recovered? For in that they committed themselves to the art they showed their unwillingness to behold nothing but the reality of luck, so that while freed from dependence upon luck they are not freed from dependence upon the art. For in that they committed themselves with confidence to the art, they thereby acknowledged also its reality, and when its work was accomplished they recognized its power.[22]

While making a slight concession to his adversaries and granting that luck may sometimes play a role in the physician's success, or ill-luck in the case of failure, the author strongly affirms the reality and the power of the art, which generally leads to success if correctly applied, but, if incorrectly applied, leads to failure. This way of minimizing the role of luck and of affirming the power of science is encountered also at the end of the treatise *Places in Man* in connection with a general argument about the art of medicine: "For anyone who has an understanding of medicine in this way depends very little upon good luck, but is able to do good with or without luck. For the whole of medicine has been established, and the excellent principles discovered in it clearly have very little need of good luck. Good luck is arbitrary and cannot be commanded, and even prayer cannot make it come; but understanding can be commanded, and of itself represents good luck, whenever the person who has knowledge employs it."[23]

Despite the technical character of this discussion, the notions of science (or "understanding") and luck are not totally abstract. Indeed, they are personified here, being compared to two women, or possibly two goddesses, of opposed temperaments: the one is dominating and does not allow herself to be swayed even by prayer, whereas the other is easily swayed, at least by one who knows how. In fact, the Greek term *tuchè*, which corresponds to our words "chance," "luck," "fortune," was later to come to designate a deity.[24] What one finds in embryonic form here is the celebrated passage in which Galen opposes the goddess Fortune, surrounded by her adherents, to the god of the arts, Hermes, accompanied by his followers. A few excerpts will give an idea of this apologue:

Is it not therefore shameful to scorn the culture of the arts to attach ourselves to Fortune? In order to reveal the perversity of this spirit, the ancients, not content to represent it, whether in painting or in sculpture, with the features of a woman (and that was already a rather significant symbol of unreason), have put a rudder in her hands, placed a spherical pedestal beneath her feet, and covered her eyes with a blindfold, wishing by all these attributes to show us her instability. . . . See by contrast how different from those of Fortune are the attributes that painters and sculptors have given to Hermes, the master of reason and the universal artist: he is a fresh-faced young man whose beauty is neither borrowed, nor enhanced by ornaments, but is only the reflection of the virtues of his soul. His visage is smiling, his eyes are piercing, his pedestal has the most solid form, that of a cube. . . .

Examine the followers of Fortune, [and] you will find them all idle and unskilled in the arts; borne by hope, they run after the swift goddess, these ones near, those ones far, some even hanging from her hands. . . . But the other procession, that of Hermes, is composed only of men who are decent and cultivate the arts; one sees them neither run, nor shout, nor argue among themselves. The god is in their midst; all are ranged in order around him; each one occupies the place that has been assigned to him. Those who are nearest to Hermes, who immediately surround him, are the geometers, the mathematicians, the philosophers, the physicians.[25]

In Hippocrates' time, obviously, so detailed and unflattering an image of Fortune remained something yet far off in the future; but the notion of chance was well understood, and the pejorative sense that was already attached to it could be used to bring out the contrast with what was more positively implied by the notion of art or science.

Conditions for the Existence of Science

What, for the Hippocratic physician, were the criteria that demonstrated the existence of science and opposed it to chance?

Signifying the opposite of indiscriminate chance, science was defined first by the possibility it offered of making normative distinctions. To know was to be able to discriminate between what was correct and what was not. The author of *The Art* expresses this point very clearly: "Now where correctness and incorrectness each have a defined limit, surely there must be an art. For absence of art I take to be absence of correctness and of incorrectness; but where both are present art cannot be absent."[26] Even error, in this perspective, has a positive value: "Again, mistakes [in regimen], no less than benefits, witness to the existence of the [medical] art."[27]

To this theoretical distinction between what is correct and what is not corresponds a difference in the real world between good and bad practitioners of medicine. This difference was likewise used as a criterion of the existence of medical science, as the following passage from *Ancient Medicine* testifies: "Some practitioners are poor, others very excellent; this would not be the case if an art of medicine did not exist at all, and had not been the subject of any research and discovery, but all would be equally inexperienced and unlearned therein, and the treatment of the sick would be in all respects haphazard. But it is not so; just as in all other arts the workers vary much in skill and in knowledge, so also is it in the case of medicine."[28]

The proof that the distinction between good and bad practitioners was indeed an essential criterion of the existence of the art is that its absence was generally accepted as evidence that the art did not exist. The author of *Ancient Medicine*, it will be recalled, sought to trace the beginning of the art of medicine to the discovery of the diet suitable to persons in good health. Having run up against the common opinion that cooking was not to be considered an art, however, he found himself obliged to admit that this opinion was not entirely without foundation:

To this discovery [of healthy diet] and research what juster or more appropriate name could be given than medicine, seeing that it has been discovered with a view to the health, saving, and nourishment of man, in the place of that mode of living from which came the pain, disease and death?

That it is not commonly considered an art is not unnatural, for it is inappropriate to call anyone an artist in a craft in which none are laymen, but all possess knowledge through being compelled to use it.[29]

This distinction between good and bad practitioners emerges above all in the case of the most dangerous diseases. Indeed the author of *Breaths* states: "[T]o judge of the most obscure and difficult diseases is more a matter of opinion than of art, and therein there is the greatest possible difference between experience and inexperience."[30] The author of *Ancient Medicine* develops this theme more amply and more brilliantly in comparing the physician to the captain of a ship:

For most physicians seem to me to be in the same case as bad pilots; the mistakes of the latter are unnoticed so long as they are steering in a calm, but, when a great storm overtakes them with a violent gale, all men realize clearly then that it is their ignorance and blundering which have lost the ship. So also when bad physicians, who comprise the great majority, treat men who are suffering from no serious complaint, so that the greatest blunders would not affect them seriously—such illnesses occur very often, being far more common than serious disease—they are not shown up in their true colours to laymen if their errors are confined to such cases; but when they meet with a severe, violent, and dangerous illness, then it is that their errors and want of skill are manifest to all. The punishment of the imposter, whether sailor or doctor, is not postponed, but follows speedily.[31]

Thus, therefore, while chance represents the reign of the undifferentiated, art manifests itself through a distinction among values and a hierarchy of competences that are revealed in decisive moments. The reign of science is the reign of difference. "A healer is a man worth many men in his knowledge," as had already been said in the *Iliad*.[32] This traditional notion of the superiority of the man of science was built into the very definition of science from the moment it began. And science, to the extent that it was not equally distributed among the citizens of a polity, was not regarded as a political virtue. This is the point made at the end of Protagoras's version of the myth of Prometheus, as recounted by Plato, where the phase of human history in which the arts were discovered, which is to say the era of difference, was to be completed by the acquisition of political virtues, which is to say by the era of equal distribution among men:

Zeus was afraid that our whole race might be wiped out, so he sent Hermes to bring justice and a sense of shame to humans, so that there would be order within cities and bonds of friendship to unite them. Hermes asked Zeus how he should distribute shame and justice to humans. "Should I distribute them as the other arts were? This is how the others were distributed: one person practicing the art of medicine suffices for many ordinary people; and so forth with the other practitioners. Should I establish justice and shame among humans in this way, or distribute it to all?" "To all," said Zeus, "and let all have a share. For cities would never come to be if only a few possessed these, as is the case with the other arts."[33]

Causality and Science

The world of science is not only one in which values and human beings are differentiated; it is also one in which the coherence of things is perceived. While chance is synonymous with disorder and apparent spontaneity, science by contrast discovers the natural order of things. One of the greatest virtues of the physicians of the Hippocratic Collection is to have stated, in its most universal form, what was later to be called the principle of determinism. All that occurs has a cause. It is in the treatise of *The Art* that the most theoretical statement of this principle is to be found: "Indeed, under a close examination spontaneity disappears; for everything that occurs will be found to do so through something [*dia ti*], and this 'through something' [*dia ti*] shows that spontaneity is a mere name, and has no reality. Medicine, however, because it acts 'through something' [*dia ti*], and because its results may be forecasted, has reality, as is manifest now and will be manifest for ever."[34]

This Hippocratic physician was probably not the first person in classical Greece to have formulated the idea of the necessary linking of cause and effect. Leucippus, the founder of atomism and Democritus's teacher, had earlier said in his treatise *On Mind*: "No thing happens in vain, but everything for a reason and by necessity."[35] Here one finds the philosopher, like the physician, denying the operation of chance insofar as this is understood as an inexplicable or spontaneous production of reality. Nonetheless, Leucippus's remark does not convey his precise meaning, for it has come down to us out of context. The Hippocratic text comes nearer in any case, by its very formulation, to prefiguring Aristotle's claim that art is defined by knowledge of a "why" (literally, a "through something").[36] What the Hippocratic author contributes that is new and remarkable is that the notion of causality is already linked to that of prediction.

But if the knowledge of causes appeared indispensable to the physicians of the *Corpus Hippocraticum*, this was above all because it allowed a correct and natural treatment to be decided upon. As the author of *The Art* puts it: "[F]or the same intelligence is required to know the causes of diseases as to understand how to treat them with all the treatment that prevents illnesses from growing worse."[37]

The author of *Breaths* begins his discourse by a series of general consider-ations that point in exactly the same direction: "For knowledge of the cause of a disease will enable one to administer to the body what things are advan-tageous [using opposites to combat the disease]. Indeed this sort of medicine is quite natural."[38] From this last passage it is clear that the causal method is the indispensable condition of a true medical art.

The treatise *Ancient Medicine*, finally, insists that the man of science must not limit himself to a descriptive or prescriptive statement of an illness, but must go beyond this to the next stage, which involves making an interpretive statement once the causes have been taken into account. The passage is famous. After having defined the task of the physician, who has to study the influence of foods and the different elements of regimen upon human beings, the author takes the example of cheese: "It is not sufficient to learn simply that cheese is a bad food, as it gives a pain to one who eats a surfeit of it; we must know what the pain is, the reasons for it [*dia ti*], and which constituent of man is harmfully affected."[39]

Science must therefore be causal or it is not science. In these earliest epistemological texts of ancient Greece, some of the leading concepts that were to guide the development of science for centuries afterwards can be seen to emerge with quite stunning clarity from reflection upon the art of medi-cine. There remains, of course, a gap between theoretical assertion and practi-cal application. The author of *Ancient Medicine*, for example, despite his fine statements about the need for causal knowledge, does not proceed to try to carry out his program through experimental investigation. But a certain conceptual architecture was nonetheless now in place. In particular, the do-main of science, characterized by distinction, unification, and prediction, was now held to be marked off from the domain of chance, ruled instead by the indistinct, the unexplained, and the unforeseeable. Thus came into being the cognitive paradigm of order and the exclusion of disorder, which was to serve as the basis of the deterministic conception of science up to the point when it came under attack by modern epistemology.

From Hippocratic Epistemology to Platonic Epistemology

That the Hippocratic Collection should have been the sole corpus of Greek literature of the fifth century B.C. to have preserved in its entirety a treatise devoted to epistemological problems is in large measure itself the result of chance. Medicine, as we have seen, was not the only activity to establish itself consciously as a discipline in the second half of the fifth century.

Rhetoric did so as well. The pressing need to employ this useful skill with the greatest possible effectiveness seems to have contributed to its being formally constituted as an art. In any case, with the development in the fifth century of private trials in the democratic cities, judicial rhetoric came to seem as indispensable to the safety of citizens as medicine to the safety of people in general. For if medicine was a way for people to escape illness and, in the most critical cases, death, rhetoric was a way for citizens to avoid the various harms that threatened their property or their persons, and, in the most serious cases, the penalty of death. While allowing for obvious differences, a similarity between these two activities may therefore also be observed. The logographer who, for a fee, composed courtroom speeches for a client risking his life at trial in effect prescribed argumentation that in his judgment was most likely to remove his client from all danger, just as the physician prescribed for his patient, again for a fee, the most effective medicines for eliminating the risks of disease and illness. The situation facing these two practitioners, the logographer and the physician, was at bottom much the same. It is not surprising, then, that at the same time as physicians were composing theoretical works (*technai*) about medicine there should have begun to appear other such works devoted to the art of rhetoric. As it happens, the names of the first authors of these rhetorical manuals are known to us. Cicero, citing the authority of Aristotle, says that the first ones to have written down the rules of rhetoric were two Sicilians, Corax and his pupil Tisias, and that they were prompted by the proliferation of private trials in the wake of the abolition of tyranny in Sicily.[40] Unfortunately, none of these treatises on forensic oratory has survived. There is a risk, then, of overstating the importance of the role played by the physicians of the fifth century in advancing epistemological inquiry and, correspondingly, of underestimating that of the rhetoricians. However, the importance assigned by Plato to the comparison with the art of medicine, and more particularly with the medicine of Hippocrates, in his epistemological reflections upon the art of rhetoric indicates that the epistemological analysis of the physicians of the fifth century was regarded by their contemporaries as pioneering work. It was also transferable: Plato was to borrow the epistemological model of medicine, the science of the body, and apply it to rhetoric, the science of the soul.

There are points of similarity, in fact, between Hippocratic epistemology and Platonic epistemology. If we confine our attention to the two dialogues in which the Athenian philosopher criticizes the rhetoric of his time in an attempt to provide a foundation for a true art of rhetoric, we find precisely the Hippocratic idea just noted that scientific knowledge is causal knowledge.

In the *Gorgias*, Plato has Socrates show that knowledge of causes is the distinctive criterion for deciding what is art and what is not. To establish this distinction, he contrasts cooking with medicine:

And I say that [pastry baking] isn't a craft [*technè*], but a knack [*empeiria*], because it has no account of the nature of whatever things it applies by which it applies them, so that it's unable to state the *cause* of each thing.[41] . . . I was saying, wasn't I, that I didn't think that pastry baking is a craft [*technè*], but a knack [*empeiria*], whereas medicine is a craft. I said that the one, medicine, has investigated . . . the *cause* of the things it does, and is able to give an account of each of these. The other . . . proceeds towards its object in a quite uncraftlike way, without having at all considered . . . its *cause*.[42]

Then in the *Phaedrus*, in order to ground a true art of rhetoric, Plato takes medicine as his model and makes explicit reference to the Hippocratic method.[43] Just as the physician established causal relations among the effects produced by different types of foods or medicines on different types of bodies to heal them and strengthen them, so the philosopher was to establish causal relations among different types of discourses and different types of souls in order to know how to persuade them: "[H]e will classify the kinds of speech and of soul there are . . . and explain what causes each. He will then coordinate each kind of soul with the kind of speech appropriate to it. And he will give instructions concerning the reasons why one kind of soul is necessarily convinced by one kind of speech while another necessarily remains unconvinced."[44] Causal knowledge was therefore a necessary condition for the existence of science in both Plato and the writings of the Hippocratic physicians.

But discrepancies between Platonic and Hippocratic approaches to epistemology were to force a rearrangement of the concepts on which the contrast between science and its opposite was predicated. In Plato, as in the Hippocratic Collection, one does indeed find a distinction made between science (*technè*) and nonscience (*atechniè*).[45] But while nonscience for the Hippocratics was synonymous with luck or chance (*tuchè*), Plato tended in both the *Gorgias* and the *Phaedrus* to substitute for this the term "empirie" (*empeiria*), or practice without knowledge of principles. In the former case, one need look no further than the passage just cited on cooking, which is said not to be an art (*technè*) but an empirie (*empeiria*). In the *Phaedrus*, art (*technè*)—both medical and rhetorical—is opposed to empirie (*empeiria*) and to routine.[46] By contrast, in the Hippocratic corpus, experience (*peirè*) is the mark of the man who knows. It is synonymous with competence, and always carries a positive connotation. The point of this brief comparative sketch of Hippocratic and Platonic etymology is that it allows us to look beyond the obvious resemblances of the two accounts and actually see the emergence of a conceptual shift that was to have important implications for the theory of scientific knowledge.

For in revising the concept of experience in this way, Plato introduced into the history of ideas the pejorative sense that was long to be attached to empirical knowledge and established a ranking among types of knowledge, placing rational knowledge—the only kind capable of explaining its own development—above empirical knowledge, which involved only routine and memory.[47] This novel rearrangement carried with it the seeds of the distinction between two modes of knowledge: empirical knowledge, which was to be rehabilitated by the sect of empiricist physicians, and the logical knowledge advocated by physicians of the dogmatic sect. Both sects, though they were rivals, claimed Hippocrates as their authority, scouring the collection for what they wanted to find there. But the distinction between these two modes of knowledge was foreign to Hippocratic epistemology. Here, as also in other contexts, Hippocrates has often been interpreted in terms of a conceptual distinction that did not yet exist in his own time.

ELEVEN

Medicine in Crisis and the Reaction against Philosophy

In the face of external attacks made by those who wished to deny the reality of medicine, physicians had to form a united front to defend it as an art in the manner suggested by the Hippocratic treatise of this very name—*The Art*. But when it was a question not of the existence of the medical art, but of the methods proper to it, specialists found themselves divided. The internal quarrels could be as bitter as the disputes with critics outside the profession. Among physicians themselves, the essential problem of method that was debated had to do with the relation of medicine to philosophy. For there existed a philosophical style of medicine, which had its partisans and its adversaries; and although the external enemies of medicine are known to us only indirectly, through the account of the treatise *The Art*, the debate over medicine and philosophy is at the very heart of the Hippocratic Collection as a whole. Owing to its diversity, the collection preserves works representing each of the two camps. It therefore provides a vivid description of a crisis in medicine—a crisis in the sense in which the Hippocratic physicians spoke of crisis in the context of disease, that is, a decisive moment—when the medical art began to assert its autonomy in relation to philosophy.

The Pre-Socratic Philosophers of the Sixth Century and Cosmology

Already a century before the oldest Hippocratic treatises were composed, philosophy had begun to flourish in Ionia. The first of those who today are called the pre-Socratic philosophers, Thales, Anaximander, and Anaximenes, lived at Miletus. Also active in the sixth century was Pythagoras, born on the island of Samos and a contemporary of the famous tyrant who ruled the island, Polycrates, as well as Xenophanes, born at Colophon in Ionia and a contemporary of Anaximander. Greek philosophy was indeed born in Ionia in the sixth century, even if it very soon spread through the Occident with the departure of Pythagoras and Xenophanes for southern Italy, the former to Croton, the latter settling at Elea after a tour of Sicily. But the philosophy of the first Milesians was primarily a cosmology—that is to say, a series of speculations about nature. In their works, particularly those treatises traditionally entitled *On Nature*, they sought to give as rational an explanation as they could for subterranean, terrestrial, and celestial phenomena. The goal of philosophy, in their view, was to attain universal knowledge. Not everyone agreed. "Much learning does not teach understanding," Heraclitus was to remark archly in the next century, "or it would have taught Hesiod and Pythagoras, as well as Xenophanes and Hecataeus."[1]

Why Is Seawater Salty?

It is difficult for us to imagine the multiplicity of problems that fascinated the pre-Socratics, things both small and large, having to do with earth, water, air, and fire. One such problem, among a host of others, needs to be mentioned for its effect upon one of the Hippocratic treatises. For the first philosophers of Miletus, a great port city, one of the many phenomena needing to be explained was the existence of a saltwater sea next to freshwater springs. How was the ocean formed and why is it salty? This is just the sort of question that characterized the "natural philosophy" of the ancients: it sought to explain a natural phenomenon in terms of a theory about its genesis. Anaximander of Miletus is the earliest philosopher whose answer to this question has been preserved, in the form of a summary: "Anaximander says that the ocean is the residue of the first wetness, the greatest part of which was dried up and drawn upwards by the fire [of the sun] and the remaining part of which was transformed on account of the complete coction."[2] The saltwater ocean is explained therefore by the dual phenomenon of evaporation and coction. His contemporary Xenophanes of Colophon was also familiar with the phenomenon of the evaporation of saltwater, and had managed to explain correctly the formation of clouds and why rain falls in the form of freshwater by means of such evaporation: "Xenophanes declares that it is due to the heat of the sun, as initial cause, that celestial phenomena arise. For the wet being drawn upwards from the sea, the fresh part, becoming separated owing to the fineness of its particles, forms clouds in darkening and falls back [to earth] in the form of rains by condensation."[3] Anaximander's theory was to be adopted in the following century by a philosopher who enjoyed a certain celebrity during the period, Diogenes of Apollonia.[4] Now this is precisely the sort of explanation that was adopted by the Hippocratic author of *Airs, Waters, Places* in dealing with the influence of waters upon health. In fact, to show why rainwater is the lightest and freshest of waters, he retraces the formation of rain in a passage that, despite its length, deserves to be quoted almost in full, for quite exceptionally it preserves a complete and authentic account of this phenomenon, whereas the opinions of the pre-Socratic philosophers are known only indirectly through later, more or less simplified summaries:

Rain waters are the lightest, sweetest, finest and clearest. To begin with, the sun raises and draws up the finest and lightest part of water, as is proved by the formation of salt. The brine, owing to its coarseness and weight, is left behind and becomes salt; the finest part, owing to its lightness, is drawn up by the sun. Not only from pools does the sun raise this part, but also from the sea and from whatever has moisture in it—and there is moisture in everything. Even from men it raises the finest and lightest part of their juices. The plainest evidence thereof is that when a man walks or sits in the sun wearing a cloak, the parts of his skin reached by the sun will not sweat, for it draws up each layer of sweat as it appears. But those parts sweat which are covered by his cloak or by anything else. For the sweat drawn forcibly out by the sun is prevented by the covering from disappearing through the sun's power. But when the man has come into a shady place, his whole body sweats alike, as the sun no longer shines upon it. . . . Furthermore, when it has been carried away aloft, and has combined with the atmosphere as it circles round, the turbid, dark part of it separates out, changes and becomes mist and fog, while the clearest and lightest part of it remains, and is sweetened as the heat of the sun produces coction, just as all other things always become sweeter through coction. Now as long as it is scattered and uncondensed, it travels about aloft, but as soon as it collects anywhere and is compressed into one place owing to sudden, contrary winds, then it bursts wherever the most compression happens to take place. For this is more likely to occur when the clouds, set in motion and carried along by a wind that allows them no rest, are suddenly encountered by a contrary blast and by other clouds. In such cases the front is compressed, the rear comes on and is thus thickened, darkened and compressed into one place, so that the weight bursts and causes rain.[5]

The reasons given by the Hippocratic physician are substantially the same as those of the pre-Socratic philosophers: the lightest part of the saltwater, in salty marshes as in the sea, is drawn up by the sun and softened by the coction of the sun; then it condenses and falls in the form of precipitations of freshwater. The main thing to note about the physician's account is that he was perfectly familiar with the theories of the natural philosophers. More than this, his account appears to constitute an advance over the explanations of the philosophers, at least to judge from the summaries that have come down to us, to the extent that it makes a novel argument, relating to sweat, which serves to confirm the law that the sun attracts all liquids. Thus, in the Hippocratic account, observation of biological phenomena is used to confirm a cosmological theory.

The Pre-Socratic Philosophers of the
Fifth Century and the Development of Biology

It may be thought natural enough that a physician of the sixth century should have devoted attention to man; less so, perhaps, in the case of a philosopher. But this interest was not foreign to the concerns of the pre-Socratic philosophers of the fifth century. From the sixth century until the second half of the fifth, one witnesses a shift in the focus of philosophical interest. In the sixth century, philosophers were essentially cosmologists. The first Milesians—Thales, Anaximander, and Anaximenes—were concerned more with astronomy and physics than with anthropology and medicine; only the Pythagoreans who had settled at Croton, where there existed a medical tradition,[6] departed from their example. It is in any case in the city of Croton that we find the first known example of a philosopher-physician— Alcmaeon, who, if he was not actually a Pythagorean, was at least closely associated with the circle of Pythagoras's disciples.[7] He was young when Pythagoras was already old.[8] Aristotle mentions him as a philosopher in his *Metaphysics*.[9] But Alcmaeon was chiefly a physician.[10] In the history of medical ideas, he occupies a place of the first rank: it is to him we owe the most ancient definition that has come down to us of health and illness. According to this definition, health results from the balance and mixture of the constitutive qualities of man (wet, dry, hot, cold, bitter, sweet, and so on); illness, by contrast, is caused by the predominance of one of them.[11] This conception was in large part to be adopted by the Hippocratic physicians.

What is of greatest interest to us at the moment, however, is the way in which philosophers came to pay greater attention to the domain of living things during the course of the fifth century.

Empedocles and Medicine

The most celebrated of the philosophers representing this new tendency was Empedocles, a native of Agrigentum in Sicily. It is true that the incipient symbiosis between cosmology and biology was all the more natural in his case to the extent that he was, like Alcmaeon of Croton, both a philosopher and a physician. While his medical activity is now much less known than his philosophical work, it is well attested by ancient accounts. Galen, in fact, cites Empedocles as one of the three leading physicians of Sicily, rivals to the Asclepiads of Cos and those of Cnidus;[12] the two others were Philistion and Pausanias. Now it was precisely this Pausanias to whom Empedocles dedicated his great philosophical poem *On Nature*. Empedocles also wrote a work on medicine that has not come down to us.[13] A good many more or less credible anecdotes are reported of his medical activity. He is said to have healed a woman of Agrigentum, Pantheia, after other doctors had given up on her.[14] He put an end to a pestilence in the neighboring city of Selinus by diverting the healthful waters of one river into another, whose emanations were the cause of the pestilence.[15] He was nicknamed the Windstopper for having arrested a pestilence caused by an unhealthy wind from the south, either by walling up the crevice of a mountain through which the wind blew onto the plain[16] or by having asses' hides hung around the town.[17] The most extraordinary case is that of a woman whom he is said to have kept in a state of apnea, or suspended breathing, for thirty days.[18] One may be tempted to suspect the authors of these anecdotes of pure invention. But Empedocles himself was the source of this image of the doctor-magician, as when he proclaimed:

> What drugs there are for ills and what help against old age
> you will learn, since for you alone shall I accomplish all this.
> And you will stop the power of the tireless winds which sweep over the earth
> and destroy the crops with their breath,
> and again, if you wish, you will bring on compensating breezes.
> And after black rain you will produce a seasonable drought
> for men, and after the summer drought you will produce
> tree-nurturing streams . . .
> And you will lead from Hades the power of dead men.[19]

Empedocles apparently did not manage to make a clear distinction between magic and medicine, as the Hippocratic physicians were to do some years later. Even if allowances are made for the prophetic tone that is characteristic of the poetic genre, one cannot help but see that his promises are scarcely compatible with Hippocratic thought; indeed, they expose him to the accusations made by the author of *The Sacred Disease*, who castigates those who claim to know how to "make storm and sunshine" by "magic and sacrifice."[20] But the image of the all-powerful magician that Empedocles wished to create for himself did not prevent him, in *On Nature*, from approaching not only cosmological questions in a rational spirit, but also the great biological problems debated during his time, such as generation, digestion, breathing, sensory perception, thought, sleep, and death. In particular, his explanation of how breathing works—through the alternating motions of blood within the body and of air outside—has remained famous, mainly because he illustrates it by a lovely poetical comparison with the alternating motions of water and air in a clepsydra, the vase used for telling time that, since its base was pierced with holes, archeologists call a "watering can."[21]

Anaxagoras and Biology

This tendency to integrate biological and cosmological inquiry was perhaps still more profound in Anaxagoras, although he was not a physician like Empedocles. Originally from Clazomenae in Asia Minor, Anaxagoras was older than Empedocles, though his work dates from a later period.[22] Both held that the world was to be explained on the basis of primary elements. But while the primary elements in the case of Empedocles—fire, air, water, and earth—emerged directly from cosmological inquiry, those of Anaxagoras seemed to issue instead from biological research. "[T]he homoeomerous substances (e.g. flesh, bone and so on)," Anaxagoras maintained, "are the elements."[23] Although in principle there are an infinite number of homeomeries [*homoiomerei*], or substances formed of like parts, Anaxagoras liked to cite those that constituted the human body.[24] This was because he had reflected at length, and in particular, upon the principle of generation. He maintained that the human seed contains indiscriminate mixtures of all the homeomeries that make up the body: flesh, bone, blood, nerves, blood vessels, nails, even hair. To prove this, he posed the following question: "For how . . . could hair come into being from what is not hair, or flesh from what is not flesh?"[25] His answer was that the parts of the seed are invisible, owing to their smallness; but that, upon growing in size, they are separated and become visible. It is this biological model of generation that Anaxagoras seems to have transposed to cosmology. Thus, for example, familiar cosmological substances such as fire and air were no longer primary elements for Anaxagoras, as they were for Empedocles, but mixtures.[26] It may be assumed that the general public understood nothing of these subtleties. For the citizens of Athens, Anaxagoras was the philosopher who had the audacity to claim that the sun was not a god but an incandescent mass; and, although he was the teacher and friend of Euripides, and above all of Pericles, he fell victim to popular superstition and was condemned for impiety.[27] Nonetheless, his interest in biology is attested not only by the indirect influence it had on his cosmological theories but also by the experiments that he carried out upon animals. One anecdote reported by Plutarch testifies to this.[28] During Anaxagoras's stay at Athens, a one-horned ram was brought to Pericles from his estate. The seer Lampon interpreted this anomaly as a sign of Pericles' impending victory over his rival Thucydides in the struggle for political control of Athens. But Anaxagoras, who was also present, had the skull of the animal opened and showed all who were there that the anomaly was due to an atrophy of the brain: instead of occupying the whole cranium, the brain ended in an egg-like point at the root of the single horn. Anaxagoras was immediately praised for his learning on all sides. (Plutarch adds, not unmaliciously, that the seer Lampon was later praised on all sides when his prediction proved to be correct.) The anecdote demonstrates, in any case, Anaxagoras's scientific cast of mind in relying on observation in order to interpret biological facts rationally. His approach in this instance is comparable to that of the author of *The Sacred Disease*, who opened the skulls of animals affected by epilepsy to note the pathological state of the brain and to show that the cause was not divine: "The truth of this is best shown by the cattle that are attacked by this disease, especially by the goats, which are the most common victims. If you cut open the head you will find the brain moist, very full of dropsy and of an evil odour, whereby you may learn that it is not a god but the disease that injures the body."[29]

In the final analysis, the philosopher of Clazomenae must be judged to have been closer to the spirit of Hippocratic thinking than the medical philosopher of Agrigentum. Is it any surprise, then, that the same Hippocratic treatise should take sides against Empedocles[30] and in favor of Anaxagoras?

Medicine and Philosophy in Diogenes of Apollonia

The importance assumed by medical knowledge in philosophical reflection can best be gauged, however, by considering the work of a contemporary of Anaxagoras, Diogenes of Apollonia, in Crete. While Diogenes upheld the old cosmological theory of his teacher, Anaximenes, his broader interests in biology and medicine enabled him to revitalize and extend it.[31] He adopted the basic hypothesis of Milesian philosophy—namely, that everything derives from a single principle (for him, as for Anaximenes, this principle was air)—but his knowledge of man was much more precise. Diogenes devoted an entire book to the nature of man;[32] and even in his great work *On*

Nature he displays a striking knowledge of human anatomy in examining the biological problem of generation. In connection with his view that the seed consists of warm, foaming blood, he gives a long description of the anatomy of human blood vessels whose scientific sophistication is not inferior to that of the Hippocratic Collection. The proof of this is that Aristotle cites Diogenes' account in its entirety alongside that of Polybus, Hippocrates' disciple and son-in-law, in describing the state of anatomical knowledge among his predecessors.[33] What clearer evidence could one ask for that philosophers and physicians were seen as rivals in the field of human biology?

What is more, the boundaries between philosophy and medicine became blurred in this period, to the point that it is sometimes difficult to know whether a philosopher was simply acquainted with medicine or whether he was himself a physician. One may wonder, in particular, whether in fact Diogenes of Apollonia was not a physician, for we possess other evidence of his medical competence. The tongue, which according to him was the point at which all the blood vessels converged, was the source of a great deal of information about illnesses.[34] He was known for having assigned great importance to a patient's complexion in both the diagnosis and prognosis of disease.[35] Given that this last piece of information has come down to us as part of traditional medical lore, it is not impossible that Diogenes of Apollonia was considered in antiquity not only as a philosopher but also as a physician.

The Medical Theories of Two Fifth-Century Philosophers: Hippon and Philolaus

New light was shed on the relations between pre-Socratic philosophy and medicine with the discovery at the end of the nineteenth century of the *Anonymus Londinensis.*[36] The original source of this papyrus, as we have seen, was the encyclopedia of physicians that had been composed by the Aristotelian school and attributed to one of Aristotle's pupils, Meno. One of the surprises was the information it contained about the medical theories of two thinkers who until then were known only as philosophers.

The first was Hippon. A native of Samos, Hippon lived in southern Italy at Rhegium, Croton, and Metapontum.[37] He was apparently well known in Athens, for he figures in a comedy by Aristophanes' great predecessor, Cratinus, entitled *Panoptai* (or *The All-Seeing Ones*). In this play, staged well before Aristophanes' *Clouds*, Cratinus satirizes philosophers.[38] Hippon of Samos had adopted Thales' old theory, holding that water is the primordial substance of the universe. He was well known to have taken an interest in biological problems, particularly ones related to generation and growth, with regard to which he introduced an arithmology based on the numbers seven and ten.[39] But the *Anonymus Londinensis* gives a clearer account of the way in which he explained diseases in terms of his basic hypothesis: the onset of illness is triggered by the innate moistness of the body, either through an excess or a lack of it. As for death, this was caused by a complete drying out of moisture, or, as we would say today, by dehydration. Hippon does not seem to have been a great mind. Aristotle, in any case, judged him harshly, describing him as a second-rate thinker.[40]

The second philosopher whose medical theories came to light through the *Anonymus Londinensis* was Philolaus of Croton. With Philolaus we are back in the world of Pythagoreanism. He belonged to the generation that experienced the dramatic end of the Pythagoreans' political dominance at Croton, and went into exile, first in Lucania and then at Thebes, where the Pythagorean community had taken refuge. Plato refers to his teaching there in the *Phaedo*, mentioning two of Philolaus's disciples, Simmias and Cebes, who were present during Socrates' last moments in prison.[41] According to the *Anonymus Londinensis*, Philolaus believed that the human body is solely constituted by heat, while the air that it inhales is cold.[42] As for diseases, these were caused by three humors, blood, bile, and phlegm, and were favored by every excess or lack of heat, food, and cold.[43] His conception of the nature of man seems to have been related to his cosmological theory, according to which fire occupied the center of the universe and was the guiding principle of it.[44] Nonetheless, it is hard to see how he managed to reconcile the details of his biological theory with his fundamental hypothesis, which consisted in explaining the world through the harmony of two contrary principles, the illimited and the limited.[45] This information about the interest shown by Philolaus in medicine seems to confirm what was already known from Alcmaeon; namely, that the connection between philosophy and medicine was close in the Pythagorean tradition at Croton.

Democritus

Before concluding this rapid review of philosophers who took an interest in biology and medicine before and during Hippocrates' time, we must once again mention Democritus, who, it will be recalled, was a native of the city of Abdera on the Thracian coast. He may be situated chronologically in relative terms: we know he was young when Anaxagoras was old. He was dubbed Science—a nickname that was well deserved. Indeed his range of interests was universal, and he took up many questions that touched on biology (and, in connection with this, ethics) in addition to cosmology. His immense work comprised even more treatises than are gathered together under the name of Hippocrates; all of it, apart from a few fragments, has disappeared. But of the list that has been preserved of the seventy treatises that make up this body of work, a number of titles attest to his interest in human biology (*On the Nature of Man* [or *On the Flesh*], *On the Intellect*, *On the Senses*, *On Flavors*, *On Colors*) and in medicine (*Prognostication*, *On Diet* [or *Dietetics*], *Medical Knowledge*, *On Fever and Those Who Are Made to Cough by Illness*).[46] Though we lack these treatises, many accounts inform us of the various biological questions that he tackled and of the answers that he gave to them. The abundance of evidence recorded by Aristotle and his school is a sign of Democritus's very great historical importance. His atomic theory of matter, for which he remains best known, exercised an influence outside philosophy on the medicine of the Hellenistic period, notably upon Erasistratus (third century B.C.) and upon Asclepiades (first century B.C.).

One tradition maintains—apparently on the principle that more shall be given unto those that have—that Hippocrates was a disciple of Democritus,[47] or even a disciple of a disciple of Democritus, Metrodorus of Chios.[48] This tradition, transmitted by a Byzantine encyclopedia, is improbable, because it gets the relative dates of Democritus and Hippocrates badly wrong. By its accounting, Hippocrates would have been young when Democritus was quite old;[49] in fact, they were close contemporaries.[50] Nonetheless, this tradition attests in its own way to the fact that belief in the influence of pre-Socratic philosophy upon Hippocratic medicine is not the invention of modern scholarship.

Hippocratic Physicians and Philosophy

The philosophers of the fifth century, whether they were predecessors or contemporaries of Hippocrates and the most ancient Hippocratic writings, therefore concerned themselves with biological and anthropological problems. Consequently, it is not surprising that a rather large number of similarities have been noted between the pre-Socratics and the Hippocratics. But not all of these similarities are necessarily to be explained in the same way. Some of them occur within the framework of biological problems that physicians dealt with strictly in the terms of their own profession; in such cases, one need not assume, as is too often done, any systematic influence of philosophy on Hippocratic thought. Other such similarities are found, by contrast, in treatises whose physician-authors associated their anthropology with a cosmology. It is mainly with reference to these cases that one can legitimately speak of a philosophically minded medicine.

Biological and Embryological Problems as Seen by Physicians and Philosophers

A whole series of biological problems was framed within a medical as well as a philosophical perspective. We may list a few of the questions they involved: What is the nature of man? Of the human body and soul? How are sensations and intelligence produced? The voice? Breathing? Sleep and dreams? How does generation occur? Growth and death? What is responsible for health and disease? Of all these questions, the one that perhaps was the source of the greatest difficulty, and the one that was the most heatedly debated by physicians and philosophers alike, concerned generation, or, as we would say today, embryology. The fascination with embryology, at least among the philosophers, was part of a larger fascination with the origins of man and the universe—what at the time was called an "inquiry into nature." Embryological research was broken down into a variety of problems, of which the principal ones were these:

1. What is the nature of the human seed? From what part of the body does it come?
2. Does the seed come from the man and the woman or from the man alone?
3. What explains the formation of a boy and a girl? the resemblance of a child to his parents?
4. How does the embryo develop in the womb? How are the parts of the body formed?
5. At what moment is the embryo viable?
6. What explains sterility in women or men? the birth of twins? superfoetation?

Remarks on all these problems are found scattered throughout several of the major treatises of the Hippocratic Collection. But the collection also contains works devoted solely to the subject of embryology. Contrary to what is still believed by some eminent embryologists today, the first treatise on embryology is not due to Aristotle. Treatises exclusively devoted to this subject existed prior to Aristotle, as part of the Hippocratic Collection.

When Is the Foetus Viable?

One of these embryological treatises, entitled *Eight Months' Child*, was concerned with a type of problem that to us now seems curious: why is the foetus viable from the seventh month but not from the eighth? Such questions were also discussed by the pre-Socratics. We have the opinion of Empedocles, who sought to explain why foetuses born after seven months, like those after ten, were viable. His reasoning is oddly fanciful, and closely connected with the concerns of cosmology: "According to Empedocles, when the race of men was born of the earth, the length of the day, on account of the slowness of the transit of the sun, was equal to what now is a period of six months; but as time went by, the day was equal to what is now a period of seven months; this is why the foetuses of ten months and of seven months are viable, the nature of the universe being used to making the foetus grow in a single day after the night when it was conceived."[51] The answer given by the Hippocratic author is somewhat less fanciful and, in any case, free of all cosmological considerations. This physician believed that the child is subject to pain and suffering for forty days around the eighth month, whether or not it is in the womb. If a foetus born in the eighth month does not survive, it is because it is exposed to two shocks, one right after the other: the suffering of the eighth month and the pain of birth. By contrast, the foetus born at seven months survives more easily because by the time of its birth it has not yet experienced the suffering of the eighth month; and the foetus of ten months is viable because the suffering of the eighth month is already well passed by the time it is exposed to that of delivery. While the role played by arithmology in this explanation cannot be denied, we may nonetheless appreciate the physician's fine analysis of the changes undergone by the child at birth, when it is forced to give up a familiar and comfortable environment for a foreign and rather harsher world:

In place of breaths and liquids so closely related, as they must always be in the womb on account of the bonds of familiarity and benevolence, the newborn takes in only foreign products, rawer, drier, less human, which necessarily provokes much suffering and many deaths; for even among adults changes of location and regimen often bring on illnesses. The same reasoning holds for clothes: instead of being enveloped by flesh and warm humors, moist and related, the newborns are wrapped in the same garments as adults.[52]

The treatise *Eight Months' Child* contemplates only the final phase of development of the embryo. There exists in the Hippocratic Collection, however, a work that sets out to follow the development of the embryo from the moment of insemination until its delivery into the world; manuscript tradition has wrongly split it into two treatises, entitled *Generation* and *Nature of the Child*. A few remarks about the content of this work, accompanied by a brief commentary, will give an overview of the embryological problems addressed and the sort of solutions given to such problems in Hippocrates' time.

Where Does the Seed Come From?

According to the author of *Generation / Nature of the Child*, the seed comes from both the man and the woman. This opinion was widely shared among Hippocratic physicians.[53] Opposed to it was the ancient belief that the woman is only the receptacle of the man's seed. The clearest statement of this view is to be found not in a technical account but in a play, the *Eumenides* of Aeschylus.[54] According to the Hippocratic author, however, the seed comes from every part of the body and from all of the humors. Other Hippocratic physicians subscribed to such a theory, which modern scholars call "pangenesis," particularly the author of *Airs, Waters, Places* and *The Sacred Disease*.[55] This pangenetic theory is usually contrasted with an older "encephalomyelitic" theory, so called because it holds that the seed is derived from the brain and the spinal cord. But the reality was more complex than the cut-and-dried distinctions of modern scholarship would seem to imply. The Hippocratic author, while he affirmed that seed comes from all parts of the body, had it passing through the brain and the spinal cord. This passage of the seed is related to a curious belief according to which men become impotent following an incision behind the ear: "Those who are incised around the ear can have sexual relations and ejaculate, but the seed is of small amount, weak, and sterile. This is because the majority of the seed travels from the head down past the ears toward the spinal cord. This path, on account of the healing of the incision, is filled in [i.e., blocked]."[56]

This belief is all the more curious since it passed for a scientific truth. It served even to combat a belief that in another treatise was judged popular. Criticizing the idea that the impotence of the Scythians known as Anaries was caused by a deity,[57] the author of *Airs, Waters, Places* remarks that the treatment employed by those who suffered from this condition could only make it worse: "They cure themselves in the following way. At the beginning of the disease they cut the vein behind each ear. . . . Now, in my opinion, by this treatment the seed is destroyed. For by the side of the ear are veins, to cut which causes impotence, and I believe that these are the veins which they cut."[58]

If one compares this passage with the preceding one, it is clear that for the author of *Airs, Waters, Places*, no less than for the author of *Generation/Nature of the Child*, the seed comes from the brain and descends alongside the ear; and as the author of *Airs, Waters, Places* also believes that the seed comes from the entire body, it follows that neither of these two physicians understood the distinction that modern scholars have sought to introduce between an "encephalomyelitic" theory and a "pangenetic" theory.

Conception of the Child and Growth of the Embryo

The conception of the embryo, according to the author of *Generation / Nature of the Child*, occurs when the seed of the man is retained in the womb and mixed with the seed that issues from the woman. The sex of the embryo thus formed is determined by the nature of the two seeds: if they are strong, they give birth to a boy; if they are weak, to a girl. As for resemblances between child and parents, these are explained by the predominance of one of the two seeds over the other. The fact that a boy may more closely resemble his mother, or a girl her father, is seen by the author as confirmation that the embryo is the product of the union of two distinct seeds, issuing respectively from the father and the mother. He goes on next to explain how the embryo develops. Being hot, it breathes by receiving the cool air of the mother, and it is fed by the blood of the mother, which descends into the womb—in both cases by means of the umbilical cord. The author is to be congratulated for having gotten the role of the umbilical cord right. For the manner in which the embryo breathed and took nourishment was an open question at the time; another Hippocratic physician maintained, in fact, that the embryo took nourishment through the mouth. This was the author of *Fleshes*, who relied upon an exact observation to draw a confident, but false, conclusion:

For example the fetus in the belly continually sucks with its lips from the uterus of the mother and draws nourishment and breath to its heart inside. . . . If anyone asks you how you know that the fetus draws and sucks in the uterus, you may reply as follows. Both humans and animals have faeces in their intestines at the time of birth, and immediately at birth pass stools—but there would be no faeces, if the fetus did not suck in the uterus. Nor would a baby know how to suck from the breast immediately at birth, if it did not also suck in the uterus.[59]

If the embryo is nourished by its umbilical cord, how then does it grow? Growth occurs by coagulation of the blood, which turns into flesh. The author of *Generation/Nature of the Child* connects this transformation of blood into flesh with the halt of menstruation during pregnancy. In the course of growth, the various parts of the embryo become differentiated under the influence of breathing, with like parts tending toward like. The male foetus is formed faster than the female foetus. The author goes so far as to specify the number of days: a maximum of thirty days for the male, forty-two for the female. The reason, according to him, is that the female seed is weaker and more moist than the male seed. The view that the female was formed in the womb less rapidly than the male was widely held in ancient embryology. This was not only a Hippocratic prejudice; Aristotelians subscribed to it as well.[60] The last stage of the development of the foetus is marked by the ramification of the extremities, fingers on the hands and toes on the feet, with the growth of nails and hair. Next, the foetus begins to move. Here again, of course, the boy is more advanced than the girl. The physician supplies the figures: the boy at three months, the girl at four. The growth of the embryo is altogether comparable to that of a plant, the mother being to the child what the earth is to the plant—a comparison developed by the author at length. Finally, the moment of birth arrives in the tenth month: the foetus frees itself from the womb by pushing against and rupturing the membranes that surround it. The author concludes his account by considering the case of twins. According to him they are born of a single act of intercourse and develop in two different pockets of the uterus. The problem of twins was one of the obligatory questions for embryology. The Hippocratic physicians were agreed in regarding twins as the result of a single act of intercourse.[61] But at this time there were probably other thinkers who held that two instances of coitus were necessary and that the development of twins was analogous to a superfoetation.[62]

Hippocratic versus Pre-Socratic Embryology

Since all these problems of embryology were addressed not only by physicians of the period but also by pre-Socratic philosophers, scholars have sought to compare their opinions, usually with a view to estimating the influence of the philosophers upon the physicians. Thus, for example, in attempting to account for the ideas of the physician who wrote the first complete treatise of embryology—*Generation/Nature of the Child*—scholars have cited the names of almost all the philosophers mentioned in our previous discussion of the pre-Socratics and medicine: Empedocles, Anaxagoras, Diogenes of Apollonia, the Pythagoreans, and Democritus. Credit currently goes to Democritus, particularly since for him and the author of the Hippocratic treatise alike the seed comes from all parts of the body.[63] But there is no trace of atomism in the Hippocratic treatise; nor does anything point to Democritus as the originator of the pangenetic theory. When Aristotle refers to this theory, he associates it with no name in particular.[64] It seems therefore that modern scholars have been deceived, still more than the ancient Greeks themselves, by the mirage of a first inventor. Without wishing to involve the reader in a quarrel among experts, it must be emphasized that our knowledge of the embryology of the pre-Socratics is very indirect and fragmentary; it is accessible to us only through later, and often distorting, accounts that report opinions out of context. All this surely counsels prudence in searching for possible influences of philosophical thought upon the Hippocratic physicians—all the more since the flowering of embryological inquiry among the pre-Socratic philosophers might just as easily be explained by the influence of medical thought upon them. In all likelihood there were reciprocal influences that today can no longer be disentangled.

The First Observations in Embryology:
The Embryo and the Egg

The search for sources has its limits. Sometimes it risks masking the essential point. One has only to read this first manual of embryology straight through to be struck by its personal quality, derived from actual experience of medical practice, and by the remarkable coherence of its argument. Instead of shaking the tree of doxography in the hope that a few dessicated fruits will fall into our hands, we are better off savoring the delightful way in which the author of *Generation/Nature of the Child* observes—or believes he has observed—a seed six days old, comparing it to an egg:

Besides, I have seen myself seed that remained six days in the womb and that then fell out of it. . . . I am going to recount how I came to see this six-day-old seed. A woman of my acquaintance possessed a highly valued singer, who had intercourse with men: she could not become pregnant, lest she lose her value. This singer had heard what the women said among themselves: for a woman to become pregnant, the seed must not come out, but must stay inside. Having heard these things, she noted them and always remembered them. So when she realized that the seed was not coming out, she confided in her mistress, and word made its way to me. And I, on receiving the news, ordered the singer to jump, bringing her heels up as high as her buttocks; she had already made seven jumps when the seed landed on the ground with a muffled sound. On seeing this, the singer reflected and was surprised. How it appeared I am going to explain. It is as though one had entirely removed the shell of a raw egg and through the interior membrane the liquid inside was transparently visible. This is what it looked like, to be concise. Moreover, it was red and rounded. In the membrane there appeared thick white fibers, and around the membrane, on the outside, clots of blood. From the middle of the membrane there jutted out something slender that seemed to me to be the umbilical cord, by which breath is first drawn in and exhaled. And the membrane, extending from that, was stretched all around, enveloping the seed. Such was the seed of six days that I saw.[65]

This is clearly a classic performance. Five centuries later, in fact, Galen was to cite the entire passage in his treatise *On the Seed*, and again in his treatise *On the Formation of the Foetus*. "This is a passage," Galen tells us, "that instructs us by the exactitude of the observation and diverts us"[66]—a splendid tribute from the greatest physician of the Roman period to his illustrious precursor.

The Hippocratic author concludes this anecdote by announcing that a little further on he will report another observational result that establishes the validity of his entire position on the seed and the development of the embryo. In the event, he keeps his promise. It turns out to be the occasion of a second bravura passage, which has remained celebrated in the history of the sciences because it marks the first time that the development of a chicken's egg is used in human embryological research:

I am now going to describe, as I promised a bit earlier, how anyone who wishes to have knowledge of this subject may discern, within the limits of human intelligence, that the seed is in a membrane, that in the middle of it is found an umbilical cord, that this seed first draws in breath to itself and expels it to the outside, and that from the umbilical cord extend the membranes. And for all the rest of the growth of the child that I have described, one will find that it goes on until the end in its entirety as I have shown in my accounts of it, if one wishes to refer to the proofs that I am going to give. One may put twenty eggs or more to hatch under two hens or under several and each day, beginning on the second day [and continuing] until the last, when the egg hatches, take away an egg and break it open: one will discover by examination that everything agrees with what I have said, as far as the growth of a bird may be compared with the growth of a man. In fact, the membranes are stretched from the umbilical cord and all that I have said about the child is found to be so in the bird's egg: this is what one discovers from the beginning until the end. Of course, if one has not seen it before, one will be surprised that there is an umbilical cord inside a bird's egg; however, it is so. This, then, is what I had to say on this subject.[67]

It is plain from such passages that the author's knowledge was not derived mainly from books. Here it rests on observation, whether owing to a happy chance, as in the case of the singer-prostitute, the slave of one of his friends, or taking the form of a rudimentary experiment, as in the case of the chicken eggs. It is in any case on the strength of such personal observation that he claims validity for his explanations. This scientist well deserves to be admired for his ingenuity, and for his pride in the proofs that he advances, but his sense of modesty should be appreciated as well, for he is conscious of the limits of human knowledge.

Toward a Philosophical Medicine

But alongside this approach to embryology, which was developed from a medical perspective, there exists another treatise in the Hippocratic Collection—the *Regimen*—that presents an embryology very closely tied to cosmological considerations. The tone is different; speculation gains the upper hand over observation. Here one is dealing with philosophical medicine. Given that man, like the universe itself, is constituted of two primordial elements, fire and water, the author of the *Regimen* treats the development of the embryo in terms of that of the universe:

In a word, all things were arranged in the body, in a fashion conformable to itself, by fire, a copy of the whole, the small after the manner of the great and the great after the manner of the small. The belly is made the greatest, a steward for dry water and moist, to give all and to take from all, the power of the sea, nurse of creatures suited to it, destroyer of those not suited. And around it a concretion of cold water and moist, a passage for cold breath and warm, a copy of the earth, which alters all things that fall into it. Consuming and increasing, it made a dispersion of fine water and of ethereal fire, the invisible and the visible, a secretion from the compacted substance, in which things are carried and come to light, each according to its allotted portion. And in this fire made for itself three groups of circuits, within and without each bounded by the others: those towards the hollows of the moist, the powers of the moon; those towards the outer circumference, towards the solid enclosure, the power of the stars; the middle circuits, bounded both within and without. The hottest and strongest fire, which controls all things, ordering all things according to nature, imperceptible to sight or touch, wherein are soul, mind, thought, growth, decrease, mutation, sleep, waking. This governs all things always, both here and there, and is never at rest.[68]

In this passage, which contains certain enigmatic formulations—perhaps intentionally so, after the fashion of Heraclitus—the fundamental notion is that of imitation (*mimesis*). The body is a copy of the Whole.[69] Embryology, rather than being considered an observational science, becomes a branch of speculative philosophy whose reconstruction is guided solely by the belief that human anatomy and physiology reproduce the organization and unfolding of the universe. Moreover, read out of context, this passage can be interpreted as an argument not about the formation of the embryo (embryogenesis) but about the origin of man (phylogenesis).

The Origin of Man

The origin of man, and more generally of living beings, was the province in the fifth century of the pre-Socratic philosophers and treated on the same level as the formation of the universe. It suffices to recall the pre-Socratic style of inquiry into nature, as reported by Plato in the *Phaedo*, where Socrates recollects his youthful enthusiasm for this kind of research:

When I was a young man I was wonderfully keen on that wisdom which they call natural science, for I thought it splendid to know the causes of everything, why it comes to be, why it perishes and why it exists. I was often changing my mind in the investigation, in the first instance, of questions such as these: Are living creatures nurtured when heat and cold produce a kind of putrefaction, as some say? Do we think with our blood, or air, or fire, or none of these, and does the brain provide our senses of hearing and sight and smell, from which come memory and opinion, and from memory and opinion which has become stable, comes knowledge? Then again, as I investigated how these things perish and what happens to things in the sky and on the earth, finally I became convinced that I had no natural aptitude at all for that kind of investigation.[70]

The aim of these philosophers amounted therefore to explaining how man was originally formed on the basis of first principles. Now there exists in the Hippocratic Collection a treatise that corresponds perfectly to the program recollected by Socrates in Plato's dialogue. This is the treatise on *Fleshes*, the title of which moreover calls to mind that of Democritus's treatise *On the Nature of Man* (or *On the Flesh*).[71] Indeed, the Hippocratic treatise is of inestimable value, for the treatises of the pre-Socratics either have been lost or are preserved only very fragmentarily, and this constitutes the sole wholly preserved example of the inquiry into nature that so delighted the young Socrates. While it is perfectly true that the author presents his work as a treatise of medicine,[72] there is no longer any distinction made between problems of medicine and philosophy; what he recounts in this treatise is the first formation of human life on the basis of its constituent elements rather than the formation of the embryo from the seed, as was still the case in the treatise on *Regimen*.

The author of *Fleshes* proposes, as he says in his preamble, to show "how man and the other animals are formed and come into being."[73] Does this not precisely match the philosophers' program of natural inquiry as Socrates describes it at the beginning? In view of the fact that man has been formed from certain elements of the universe, the author feels obliged to begin with a discussion of the formation of the universe. His anthropology therefore relies upon a cosmology. The only difference between the physician and the philosopher is the relative weight each gives to the discussions of cosmology and anthropology. The author of *Fleshes* has no interest in discussing cosmology for its own sake, but wishes only to briefly establish those elements involved in the formation of the universe that are necessary for the purposes of anthropology. The universe, according to his account, was formed in the aftermath of a general upheaval of matter, which was initially mixed together, by the separation of three elements: heat rose into the upper part and formed the aether; earth, the cold and dry element, occupied the lower part; and the part in between was taken up by the thick and moist air. The author then devotes the main part of his preliminary discussion to explaining how the different parts of man were formed out of earth. When the earth became separated from the heat, its isolation was not complete; it still contained pockets of heat of varying size. The action of this residual heat upon the earth led to the formation of the different tissues of the human body by a process that, interestingly, recalls the theory to which Socrates alludes in the *Phaedo* in order to explain the origin of living things: everything begins by means of that famous "putrefaction" that results from the action of the heat upon the cold of the earth. Here is how the author explains the initial formation of living tissues through putrefaction, which follows directly upon his statement regarding the formation of the universe:

Now while these [elements of the universe] were mingled with one another in a state of turbulence as they rotated, much heat was left behind at various places in the earth, in some places great amounts, in others lesser amounts and in still others very small amounts, but these many in number. As with time the earth was dried out by this heat, the materials left behind engendered putrefactions about themselves, which had the form of tunics [i.e., membranes]. Now what was heated for a great time and happened to arise from the putrefaction of the earth as fat, and containing the least moisture, quickly burnt up and became bones. That, on the other hand, which happened to be more gluey and to contain cold could not be burnt up on being heated or become dry, since it contained neither any fat that could be burnt up nor any moisture that, on being burnt up, could become dry; for this reason it took a form rather different from the other things, and became cords and vessels. The vessels were hollow and the cords solid owing to the fact that in the cords there was not much cold; in the vessels, on the other hand, cold was present, so that in the case of the vessels the part of this cold around the outside that was most gluey was baked through by the heat and became membraneous, while the cold in the inside, on being mastered by the heat, dissolved and became liquid.[74]

Thus the bones, tendons, and vessels of the body were formed, in a sort of gigantic kitchen, where fire burned and roasted and liquefied the earth. Reading passages like this one, we begin to understand why Socrates should have racked his brains contemplating such questions and why, in the end, he should have declared himself totally incompetent to decide them. Unperturbed, however, the author carries on, and with great learning shows how all the parts of the body are formed out of these two substances, the fatty and the gluey, themselves having been generated by the putrefaction of the earth under the influence of the heat that remained trapped in it. In this way he explains the formation of the throat, esophagus, intestines, bladder, brain, spinal cord, heart, lungs, liver, spleen, kidneys, flesh, joints, nails, teeth, and finally hair on the head and body. The author, with his theory of the fatty and the gluey, has an answer for everything: "You may perhaps wonder that there is much hair in the axillae and on the pubis, and in fact over the whole body. The same explanation holds there: in any part of the body where anything gluey happens to be present, there hair occurs because of the effect of heat."[75]

The Explanation of Thought and the Senses

The philosophers' inquiry into nature, as outlined by Socrates in the *Phaedo*, did not consist solely in retracing the genesis of living things, but also in giving an explanation for thought and the senses. This part of the program is also carried out in the *Fleshes*. Socrates joined various of his predecessors in wondering whether blood was the source of thought, or air, or fire, or else the brain. The answer given by the physician of the Hippocratic treatise is similar to the third solution mentioned by Socrates. According to him, it is heat: "I believe that what we call heat is in fact immortal, that it perceives all things, and sees, hears and knows all that is and all that will be."[76]

This is not, it should be pointed out, the answer that was to be attributed to Hippocrates by posterity. The richness and variety of the treatises of the Hippocratic Collection are such that most of the possible solutions mentioned by Socrates are upheld by one or another of them. According to the *Breaths*, blood is the source of thought.[77] The author of *The Sacred Disease*,[78] in a celebrated passage refuting those who locate the source of intelligence in the diaphragm and the heart, opts without hesitation for the brain. It is with this latter theory that the name of Hippocrates was later to be associated.

As for the explanation of the different sensations, this occupies an important place in the *Fleshes*, where it comes immediately after the discussion of the genesis of living things.[79] The author first explains hearing, then smell, vision, and finally speech, which the Hippocratics ranked among the senses.[80] He goes on to criticize the theory of those who held that hearing was to be explained by the brain—one of the theories noted by Socrates in the *Phaedo*—specifically identifying them as the authors of well-known treatises on nature: "There are some writers on nature who have said that it is the brain which echoes, but this cannot be so; for the brain itself is moist, and the membrane around it is moist and thick, and around the membrane there are bones; now nothing moist echoes, but rather what is dry, and it is what echoes that gives rise to hearing."[81]

In keeping with a quite admirable custom of scientific debate, men of learning in the Periclean Age refrained from citing each other by name, above all while they were still alive. Naturally, to historians of antiquity this habit seems deplorable. The authors of the treatises on nature whom the physician criticizes remain anonymous ("There are some writers on nature who . . . "). Similarly, the Socrates of the *Phaedo*, reporting the theory of the birth of living things by putrefaction, adds the qualification "as some say . . . "—not much help, that! It assuredly does not satisfy modern scholars, who, abhorring a vacuum, have patiently scoured the doxography of the pre-Socratics in the hope of being able to provide the anonymous with names; more particularly, they have sought to identify which pre-Socratic philosophers were the source of the theories expounded by the author of the *Fleshes*. Here again we encounter the same cohort of philosophers whose interest in biology we have already noted—Empedocles, Diogenes of Apollonia, Anaxagoras—along with the disciples of Heraclitus, Archelaus of Athens, and a few others.

But the *Fleshes* is not a mere compilation of philosophical works on nature. At least such a conclusion is not supported by the author's own statement of what he set out to do: "From here on, then," he says in his preamble, "I present opinions that are my own."[82] Why should we not believe him? This does not mean that everything found in the treatise is original. It is well to keep in mind that the ancients did not have the same conception of originality that we have. Even so, the coherence and novelty of his principle of explanation needs to be acknowledged: the fatty and the gluey, that fabulous pair, does indeed appear to have been his invention; there is no equivalent in the surviving doxography of the pre-Socratics. But still more than this, the role played by the personal experience of the author must be emphasized. To justify certain of his explanations (which, while sometimes correct, are often wrong), he appeals in a pertinent way to real life. Consider, for example, his passage on voice and speech, the interest of which will not be lost on linguists today. It is the earliest account of the physiology of voice and speech that has been preserved in its original form, and the only one we know of prior to Aristotle:

Speech takes place through air, by a person drawing it inside his whole body, but mostly into his hollow parts; as this air is forced out through the empty space, it produces sound through the resonance of the head. The tongue articulates by touching: as the tongue encloses the air in the throat and touches the palate and the teeth, it gives the sound clarity. If the tongue does not articulate by touching each time, the person does not speak clearly, but utters, as they all are by nature, mere sounds. A proof of this is that persons deaf from birth do not understand how to speak, but utter only mere sounds. Nor is it possible to speak, if you try to after breathing out. This is clear: when people wish to speak loudly, they draw in breath which they then force out and shout loudly as long as their breath lasts; then their voice dies away. Those who sing to the accompaniment of the lyre, when they must sing an extended passage, first forcefully draw in their breath as much as possible, and then greatly extend their delivery, and recite and sing loudly as long as they still have breath; when their breath is gone, they stop. From these examples, it will be clear that it is the breath that speaks. I have seen persons that have cut their own throats sever the throat completely: these may live, but they cannot speak, unless someone closes their throat: then they can speak. From this, too, it is clear that the person cannot draw his breath into the hollow spaces, because his throat has been cut, but instead sends his breath out through the cut. So it is with voice, and likewise with speech.[83]

The author is plainly more persuasive when he reports his own observation than when he is toying with philosophical notions such as the fatty and the gluey. His point with regard to the distinction between voice and speech is well taken. He is not to be reproached for not knowing of the vocal cords—Aristotle did not know of them either. The author of the *Fleshes* was a trained and careful observer. In the last case that he cites, having to do with patients whose throats had been cut, one is conscious of the extent to which philosophical discussions of nature are enriched by the physician's attention to detail.

This nonetheless is a singular and curious treatise of medicine, which speaks of diseases only in passing, and then only to tell us that they obey a septenary rhythm.[84] Its author was seduced by the same mirages that seduced the young Socrates. But how can we hold this against him? His work remains the only entirely preserved piece of evidence we have regarding the pre-Socratic inquiry into nature. If it has survived the ravages of time, paradoxically this is due to the fact that its author was a physician. But at this early stage in the development of anthropology, there was no longer any real difference between a philosophical physician and a medical philosopher.

Reactions against a Philosophical Medicine

The diversity of the Hippocratic Collection appears perhaps most clearly in connection with this question of the relation between philosophy and medicine.

To begin with, the philosophically minded treatises—that is to say, the ones that draw upon cosmology for their conception of the nature of man—are themselves a diverse lot. The theories they contain of man and the universe are as varied as those of the pre-Socratic philosophers. A century later, Isocrates was to scoff at the diversity of opinions among the "ancient sophists" (as he called the pre-Socratics) "who maintain, some of them, that the sum of things is made up of infinite elements; Empedocles that it is made up of four, with strife and love operating among them; Ion, of not more than three; Alcmaeon, of only two; Parmenides and Melissus, of one; and Gorgias, of none at all."[85]

One may say the same thing about the philosophically inclined physicians of the Hippocratic Collection. One of them is committed to monism: air, for the author of the *Breaths*, is the primordial element in both the universe and man, and the sole cause of all diseases. Another adopts a dualist solution: the author of the *Regimen* retains two opposed and complementary elements, fire and water. Another, the author of the *Fleshes*, advocates a cosmology involving three elements, heat, earth, and air; and still another, the author of the *Sevens*, is partial to the number seven and holds, in particular, that the soul-seed of man has seven natural parts: heat, cold, wet, blood, sour, sweet, and salty.[86]

But the diversity of opinion in the Hippocratic Collection regarding the relation between medicine and philosophy has to do mainly with the fact that it contains the traces of a quarrel over method, pitting the partisans of a philosophical medicine against opponents of such an approach.

Two treatises reacted vigorously against the philosophical tendency in medicine, affirming the autonomy of the medical art. The first was *Ancient Medicine*. This treatise has the great merit of posing the problem of method with supreme clarity. We have already seen how its author, a defender of traditional medicine, reconstructed the "archaeology" of his art.[87] The primary inspiration for this apologetic history was disagreement with those innovative physicians who aspired to found a new medicine on the basis of simple postulates, such as heat, cold, dryness, or moistness, in order to explain diseases.[88] These innovators were no doubt reacting against an excessive empiricism, wishing to base the art of medicine instead on one or two simple and clear principles, just as the philosophers relied upon a small number of fundamental elements to account for the diversity of the real world. But in the eyes of the author of *Ancient Medicine*, these simple postulates were too simple—they oversimplified reality, and so failed to explain it. He goes on next to broaden his attack to take in the entire movement of philosophical medicine. This brings him to the crucial moment of the treatise, where he scrupulously characterizes the method of his opponents and lucidly contrasts it with his own method. Let us listen first to the statement of his opponents' method: "Certain philosophers and physicians assert that nobody can know medicine who is ignorant what a man is; he who would treat patients properly must, they say, learn this. But the question they raise is one for philosophy; it is the province of those who, like Empedocles, have written on natural science, what man is from the beginning, how he came into being at the first, and from what elements he was originally constructed."[89]

In laying out the position of his adversaries, among whom he numbers Empedocles, the author of *Ancient Medicine* has the great virtue of taking it seriously and of emphasizing that it was based upon a methodological requirement. Medicine for these thinkers was not an autonomous science, for it presumed a prior knowledge of man. But what kind of knowledge was demanded? The reference to Empedocles already gives us a clue; and the questions needing to be answered that come next leave no doubt about the matter. The knowledge that was required—about the original formation of human life and about the basic constitution of human beings—was the very same knowledge demanded by the "inquiry into nature" that Socrates describes in the *Phaedo*.[90] In the minds of the Hippocratic author's opponents, medicine therefore presupposed a prior philosophical anthropology. It depended, in other words, upon cosmology.

By a rather extraordinary coincidence, the Hippocratic Collection itself preserves a passage in which a partisan of the philosophical approach to medicine affirms the methodological requirement mentioned by the author of *Ancient Medicine*, and in terms that are very similar to the ones used there. The passage in question is part of a prefatory statement by the author of the *Regimen*: "I maintain that he who aspires to treat correctly of human regimen must first acquire knowledge and discernment of the nature of man in general—knowledge of its primary constituents and discernment of the components by which it is controlled. For if he be ignorant of the primary constitution, he will be unable to gain knowledge of their effects: if he be ignorant of the controlling thing in the body he will not be capable of administering to a patient suitable treatment."[91] This coincidence is not necessarily to be explained by any direct connection between the two treatises; but it does, in any case, attest to the exactitude of the author of *Ancient Medicine* in characterizing the argument of his adversaries.

Immediately after having presented this thesis, the author states his own position. His argument against philosophical medicine amounts to turning the argument of his adversaries on its head by a simple inversion of terms. On his view, medicine does not need to be based on a prior knowledge of human nature; to the contrary, medicine—properly understood—is itself the source of knowledge of the nature of man:

I also hold that clear knowledge about natural science can be acquired from medicine and from no other source, and that one can attain this knowledge when medicine itself has been properly comprehended, but till then it is quite impossible. . . . Since this at least I think a physician must know, and be at great pains to know, about natural science, if he is going to perform aught of his duty, what man is in relation to food and drinks, and to habits generally, and what will be the effects of each on each individual. It is not sufficient to learn simply that cheese is a bad food, as it gives a pain to one who eats a surfeit of it; we must know what the pain is, the reasons for it, and which constituent of man is harmfully affected.[92]

This simple inversion of the premises of the problem entailed a considerable change in the method of knowledge to be employed and in the corresponding epistemological status of medicine. The physician was no longer to attempt to recreate man on the basis of certain basic elements, as a painter represents man using certain fundamental colors; he was to set himself the task, instead, of observing the various reactions of the human body to different influences of regimen (whether in the form of food, drink, or exercise). By means of this sort of causal analysis, of action and reaction, it became possible for the physician to determine the different categories of human nature. For the general notion of human nature, which fell under the head of philosophical knowledge (*phusis*), the physician substituted the various categories of human nature obtained by careful observation (*phusies*—the plural of *phusis*). The status of medicine as a branch of knowledge was thus altered as well. No longer was medicine obliged to tag along behind philosophical anthropology; medicine was now itself the science of man.

The second assault upon philosophical medicine is found at the beginning of the treatise *Nature of Man*. From the very first sentence, Polybus, Hippocrates' pupil and son-in-law, sharply attacks those who treat human nature as something beyond the limits of medicine: "He who is accustomed to hear speakers discuss the nature of man beyond its relations to medicine will not find the present account of any interest. For I do not say that a man is air, or fire, or water, or earth, or anything else that is not an obvious constituent of a man; such accounts I leave to those who care to give them."[93]

From the very outset, then, the motivation is analogous to that of *Ancient Medicine*, for the author of *Nature of Man* is prepared to challenge all knowledge of human nature whose source lies outside medicine; and the examples that he chooses clearly indicate that he is taking aim at philosophical conceptions of human nature derived from cosmology. But the argument takes a different direction to the extent that Polybus limits his attack to philosophical monists, which is to say to those philosophers who reduce everything to a single principle. He exploits the differences among their theories in such a way as to make them nullify each other, humorously allowing Melissus of Samos, the most celebrated of the monists, who was later to be cited by Isocrates as the paragon of this style of philosophy, to triumph over his rivals.[94] But Melissus, a disciple of Parmenides, thought that the unique element was neither air, nor fire, nor water, nor earth—which is to say that his principle was still less obvious than that of the other monists. Polybus goes on next to criticize those physicians who believed that man was constituted of a single humor, in order to establish that human nature is made up of four humors: blood, phlegm, yellow bile, and black bile.

This reaction by medicine against philosophy was not grasped by the two great philosophers of the fourth century. Plato, in the *Timaeus*, gives an account of philosophical medicine; and Aristotle, in his treatise *De sensu et sensibilibus*, emphasizes the close relation between philosophy and medicine: the good philosopher who studies nature, he says, studies medicine last, while the good physician who approaches his art in a sufficiently philosophical manner (*philosophôtérôs*) starts off by studying nature.[95] In the debate over method, Aristotle plainly takes the side of philosophical medicine.

Later, by contrast, Hippocrates' reaction against philosophical medicine was to be considered, at least by some authorities, to be the greatest of his virtue.[96] The Latin encyclopedist Celsus, in the preface to his *De medicina*, describes the birth of medicine in Greece in the following terms: "At first the science of healing was held to be part of philosophy. . . . Hence we find that many who professed philosophy became expert in medicine, the most celebrated being Pythagoras, Empedocles and Democritus. But it was, as some believe, a pupil of the last, Hippocrates of Cos, a man first and foremost worthy to be remembered, notable both for professional skill and for eloquence, who separated this branch of learning from the study of philosophy."[97]

PART IV

The Grandeur and
Limits of Hippocratism

Despite the many differences that may be detected among the works that make up the Hippocratic Collection—due to the personalities of their authors, to their belonging to different medical milieux, often indeed to different eras—and despite the internal disputes that divided some of the Hippocratic physicians—notably, as we have just seen, over the problem of medicine in relation to philosophy—one nonetheless finds a common stock of ideas and a common style of thought. The attitude these physicians share toward both patient and illness constitutes something that may be called Hippocratism.

In the middle sections of this book we have had occasion to insist upon certain important aspects of Hippocratism: the duty of the physician in his relationship with the patient, in the second part; and, in the third part, the physician's rational approach to illness and critical reflection about his work. We will not return to these matters in the fourth, and final, part that follows. It remains for us to complete our sketch of Hippocratism by insisting upon new aspects of it, such as the method of observation, the conception of health and illness, and the conception of nature; and also to judge the value of this tradition as a whole, drawing attention to its strengths without seeking to hide its weaknesses. Finally, we need to provide at least a glimpse of the richness and the complexity of the many interpretations that have been given to Hippocratism, from antiquity until our own day. Recounting the history of Hippocratism in detail is out of the question, however, for this would be as vast a project as giving a detailed account of the history of Aristotelianism.

From Observation of the Visible to
Reconstruction of the Invisible

One of the great strengths of the Hippocratic physician was his ability to observe, and then record, his observations with the most meticulous care. The patient was his chief source of observations. Observation of the patient, in turn, led him to make remarks of two kinds. Some are of a general nature and refer to the constitution common to all human beings; these may be called anatomical remarks. Others are of a particular nature and concern the clinical signs presented by each of the patients observed. While naturally these two kinds of remarks are closely related, it will nonetheless be convenient to distinguish them for purposes of analysis. Let us begin with clinical observation, which involves features that are more immediately accessible than those of internal anatomy, and therefore less in need of reconstruction on the basis of indirect evidence.

Clinical Observation

Everything that could be perceived regarding the manifestations of a disease was noted by the physician, for the least detail might provide a valuable clue.[1] Prognosis, like diagnosis, was only possible given a set of signs. Certain texts give advice regarding the manner of observing. This is to say that for the Hippocratic physician, observing was not simply a matter of looking; there was a whole art to observing. What, in his judgment, was required in order to observe properly? And what was it necessary to observe? With regard to the first question, the answer is clear. Observation was not a matter of sight alone: all the senses needed to be brought into play. Here is what one passage, a sort of surgeon's memorandum consisting of a series of concise notes, has to say about the initial phase of observation: "[Examination: look for] what is like or unlike the normal, beginning with the most marked signs and those easiest to recognize, open to all kinds of investigation, which can be seen, touched, and heard, which are open to all our senses, sight, touch, hearing, the nose, the tongue and the understanding, which can be known by all our sources of knowledge."[2]

It is difficult for us to imagine how many different interpretations this passage has inspired, from the time of the oldest commentators. From Galen, who himself commented on it, we are familiar with several of them. It is also difficult for us to imagine the lengths to which these ancient commentaries went in order to "save" Hippocrates from himself. In the passage just quoted, for example, he could not possibly have meant to write the same thing in two successive clauses—to have said not once, but twice, that the physician observes by sight, touch, and hearing. It needs to be kept in mind, however, that these were no more than rough notes, intended to recall and emphasize only the most important things. In this case the most important thing was that the physician mobilize all the means of knowledge available to him, corresponding to the five senses (sight, touch, hearing, smell, and taste) in addition to the understanding.

Two books of the *Epidemics* likewise contain advice regarding methods of observing the patient in the form of notes:

Crises, and the other things that give us knowledge, [are known] by the eyes, ears, nose, hand. [T]he ill person. [The operator] touching, smelling, or tasting, and knowing in the other ways. [Our sources of knowledge are] hair, complexion, skin, veins, tendons, muscles, flesh, bones, marrow, brain, the things from blood, the intestines, belly, bile, the other humors, joints . . . pulse, trembling, spasms, hiccups, things related to breathing, the exits, by which we know.[3]

The task is to bring the body under consideration. Vision, hearing, nose, touch, tongue, reasoning arrive at knowledge.[4]

These texts agree that observation of the patient by the physician must be made jointly by all the senses in conjunction with the understanding. If sight is put at the head of the list, this is not only because it furnishes the greatest number of observations; it is also because sight is normally the first sense to be called upon when the physician comes into contact with the patient. In some cases the physician had to formulate a tentative prognosis while yet a certain distance from the patient, and to make his initial examination by visual observation.[5] In any case, the first signs that the physician had to note in arriving at a patient's bedside were those perceptible by sight: first the patient's face, next the position assumed by the patient lying upon his bed (in technical language, the decubitus), and then the movement of the patient's hands. The author of the *Prognostic* made remarkably precise observations about all these things.

The Hippocratic Facies

The author's description of the alteration of the patient's facial features, announcing the approach of death and known as the "Hippocratic facies," was to remain the most famous description in the whole of the Hippocratic Collection. Here is what the physician says about observing the patient's visage:

First he must examine the face of the patient, and see whether it is like the faces of healthy people, and especially whether it is like its usual self. Such likenesses will be the best sign, and the greatest unlikeness will be the most dangerous sign. The latter will be as follows. Nose sharp, eyes hollow, temples sunken, ears cold and contracted with their lobes turned outwards, the skin about the face hard and tense and parched, the colour of the face as a whole being yellow or black. If at the beginning of the disease the face be like this, and if it be not yet possible with the other symptoms to make a complete prognosis, you must go on to inquire whether the patient has been sleepless, whether his bowels have been very loose, and whether he suffers at all from hunger. And if anything of the kind be confessed, you must consider the danger to be less. The crisis comes after a day and a night if through these causes the face has such an appearance. But should no such confession be made, and should a recovery not take place within this period, know that it is a sign of death. If the disease be of longer standing than three days when the face has these characteristics, go on to make the same inquiries as I ordered in the previous case, and also examine the other symptoms, both of the body generally and those of the eyes. For if they shun the light, or weep involuntarily, or are distorted, or if one becomes less than the other, if the whites be red or livid or have black veins in them, should rheum appear around the eyeballs, should they be restless or protruding or very sunken, or if the complexion of the whole face be changed—all these symptoms must be considered bad, in fact fatal. You must also examine the partial appearance of the eyes in sleep. For if a part of the white appear when the lids are closed, should the cause not be diarrhoea or purging, or should the patient not be in the habit of so sleeping, it is an unfavorable, in fact a very deadly symptom. But if, along with one of the other symptoms, eyelid, lip or nose be bent or livid, you must know that death is close at hand. It is also a deadly sign when the lips are loose, hanging, cold and very white.[6]

We need to consider the passage as a whole if we are to grasp the meaning of this account. Taken by itself, the description is of course remarkable as it stands: by means of a few observations regarding the nose, eyes, temples, ears, skin, and facial complexion (in connection with which four colors are mentioned), the physician is able immediately to provide details about the patient's condition that are at once evocative and significant; then, having given a general picture of the patient's visage as seen from a certain distance, the writer moves in for a close-up of the patient's eyes. This image corresponds to the moment when the physician draws near to the patient's bedside and takes a close look at his or her eyes, paying particular attention to their movement and to their color; with regard to their color, he looks carefully to see whether there are small black or blackish-blue veins in the whites of the eyes. But if this remarkable description is read apart from its full context, one misses the main conclusion that the author wishes to draw about the meaning of what has been observed. No particular observation or sign has absolute meaning in and of itself; its meaning, which in principle is to be interpreted in terms of the gap between health and illness in a given instance, depends in fact on a number of different variables: the individual patient with his various habits and physical particularities, the timing of the illness, the presence or absence of incidental causes, such as insomnia, diarrhea, or fasting, and the presence or absence of other signs. Information about these things, obtained by questioning the patient, thus helps to establish the relative value of the observed visual signs.

Carphology

It goes without saying that visual observation does not go beyond what can be perceived by the naked eye. Only long after the time of Hippocrates was the physician to discover the world of microbiology, thanks to the microscope, whose invention dates from the seventeenth century. But the practiced eye of the Hippocratic physician saw details that the eye of the modern physician no longer sees, since there is no longer any need to see them; modern instruments of analysis have taken its place. Several visual observations originally due to Hippocratic physicians nonetheless remain part of the inheritance of modern science, and are still associated with certain significant symptoms. The Hippocratic physicians were the first, for example, to notice what is called carphology.

The word "carphology" comes from the Greek *karphologia*, meaning "action of picking up [*legein*] whisps of straw or twigs [*karphos*]." The foundational text of carphology is to be found in the treatise *Prognostic*. It is based on an observation recorded in a brief but remarkable passage on the motion of the hands of the patient: "As to the motions of the [hands], I observe the following facts. In acute fevers, pneumonia, phrenitis and headache, if they move before the face, hunt in the empty air, pluck nap from the bedclothes, *pick up [whisps of straw] [karphologeousas]*, and snatch chaff from the walls—all these signs are bad, in fact deadly."[7]

This text can be understood only if one imagines the patient lying in a bed, one of whose long sides is against a wall made of cob, a mixture of clay and straw, and covered with blankets of rather coarse wool. The gestures of the hands, picking up or snatching at something, are noted with the most extreme precision. The patient's hand picks up a whisp of straw (or a twig) lying on the bed, or plucks bits of wool from the blanket, or snatches straw sticking out from the cob wall. Carphology, as it is described here, corresponds therefore only to that first gesture: picking up a whisp of straw (or a twig) from the bed. This is still the sense that one meets with in Galen, though there the gesture consists in picking up imaginary sticks of straw or twigs. Of the three significant gestures noted by the Hippocratic physician, the physicians of Galen's time retained only two: the gesture of picking up sticks of straw on the bed, to which they gave the name *karphologia*, and the gesture of plucking flocks of wool from the blankets, to which they gave the name *krokudismos*, from which the old technical word "crocydism" was derived. This latter term is still attested in Émile Littré's dictionary, but the definition that Littré gives is not exact, even though he had an excellent knowledge of ancient medicine, for he takes it to be synonymous with "carphology." The talent of ancient physicians for distinguishing different signs with the greatest finesse and giving them precise names no longer suits the habit of the modern mind, which looks to group things together rather than to tell them apart, with the result that the subtle distinctions of the ancients are no longer understood. Thus what were considered distinct things by the Hippocratic physician were regarded as synonymous by Littré. A further stage in the disappearance of formerly customary distinctions was reached with the removal of the word *crocydism* from modern dictionaries—so completely that the term "carphology" is currently used in a general way to denote "the activity of searching and of incessant palpation by hands and fingers observed during confused states (typhus, delirium tremens, for example)."[8] Moderns therefore group together under the term "carphology" all the manual gestures that the author of the *Prognostic* had so finely distinguished.

Digital Hippocratism

Of all the visual observations made in the Hippocratic Collection, only one—"Hippocratic fingers"—is still associated with the memory of Hippocrates in modern dictionaries of medicine. This syndrome is described in one such dictionary in the following terms:

Deformation of the fingers (and often of the toes as well) characterized by:
   1. A lateral and longitudinal incurving of the nails with the elimination and then

the inversion of the angle normally made by the plane of the nail with that of the dorsal side of the last phalanx;

2. A massive hypertrophy of the phalangette, swelling the extremity of the finger in the shape of a drumstick. Digital Hippocratism may be genetically determined through dominant autosomatic transmission. It is most often secondary to various thoracic affections, exceptionally extrathoracic affections. Digital Hippocratism may be considered a minor form of the hypertrophic osteoarthropathy [associated with the name] of Pierre Marie.[9]

It is interesting to compare this modern statement with what Hippocratic physicians actually observed. It turns out that they observed both more and less than what is included in the foregoing definition. The text that serves as the basic reference in this case is once again taken from the *Prognostic*. There the author enumerates the identifying signs of empyema; that is to say, the disease characterized by a collection of pus in the thorax and in the lung:

All sufferers of empyema may be distinguished by the following symptoms. In the first place the fever never stops, being slight during the day but more severe at night; copious sweats occur; the patient has a desire to cough, without bringing up any sputum worth speaking of; the eyes become sunken; the cheeks are flushed; the finger-nails are bent and the fingers grow hot, especially at the tips; the feet swell up; blisters rise about the body, and the appetite fails.[10]

The author does indeed mention the curvature of the fingernails as a sign of thoracic disease. But to the mind of the Hippocratic physician, this sign belonged to a larger set of signs that together were necessary for purposes of diagnosis. Tradition has therefore selected just one sign from among many. The author of the *Prognostic* nonetheless was not the only physician in the Hippocratic Collection to have noted this symptom.[11] Others likewise observed it in the case of empyema, and also in several other pneumopathies.[12] If the Hippocratic physicians remarked the incurving of the nails among the signs of thoracic disease, they did not, however, mention the swelling of the fingertips, which assume (in modern parlance) a "drumstick" shape. The author of the *Prognostic* did, of course, make an observation about the extremities of the fingers: he noted they were hot; but he did not say anything more than this. Thus the second observation that moderns subsume under the head of digital Hippocratism cannot be traced back to Hippocrates. This observation was not to be made until the first century A.D., almost five hundred years later, when it was noted by another Greek physician, Aretaeus of Cappadocia, in his remarkable description of consumption. The passage concerning fingers and nails is as follows: "[F]ingers slender, but joints thick;

of the bones alone the figure remains, for the fleshy parts are wasted; the nails of the fingers crooked, their pulps are shriveled and flat, for, owing to the loss of flesh, they neither retain their tension nor rotundity; and, owing to the same cause, the nails are bent."[13]

Aretaeus therefore noted the flattening of the pulpar extremity of the fingers, which had not been mentioned by Hippocrates. But while neither Hippocrates nor his followers noticed this symptom, they regularly recorded, along with incurvation of the nails, a swelling of the feet.[14] The significance of the link between these two symptoms was grasped by modern physicians only with the description of a new syndrome at the end of the nineteenth century by a French clinician, Pierre Marie, in connection with pulmonary diseases. Here is a part of his description: "The hands are enormous and deformed. Their dimensions are more surprising than those of acromegalics. The volume of all of the phalanges of the fingers are increased, but above all in the case of the phalangette. The nail is enlarged, lengthened; it has the Hippocratic appearance of a parrot's beak. The wrist is enlarged, forming an abrupt and enormous depression above the hand. The feet have the appearance of those of elephants."[15]

It is interesting that the modern clinician should have consciously recognized the symptom of the nail as Hippocratic (comparing it further to the beak of a parrot), probably without realizing that the swollen feet were a related symptom in the Hippocratic literature. He was surely not aware, however, that he had also rediscovered the symptom long before noted by Aretaeus in the passage just cited concerning the thickened joints of the fingers. The convergence of these symptoms in Marie's account suffices to demonstrate the superior powers of observation displayed by ancient Greek physicians. They had succeeded in observing several of the symptoms that form what modern physicians call hypertrophic osteoarthropy; on the other hand, they did not understand that these deformations—which Aretaeus explained by a diminution of flesh—were due instead to an osseous hypertrophy.

In summary, then, while the Hippocratic physicians did not note all of the signs that today are comprehended by the term "digital Hippocratism," they did anticipate the syndrome described by Pierre Marie in noting the incurvation of the fingernails together with the swelling of the feet in cases of thoracic disease.

These three examples—Hippocratic facies, carphology, and digital Hippocratism—are in any case enough to illustrate the talent of Hippocratic physicians for observing the patient by sight alone.

Observation by Touch

Following the order of the senses relevant to observation given in the surgeon's memorandum, touch came next after sight. Again, this would seem to correspond to the natural sequence of events in the physician's examination of the patient. Having begun by observing the patient at a distance, whether in the case of a person suffering from a wound or of a person affected by an acute disease, the physician drew closer in order to touch the patient. In the case of injury, the physician touched the lesion in order to be able to judge the nature of it more accurately. In the case of internal illness, the physician first palpated the hypochondria—literally, the "parts located under the cartilage"; that is to say, the lateral regions of the abdomen under the ribs. Ancient physicians attached great importance to this part of the body. It is better known today for having lent its name to an illness characterized by anxiety, the cause of which was thought to reside in the intestines lodged within the hypochondria. While this illness was not yet known in Hippocrates' time, the Hippocratic physician nonetheless showed himself to be extremely attentive to any signs noticed in this area. The author of the *Prognostic* devotes a quite long section to it, longer than that concerning any other part of the body. A few excerpts will suffice to give some idea of the prognostic value that the Hippocratic physician assigned to it, especially on the basis of tactile observation:

> It is best for the hypochondrium to be free from pain, soft, and with the right and left sides even; but should it be inflamed, painful, distended, or should it have the right side uneven with the left—all these signs are warnings. If there should be throbbing as well in the hypochondrium, it indicates a disturbance or delirium. . . . A swelling in the hypochondrium that is hard and painful is the worst, if it extend all over the hypochondrium; should it be on one side only it is less dangerous on the left. Such swellings at the commencement indicate that soon there will be a danger of death. . . . Swellings that are soft and painless, *yielding to the finger,* cause the crises to be later, and are less dangerous than those just described.[16]

The deliberate mention at the end of this passage of the physician's finger, which pushes down upon a part of the body that in turn yields to its pressure, leaves no doubt that examination in this case was by touch. Many other passages in the Hippocratic Collection also expressly refer to the finger of the physician, used to palpate parts of the patient's body as part of prognostic or diagnostic evaluation. In particular, digital examination of the vagina is often mentioned in the gynecological treatises.[17] The physician palpated a part of the body sometimes to determine whether it was sensitive to pain, but also for the purpose of soliciting other observations. Several of these deserve to be noted: for example, when the physician presses his finger upon a swelling that appears after the treatment of a fracture, "the redness is removed but quickly returns";[18] or, in a variety of ileus, when the physician presses the body with his finger lightly at any point, particularly on the feet, "it receives [its] impression there as if in dough";[19] otherwise, in a case of peripneumonia, the physician's finger irritates the tongue on touching it.[20] These were not the only parts of the body that the physician felt; he had occasion also to feel what the body rejected. One treatise mentions twice that the physician touches the pus expectorated by a patient: in one instance, a case of empyema, the pus is sticky to the touch; in another, a case of consumption, the pus is hard when pressed between the fingers.[21] The physician might also, of course, touch the patient in order to gauge the heat of the body. Thus, in the *Coan Prenotions*, mention is made of patients who "are not burning hot to the touch."[22] The reader need not be reminded that the Hippocratic physician was not yet able to quantify body temperature, knowing nothing of the thermometer, which was to be discovered only much later, at the beginning of the seventeenth century, by medical researchers at Padua.

Direct Auscultation

After sight and touch, the list of senses given in the treatise *In the Surgery* mentions hearing. The physician needed to know how to listen. Certain physicians of the Hippocratic Collection practiced direct auscultation in the case of thoracic maladies; that is, holding the ear against the chest of the patient and listening for internal sounds. One passage in particular very clearly attests this practice: "If you apply your ear for a long time and listen to the sides, it seethes inside like vinegar."[23]

In another case, a squeaking sound is heard like that obtained by rubbing leather.[24] We know now that this sound corresponds to pleural fremitus; but Hippocratic physicians, who were unaware of the existence of the pleura, could not have recognized it as such. Nonetheless, their observation was remarkably accurate, and the comparison with the noise made by leather is still employed in modern textbooks of medicine, which make reference to the rubbing of "new leather." What is more, these physicians were not satisfied merely with passive auscultation, but actually induced internal sounds of fluctuation by shaking the patient before listening in order to determine where to make an incision for the evacuation of water or of pus. The process is well described: "[S]eat him on a chair that does not move; have someone else hold his arms, and you shake him by the shoulders, listening on which of his sides there is a sound."[25] This sound is specified in other passages by a picturesque verb that denotes the sound made by an agitated liquid, one that washes up against the sides of a vase, like a wave crashing against rocks on a shore. It was therefore a fluctuating sound.[26]

The procedure of direct auscultation, whether or not accompanied by the succussion of the patient, was thereafter forgotten or only poorly known for quite a long time. It was not until the beginning of the nineteenth century that Laënnec was again to call attention to it. Laënnec was thoroughly familiar with the Hippocratic Collection, having written his doctoral thesis on Hippocrates, and recalled in his celebrated treatise *De l'auscultation médiate* that Hippocrates' passages on auscultation suddenly came to mind once more when he embarked upon his own research.[27] Moreover, he himself practiced both direct and mediate auscultation by applying Hippocrates' method of shaking the patient. In several of his case studies, or in "observations" he made on the basis of these, he makes this quite clear: "The patient having been shaken according to the Hippocratic method, a sound of fluctuating liquid was plainly heard";[28] and again: "I then announced that by shaking the torso of the patient the fluctuation of the liquid would be heard. The shock produced according to the Hippocratic procedure in fact achieved this result in the most obvious way."[29] Laënnec thus rendered homage both to Hippocrates' method and to the exactitude of his observation. This did not prevent him from criticizing Hippocrates for certain errors in diagnosis, however, in spite of the rather primitive knowledge of pathological anatomy in classical Greece. For example, he reproaches Hippocrates for not having realized that the sound of fluctuation was the result of what is now called pneumothorax, or the passage of air into the pleural cavity following the rupture of the lung wall. The founder of modern anatomopathology nonetheless remained faithful to the Hippocratic spirit—to what he called "Hippocratic empiricism, which is to say [theory] illuminated by the observation of man living and dead, the connecting of facts with one another, and a very restricted use of the inductive method."[30]

Observation by Smell and by Taste

Lastly, smell and taste are mentioned as being necessary for the proper examination of the patient. Although information about the use of these two senses is found much more rarely in the pedagogical treatises of the Hippocratic Collection, it is clear that the physician sniffed, and possibly tasted, in the course of observing the prognostic signs furnished by all bodily excretions and secretions, including sweats, stools, vomitings, expectorations, suppurations, and, in the case of women, vaginal discharges. Obviously smell was called for more often than taste. One physician sniffed the stools of adults, which he said "have the odor of the stools of small children."[31] He must have had a sensitive nose. Another such physician mentioned foul-smelling sweats.[32] Another observed a vaginal discharge that was "fetid like a rotten egg."[33] Yet another rubbed expectorated pus between his fingers and, sniffing it, noted its foul smell.[34] A foul smell was generally an unfavorable sign: according to the author of the *Prognostic*, healthy stools ought not be "over-fetid," whereas fetid ones are deadly;[35] and all foul-smelling vomits are detrimental.[36] One passage in *Diseases II* relating to the prognosis of a thoracic illness foretells the death of the patient in the event that the pus he expectorates is "livid, yellow-green and evil-smelling."[37]

Physicians plainly exercised greater discretion with regard to what they tasted. It is certain that they tasted tears, and probably other excretions as well, in order to determine whether they were very sweet or salty.[38] Did they go as far as to taste stools? A passage in Aristophanes' *Plutus* implies that they did. In the incubation scene, which we spoke of earlier in connection with miraculous healings at Epidaurus, a witness named Carion tells a woman of the coming of the god Asclepius during the night to treat the ill:

> *Woman*: And the god hadn't come to you?
> *Carion*: Not yet. Then I did something really funny. As he was approaching, I let out an enormous fart, for my stomach was bloated.
> *Woman*: Surely he took an immediate dislike to you for that?
> *Carion*: No, but Iaso, who was following him, blushed slightly and Panacea turned away holding her nose. For when I break wind, it's not incense.
> *Woman*: And the god himself?
> *Carion*: By Zeus, he didn't even notice it.
> *Woman*: Then this god of whom you speak is a lout.
> *Carion*: No, by Zeus! But he is a scatophage![39]

As an excrement-eater, then, Asclepius was said to be the equal of a dung-beetle! Was this irreverent way of characterizing the god of medicine merely an instance of exaggeration for comic effect? Or was it meant to suggest, to the contrary, that physicians actually were scatophages, that they really did go so far as to taste stools? The evidence of the Hippocratic Collection does not permit us to give a clear answer to this question.

Observation and Reason

In the pedagogical passages of the collection, where authors give advice about the way in which to conduct an examination of the patient, the list of senses is completed by mention of intelligence (*gnomè*), or reason in the sense of faculty of calculation (*logismos*). Although in such passages the authors do not explicitly describe the role of this faculty, they regarded it as being on the same level with the other senses; it had to do—at least from the point of view of an author such as that of the *Prognostic*, who represents the most authentic version of Hippocratism—with reckoning (*logizesthai*) the relative value of the observed signs. This calculation consisted, first, of determining the value of each sign as a function of the various parameters that might have an influence upon its weight in comparison with that of the others.

It suffices to take the example of the Hippocratic facies. The theoretical value of each sign depends on the gap that separates the pathological state from the normal state. But this theoretical value may vary as a function of particular circumstances (peculiar to the patient) or accidental circumstances (such as insomnia, fasting, diarrhea, and so on), which must be established by questioning the patient. Depending on the responses given, the calculation of the value of the sign may be altered. To take a specific example, when the physician sees a patient whose face is gaunt and distraught, if he learns that the patient's hunger is due to not having been given enough to eat, or to not having gotten enough sleep the preceding night, then the prognosis will be less unfavorable than otherwise.

Next, and most important, the physician's calculation consisted in arriving at a global judgment of the value attaching to the whole set of observed signs. The author of the *Prognostic* is very clear in this connection. Several general maxims can be extracted from particular passages of the treatise and from the conclusion:

You must *take into account* both the good signs and the bad that occur and from them make your predictions; for in this way you will prophesy aright.[40]

[T]he doctor must pay sharp attention to [these and] all the other symptoms also from the very first day.[41]

He who would make accurate forecasts as to those who will recover, and those who will die, and whether the disease will last a greater or less number of days, must understand all the symptoms thoroughly and be able to appreciate them, *estimating* their powers when they are compared with one another.[42]

In reality, to judge from the lists of things that the physician needed to take into account in order to form a judgment, complete knowledge of all the relevant signs was an immense undertaking. Here is the most striking such list:

The following [are] the circumstances attending the diseases, from which [we frame our] judgments, learning from the common nature of all and the particular nature of the individual, from the disease, the patient, the regimen prescribed and the prescriber—for these make a diagnosis more favorable or less; from the constitution, both as a whole and with respect to the parts, of the weather and of each region; from the custom, mode of life, practices and ages of each patient; from talk, manner, silence, thoughts, sleep or absence of sleep, the nature and time of dreams, pluckings, scratchings, tears; from the exacerbations, stools, urine, sputa, vomit, the antecedents and consequents of each member in the successions of diseases, and the abscessions to a fatal issue or a crisis, sweat, rigor, chill, cough, sneezes, hiccoughs, breathing, belchings, flatulence, silent or noisy, hemorrhages, and hemorrhoids. From these things we must consider what their consequents will also be.[43]

What is surprising about this list is both the multiplicity of the points of view needing to be adopted and the absence of a hierarchical organization. All the signs requiring examination are treated as having the same weight and are piled up one on top of another in a catalog that seems to take on epic proportions, though it was intended only as a sort of guide for the attending physician. The modern mind expects such signs to be grouped together under clearly defined heads, with the essential things being distinguished from the incidental; the modern mind, in a word, expects something more in the way of a synthesis. No matter that Aristotle did not get any further than Hippocrates in this direction—the virtues of the Hippocratic spirit are in any case to be found elsewhere: in its prodigious memory and, no less surely, in its attention to the least detail, every detail being considered as potentially significant. The sort of synthesis to which we are accustomed was not achieved in the writing of the physician, which was meant simply to recollect the various points needing to be examined, but in the practice of the physician, who in the course of actual examination needed to take into account the full range of signs in order to arrive at an evaluation of the patient's condition and to formulate a prognosis.

Case Studies of Patients

The result of this concern for even the smallest details was that the Hippocratic physicians kept records of their patients, noting on a day-by-day basis those symptoms they judged significant, from the onset of illness until its typically fatal outcome. This is the first time that case histories of patients appear in the history of medicine.

Studies of individual illnesses were known prior to Greek medicine. In Egypt, medical works were composed of a succession of brief remarks about various diseases. This style of composition also existed, as we have seen, in certain nosological treatises of the Hippocratic Collection, traditionally attributed to the Asclepiads of Cnidus. These Greek treatises display a remarkable gift for observation in their descriptions of diseases, particularly with regard to the practice of direct auscultation just mentioned.

But records of individual patients first emerged from the school of Hippocrates that earlier had left Cos for Thessaly.[44] They are preserved in the series of treatises entitled *Epidemics*. Some idea of how many case studies these contain can be had by considering that books I and III, which constitute the oldest group, by themselves contain forty-two carefully written cases. Galen counted fifty individual cases in book V.[45] If all these cases were to be brought together, they would form a tragedy in a hundred different acts. Some of these acts possess their own unity in time. Thus one patient, sustaining an injury to his liver in the morning, dies in the evening: "The one hit by a javelin at the liver was immediately suffused with a deathly color; hollow eyes; distressful restlessness. He died before the closing of the marketplace (he was struck at daybreak)."[46]

To be sure, the writing of a physician who notes with the greatest detachment what he judges significant for the instruction of his colleagues is not the same as that of the tragic author who accumulates pathetic details to impress his audience. One recalls, for example, the account in the *Medea* of Euripides of the young and beautiful bride who succumbs to the poisoned gift of her rival; nothing of that sort is to be found among the physicians. Nonetheless, emotion sometimes manages to break through the objectivity of the account. Thus the daughter of Nerius met a tragic fate:

> The pretty virgin daughter of Nerius was twenty years old. She was struck on the *bregma*[47] by the flat of the hand of a young woman friend in play. At the time she became blind and breathless, and when she went home fever seized her immediately, her head ached, and there was redness about her face. On the seventh day foul-smelling pus came out around the right ear, reddish, more than a cyathus.[48] She seemed better, and was relieved. Again she was prostrated by the fever; she was depressed, speechless; the right side of her face was drawn up; she had difficulty breathing; there was a spasmodic trembling. Her tongue was paralyzed, her eye stricken. On the ninth day she died.[49]

In mentioning the young woman's age—she was only twenty years old—the author probably had a medical reason: the long catalog of signs to be observed by the physician that we looked at a moment ago includes the age of the patient; but it certainly did not say anything about noting a patient's beauty. One can hardly fail to see a tragic contrast between the initial evocation of the beauty of this young woman, playing with her friends, like Homer's Nausicaa, and then, after an apparently harmless but in fact fatal accident, the twisted visage and fixed gaze of some eight days later. The presence of a single, medically useless adjective gives a pathetic cast to the whole description. The physician, while calmly and objectively noting the unbearably sad details of the case, is hardly insensitive to the tragedy unfolding before his eyes. But such expressions of subjective feeling as we find here, though they could be conveyed in just a word or two, are exceptional. Their absence, however, does not detract from the fascination of these descriptions, which evoke the daily experience of life and of illness in ancient Greece. Faced with so many to choose from, it is hard to select one that is representative. Here, for example, is a particularly detailed description:

The wife of Theodorus, greatly in fever, hemorrhage having occurred, in winter. The fever abated the second day; shortly afterwards she had heaviness of the right side, as from the womb. This was the first time it had happened. On succeeding days the pain in the chest was terrible. With fomentations on the right side she improved. On the fourth day, the pains; the breathing quicker. Her trachea whistled as she breathed with difficulty. She lay on her back; difficulty turning over. Towards night the fever grew more acute. There was, briefly, delirious talk. Early on the fifth day the fever seemed more mild. Sweat poured from her forehead, briefly at first, then for a long period over her whole body and feet. After this she thought the burning had grown less, and her body was cooler to the touch, but the vessels of the temples jumped more, her breath was more rapid, she talked deliriously from time to time, and all signs changed for the worse. Throughout, the tongue was extremely white; there was no cough except on the third and fifth day for a short time. There was no thirst, but expectoration. The right hypochondrium was much swollen on the fifth day but afterwards softer. Some solid excrement on the third day after a suppository. On the fifth again, a little liquid. The belly soft. Urine astringent, like [silphium] juice. The eyes as of one who is weary. She had difficulty seeing things and looking about. On the fifth day towards night, difficulty and delirious talk. On the sixth, again, at the same hour, that of the filling of the marketplace, much sweat poured from her. It went from the forehead to the whole body for a long time. She conducted herself rationally. Towards midday, however, she talked very deliriously, the chilling was similar but she had greater heaviness all over the body. Towards evening her lower leg slipped out of bed, she threatened her child irrationally and again fell silent, changed into quiescence. About the first sleep, thirst. Much delirium: she sat up and rebuked those who were there. Again she fell silent and remained quiescent. She seemed to be in a coma the rest of the night. She did not close her eyes. Towards day she answered mostly with nods, her body unmoving, reasonably alert. Again the sweat at the same hour. The eyes similarly downcast, leaning more on the lower lid, staring, torpid, the whites of the eyes yellowish and corpselike. Her whole color yellowish and dark. Mostly reaching with her hand towards the wall or the bedclothes. The gurgling occurred when she drank, and she spurted it out and brought it up through her nose. She plucked at the blankets, and kept her face covered up. After the sweats her hands were like ice. Cold sweat persisted. Body cold to the touch. She jumped up, cried out, raved. Breathing very rapid. She developed trembling in the hands. At the point of death she twitched. She died on the seventh day. She urinated a little . . . on the sixth day in the night. The urine was picked up on a twig, sticky, like semen. Sleepless all nights. After the sixth day bloody urine.[50]

This description, considering the brevity of the illness, is one of the most developed of all the studies of individual patients contained in the *Epidemics*. It tries to note the evolution of the signs not only from day to day, but also over the course of the day and throughout the night.[51] The senses of the physician are fully alert: sight, to be sure (the most extraordinary of the many visual observations being that of the leg that hangs outside the bed); touch (the hand of the physician palpating the hypochondrium and other parts of the body to gauge the degree of heat or cold); taste, or possibly smell (the urine is said to be astringent and like silphium juice); finally, hearing (the physician noting the slight whistling of air through the trachea and the heavy sounds of swallowing). His account gives the impression of being spontaneous and drawn from life: a detail like that of the woman scolding her child for no reason rings true indeed. The apparent sponteneity fails, however, to mask the fact that the physician's description is informed by prior training. It exhibits a precise knowledge of the many points needing to be examined and noted: the season, the presence of fever and of pains, the patient's breathing, her position in bed, the state of different parts of the body, the eyes, the veins in the temples, the hands, the hypochondria, as well as all secretions and excretions, including spittle, stools, and urine; also evidence of disordered states of consciousness, with a distinction being made between two degrees of confusion, incoherent talk and fits of madness.

What is more, since the description contains ellipses and leaves various things unsaid, only specialists can decipher its full meaning. The signs are noted, but their significance is generally not given. It presumes on the part of the reader a knowledge of the intrinsic value of each of these signs, corresponding to the instruction imparted by the treatise *Prognostic*, which functions for the modern student as a sort of decoding manual for the case studies contained in the *Epidemics*. In fact, echoes of much of the teaching of the *Prognostic* are to be heard here. Let us take only a few examples. With regard to the decubitus of the patient, the author notes that she is lying on her back and that she has difficulty turning over; now, according to the *Prognostic*, lying on one's back is a less favorable sign than lying on one's side, which is the position of a person in health;[52] being able to turn over easily is a favorable sign as well.[53] In respect of the eyes, the physician notes that the patient slept heavily during the night between the sixth and seventh days without the eyelids being closed; the author of the *Prognostic* notes that if the eyelids are not closed during sleep, it is an unfortunate sign, heralding death.[54] In fact, the patient dies on the seventh day. Only by knowing the intrinsic value of each of the signs can the seriousness of the symptoms be fully comprehended. On the seventh day it is noted that the patient's sweat is cold. According to the *Prognostic*, "[w]orst are the cold sweats."[55] Finally, to conclude with the movements of the hands, one recognizes in the observation of the hand that touches the wall and blanket and plucks bits of wool the famous sign of "carphology" (in the broad sense of the term), which the author of the *Prognostic* judges quite fatal.[56] Here it appears on the seventh day—the very day on which the patient dies.

Plainly, the talent of the Hippocratic physicians for clinical description was developed to a nearly perfect degree. As far as possible, they took advantage of what was perceptible by the senses and attempted, by means of the understanding, to determine its prognostic value. But the Hippocratic art of external observation was considerably limited in view of the obstacle presented by their ignorance of the invisible world inside the body.

The Reconstruction of an Invisible Internal World

Some of these physicians were aware that the passage from the visible to the invisible presented an obstacle. The one who formulated the problem most clearly was the author of *The Art*, who made a distinction between illnesses whose seat is near the surface of the skin and illnesses that reside in the cavities of the body. Whereas the former may be perceived by sight and by touch, the others are hidden from view: "Without doubt no man who sees only with his eyes can know anything of [the internal parts of the body that have] been here described. It is for this reason that I have called them obscure, even as they have been judged to be by the art."

Then, having succinctly identified the problem, he continues with excessive optimism: "Their obscurity, however, does not mean that they are our masters, but as far as is possible they have been mastered, a possibility limited only by the capacity of the sick to be examined and of researchers to conduct research. More pains, in fact, and quite as much time, are required to know them as if they were seen with the eyes; for what escapes the eyesight is mastered by the eye of the mind."[57]

From these few lines it is clear, on the one hand, that the Hippocratic physicians did not make internal observations of the human body by means of dissection, and, on the other, that they tried to get around the problem of the invisible by drawing upon the resources of the understanding.

Animal Dissection

The Hippocratic authors never directly addressed the question whether they could, or should, practice dissection on human beings. They neither spoke about it nor engaged in it. Was the subject taboo? Human dissection was not practiced in Aristotle's time either. Strictly speaking, one ought not speak of human "anatomy" during this period, if one recalls that the term signifies etymologically the "action of opening by cutting" (anatomè).[58] This activity occurred only later, as an aspect of medical practice at Alexandria during the Hellenistic era; the Greeks of the classical period had no direct experience of it. Had they themselves adopted this ritual practice—the embalming of cadavers—they would have acquired firsthand knowledge of the internal structure of the human body.[59]

This does not mean that dissection was not practiced on animals. Aristotle, in any case, clearly attests that the study of the internal parts of man was made by comparison with animals: "[T]he inner parts . . . are for the most part unknown—at least, those of man are, and hence we have to refer to those of other animals, the natural structure of whose parts those of man resemble, and examine them."[60]

In obtaining knowledge of the internal anatomy of animals, a religious rite no doubt facilitated matters. The rite of animal sacrifice, which involved opening up an animal and examining its entrails for the purpose of predicting the future, was commonly practiced in Greece during the classical era. Naturally, this practice favored the study of animal anatomy. Thus Aristotle, in order to demonstrate the surprising proposition that the heart is not liable to any serious accident,[61] explicitly makes reference to ritual observation: "Never has the heart in a sacrificial victim been observed to be affected in the way that the other viscera sometimes are. Very often the kidneys are found to be full of stones, growths, and small abscesses; so is the liver, and the lung, and especially the spleen."[62]

We may conclude then, that a form of animal anatomopathology connected with hieroscopy (literally, "examination of consecrated victims") already existed during Hippocrates' time. Moreover, a fully developed semiotics was employed by specialists in the art of inspecting the entrails of animals. The art of reading favorable or dire signs in these entrails, as a way of foretelling the future, bears comparison with the art of the Hippocratic physicians, who read the future of an illness in the visible signs, favorable or dire, presented by the patient.

Animal dissections were also no doubt carried out independently of the ritual of sacrifice as well. One recalls the opening of the skull of the single-horned goat by Anaxagoras, who observed the conformation of the brain in order to deduce from it a rational explanation that directly contradicted the interpretation of a soothsayer.[63] Aristotle, for his part, made reference to autopsies conducted on animals that had died from disease.[64] What do we find among the Hippocratic physicians? They were much more guarded than Aristotle about disclosing the sources of their knowledge about the internal structure of parts of the body. What is surprising is that they give no explanation of the way in which they came by such knowledge, even in the case of a long and detailed exposition relating to the interior of the body. For example, when Hippocrates' disciple Polybus gives an extensive description of the blood vessels in his treatise *Nature of Man*,[65] he dispenses this learning without offering any justification, as if it were all perfectly obvious. The same thing occurs when the author of *The Sacred Disease* describes at length the brain and the system of blood vessels.[66] What we find, in short, is a "magisterial" kind of authority concerning a subject which was nonetheless admitted to be obscure in principle. Galen gives a reason for this silence:

I commend Marinus, who has written on anatomical procedure, without criticizing my other predecessors who have not. For them it was superfluous to compose memoranda for themselves or others since they practiced dissection from childhood under parental instruction, as they did reading and writing. And it was not only professional physicians among our predecessors who studied anatomy, but also general philosophers. One so instructed from his earliest years would no more forget what he had learned from experience than would others the alphabet.[67]

The oral transmission of learning within the great medical families, then, is what accounted for this silence about anatomical sources. In the same passage, Galen adds that to his knowledge the first anatomical treatise was due to Diocles of Carystus, a physician of the fourth century B.C. To Galen's mind, this could only have been a treatise of animal anatomy. While the Hippocratic Collection is not entirely free of references to animal dissection, mention of it is rare, and intended not to provide a justification for a given anatomical description but rather proof of a certain opinion about pathology. The best-known passage is the one where the author of *The Sacred Disease* opens the skulls of animals affected by epilepsy to note the pathological state of the brain and to show that it did not have a divine cause.[68] Another physician takes into account the dissection that he carried out on three species of animals affected by dropsy in order to observe their lungs:

The disease also arises if tubercles form in the lung, fill up with fluid, and rupture into the chest. (That dropsy truly does also arise from tubercles, here is my proof from the cow, swine and dog. tubercles containing fluid occur most frequently among quadrupeds in the lungs of these animals, as you would very quickly discover by cutting through one, for water will run out; and it seems probable that in man such things are present much more than in animals, since we employ a more unhealthy regimen.)[69]

The merit of this passage is that it shows clearly how the author proceeds by induction. On the basis of an observation about dissected animals, he infers that man is also the victim of tumefactions in the lung.[70]

Limits of Anatomical Knowledge

Because Hippocratic physicians did not practice dissection on human beings and therefore had to reconstruct the internal structures of the human body on the basis either of what they saw or felt by means of superficial examination or of what they observed in animal dissections, it is not surprising that their knowledge of this internal world, which remained for the most part closed off to them, should have been partial, erroneous, and indeed quite odd. One often risks compounding the mistakes of these authors, however, by employing terms that assume a level of knowledge they did not possess. We must put aside all the learning of modern medicine if we wish to understand the medical knowledge of the ancients.

Even such simple words as "organs," "nerves," "veins," and "arteries" cannot be used without anachronism. The Hippocratic physicians were naturally acquainted with the principal organs, such as the brain, the heart, the lungs, the liver, the kidneys, the spleen, and the bladder, all of which were located in the two great cavities separated by the diaphragm, the "upper" cavity and the "lower" cavity. But they did not yet call them organs—this is an Aristotelian concept. They spoke instead of "structures," for they defined these parts of the body more by their form than by their function. The modern word "nerves," although it comes from the Greek *neura*, a word commonly used by the Hippocratics, no longer corresponds to what they understood by it. They confounded tendons and nerves, and did not know what we call the nervous system; for them, these were simply ligaments that served to hold the body together and to stimulate movement according to their degree of tension, which might be greater or less. Accordingly, while they were familiar with muscles, they were ignorant of their ability to be contracted. They were of course well aware of the fibrous conduits that carry the blood, but they called these *phlebes* (from which we derive our word "phlebitis") and, by and large, did not yet make a distinction between veins and arteries.[71] The word "artery" designated what we now call the trachea, which is in fact an abbreviation of the Greek *arteria tracheia*.[72] The arterial pulse had not yet been discovered, and was not to be of use in diagnosis until the Hellenistic period.[73] Throbbing veins, particularly in the temples, were well noted, but only insofar as they represented pathological disturbances.[74] In Hippocrates' time one should therefore speak instead of "vessels," with the understanding that these vessels were believed to transport not only blood but also air, and possibly other humors as well.

The arrangement of these vessels inside the body was still rather arbitrary. Each of the major descriptions contained in the Hippocratic Collection proposes its own overall system.[75] The system's starting point is apt to differ from account to account. Obviously the Hippocratic physicians had no notion of the circulation of the blood, which was to be discovered only in the seventeenth century by Harvey. One believed that the head was the point of departure for the vessels, another the liver and the spleen, still another the heart. Paradoxically, the description that since Aristotle's time has been the most famous is also the most curious. To show that his predecessors derived the vessels from the head and that he was the first to have seen that the heart is the starting point of the system, Aristotle cites as an example the long description by Polybus found in *Nature of Man*. This account, due to one of Hippocrates' most illustrious disciples, features four pairs of vessels descending from the head to the feet, with ramifications in the arms, but, remarkably, makes no mention whatsoever of the heart.

It is probably in connection with the female genital apparatus that the Hippocratic physicians displayed the most imagination. The womb, to which they rightly attributed the cause of feminine complaints,[76] was made to undergo strange travels throughout the entire body. The claim that it was liable to deviations or to different kinds of prolapse seems reasonable enough, and in fact we know it to be true; but that it was supposed to sink down into the legs, causing convulsions of the big toe, or to move in the direction of the liver, the hip, the loins, or the ribs, or to rise up as far as the heart, or even the head, is a continual source of amazement in a medicine that otherwise had succeeded in ridding itself of all traces of magic.[77] The womb seems sometimes to enjoy a life of its own in the Hippocratic writings. In one place we see a dessicated womb "run" to climb up toward the moist and throw itself upon the humor-filled liver, suffocating the woman as a result.[78] In another, a certain kind of prolapse is thought to be explained by saying that a heated womb "rushes" toward the cool of the outside.[79] Such metaphors are the holdovers of ancient mental representations in which certain parts of the body were considered to be autonomous living beings.

Not everything in the Hippocratic description of the internal world is quite this odd. For example, the disposition and form of the bones were more easily grasped than those of the vessels or of the uterus. The surgical treatises exhibit a rather remarkable knowledge of the human skeleton, and above all a clear awareness of the necessity of being perfectly acquainted with the shape of bones and ligaments in order to diagnose and correctly treat dislocations and fractures. Thus the author of *On Joints*, after having given a precise description of the spinal column,[80] denounces with both reason and emotion the ignorance of certain of his colleagues who confused the (benign) fracture of the spinous process of a vertebra with a (serious) forward displacement of the whole vertebra—that is, a slipped disk:

The spinal cord . . . would suffer, if the luxation due to jerking out of a vertebra had made so sharp a curve [forward]; and the vertebra in springing out would press on the cord, even if it did not break it. The cord, then, being compressed and intercepted, would produce complete narcosis of many large and important parts, so that the physician would not have to trouble about how to adjust the vertebra, in the presence of many other urgent complications. So, then, the impossibility of reducing such a dislocation either by succussion or any other method is obvious, unless after cutting open the patient, one inserted the hand into the body cavity and made pressure from within outwards. One might do this with a corpse, but hardly with a living patient. Why then am I writing this? Because some think they have cured patients whose vertebrae had fallen inwards with complete disarticulation; and there are even some also who think this is the easiest distortion to recover from, not even requiring reduction, but that such injuries get well of themselves. There are many ignorant practitioners; and they profit by their ignorance, for they get credit with their neighbors. Now this is how they are deceived. They think that the projecting ridge along the spine represents the vertebrae themselves, because each of the processes feels rounded on palpation.[81]

This Hippocratic physician manifestly understood the seriousness of the effects of a lesion of the spinal cord. His account shows that anatomical knowledge could vary dramatically from one physician to another, however, and that the best instructed among them were perfectly aware of the fact. The main reason for this state of affairs was the absence of any unified system of medical instruction. The perspicacity of the author of *On Joints* is proof, finally, that the most competent physicians, despite the deficiency of their anatomical knowledge in certain respects, were capable from time to time of reasoning correctly about what for them was an invisible world, inside the human body.

The Limits of Hippocratic Physiology

But when one moves from anatomy to physiology, the gaps in the knowledge of the Hippocratic physicians become still more serious and the necessity of reconstruction even more obvious. Physiological functions as vital as breathing and digestion received no satisfactory explanation. There is a great contrast between the precision with which certain physicians observed difficulties in breathing in order to deduce prognostic signs from them[82] and the explanations that others gave to account for normal breathing. They did, of course, accurately note the importance of air for life: "So great is the need of wind for all bodies that while a man can be deprived of everything else, both food and drink, for two, three, or more days, and live, yet if the wind passages into the body be cut off he will die in a brief part of a day, showing that the greatest need for a body is wind. Moreover, all other activities of a man are intermittent, for life is full of changes; but breathing is continuous for all mortal creatures, inspiration and expiration being alternate."[83]

But just as certain Hippocratic authors were able to describe the system of blood vessels without reference to the heart, certain others—and not the least important among them—were able to describe the course of air throughout the body without involving the lungs in any essential way. The same author who made these sensible remarks about the importance of air for life and who regarded air as the primordial element, in the universe no less than in man, nowhere makes reference to the lungs. It is true that he did not propose to explain the mechanism of respiration, but to demonstrate that diseases have a unique cause; namely, air.[84] But when an author does venture to provide such explanations, the results are scarcely more encouraging. Thus the author of *The Sacred Disease*, whose lucidity is rightly to be admired when he criticizes the divine conception of epilepsy,[85] proposes a physiology of breathing so far-fetched that the air breathed in by the mouth and by the nostrils is supposed to go first to the brain and then down into the belly;[86] only incidentally does it pass into the lungs. Other Hippocratic physicians clearly distinguished the esophagus, which empties into the stomach, from the trachea and the bronchial tubes, which lead to the lung—but theirs are probably more recent treatises.[87] However this may be, none of these authors had the slightest idea of alveolo-capillary gaseous exchanges, nor of the role of the circulation of the blood. They believed that air passed through the same vessels as blood. Correct observations often led to false conclusions. The author of *The Sacred Disease* correctly observed, for example, that the limbs could go numb when blood vessels were constricted; but he took this to be proof that air moves through these vessels along with blood.[88] Others believed more accurately that blood, rather than air, passes into the limbs of the body via these vessels.[89]

The phenomenon of digestion was understood in vague and metaphorical terms. What is astonishing is that in Hippocrates' time there was not yet a specific term denoting the stomach. The word "stomach" itself comes from the Greek *stomachos*. This word, derived in turn from *stoma*, meaning "mouth," was normally employed in Hippocrates' time to refer to the esophagus. Another word did exist, however, that might have been used specially to designate the stomach; namely, *gaster/gastros*,[90] from which are derived a number of modern medical terms relating to this organ. Gastroenterology, for example, is the branch of medicine devoted to the study of the stomach and intestines. But in Hippocrates' time, the word *gaster* signified not only the stomach but also in a general way the "belly," or abdomen, and could be used to indicate where a pregnant woman carried her child. What is more, physicians used yet another word, the vague term *koiliè* (cavity) to refer to the belly when they spoke of digestion.[91] The stomach proper was not yet in Hippocrates' time regarded as an important internal organ.[92] As far as digestion was concerned, this was conceived as a sort of struggle between man and food, resulting, in the case of normal digestion, in the triumph of the former over the latter; but it was also conceived as a kind of cooking in a pot, or, alternatively again, as fermentation in a vat. These three explanations were occasionally treated as one.[93] Even for Aristotle, digestion was a form of cooking.[94]

Hippocratic Humorism

The one domain of Hippocratic physiology where the imagination of certain physicians succeeded in erecting a system of perfect clarity, in order to account for an entirely obscure interior world, is that of the humors.

Observation of the different liquids that drained out of the body, in the healthy state but especially in the case of injuries and various diseases, not unreasonably inclined the ancient Greek mind to picture such liquids as "flowing" (*rhein*) within the body, since they came out of the body in a stream (in the form of spittle, urine, stools, discharges through the eyes and ears). The "more obvious symptoms, which all of us experience and will continue so to do," as one author says, are associated with a "cold in the head, with discharge [*rheuma*] from the nostrils."[95] What could be more natural than to imagine that this discharge came, like a spring, from some higher place, which is to say from the head and the brain? This conception survives still today in the French phrase for a head cold, "*rhume de cerveau*" (literally, a brain stream—"*rhume*" coming from the Greek *rheuma*). But to go beyond this rather simple metaphor, constructing on the basis of it a highly detailed system of "humors" that move up and down and around the body, involved a rather remarkable leap of the imagination. The Hippocratic imagination was equal to the task. It was chiefly from the brain that the humors were supposed to flow into the various parts of the body; but if the brain was capable of giving rise to so many humoral streams, this was because it attracted them from the rest of the body. One quite curious passage in the treatise *Ancient Medicine*, in which the author describes what we call the organs (and that he called "structures"), clearly shows the sort of role that ancient physicians were liable to assign to the various organs in connection with the motion of the humors inside the body.[96] The form and texture of these organs was held to determine their function. The ones that attracted the most humors were pear-shaped—the head, of course, but also the bladder and, in women, the womb; those that were most capable of absorbing the humors by contact were the spongy and porous organs—the spleen, the lungs, and the breasts.

Not only the internal course of the humors was reconstructed but also their number. Humors such as blood and bile were easily observable in daily experience (from wounds, sacrificial cooking, and so on) and as a result were well known before the Hippocratic age. The need for reconstruction was much greater for other humors such as phlegm and, particularly, the distinction between yellow bile and black bile. The etymology of the word "phlegm," for example, reveals a strange prehistory. In Hippocrates' time it was generally considered to be the coldest humor, predominant in winter.[97] But, etymologically, the word *phlegma* denoted fire; this was the meaning it had in Homer. It must be supposed therefore that when the term came to be employed in medicine, it initially signified an inflammation; that later it acquired the more specialized sense of a humor resulting from inflammation; and that eventually it came to denote—exactly how, we cannot say—a natural humor such as bile and, ultimately, by an unsuspected reversal of meaning, the coldest humor of the body.[98] The subsequent evolution in the meaning of the word after the Hippocratic period deserves also to be noted briefly. Persons in whom this cold humor was dominant (that is, phlegmatics) were said to have a cold and slow temperament: thus, the modern sense of "phlegmatic" and "phlegm," as well as in some languages of the colloquial variant for "laziness" (*flemme* in French, for example)—a strange fate indeed for a word that almost three millennia ago meant "fire." But it testifies, too, to the astonishing survival of the humoral theory of the ancient Hippocratic physicians in our language today. Modern medicine got rid of its humoral heritage when it became clear that it was no more than a clumsy reconstruction of reality; the humor "phlegm," as a result, has entirely disappeared from modern medical dictionaries. But these same dictionaries preserve the word "phlegmon" (from the Greek *phlegmonè*, well attested in Hippocrates and denoting an inflammation) as the name of a malady. The modern meaning of this term, which refers to an acute inflammation of the cellular tissues, has therefore remained faithful to the earliest medical sense of its etymological root.

There is no point dwelling on the various humoral theories of the Hippocratic physicians. Though they occupy a large place in many treatises, and had a quite prolonged influence on both medicine and the philosophical conception of man, they constitute the most outdated aspect of the Hippocratic heritage. For the moment it is enough to indicate that there was no single humoral theory to which all the Hippocratic physicians subscribed. Once again, the diversity of their opinions with regard to the number and kind of the humors supposed to make up human nature was equal to the diversity of opinion among pre-Socratic philosophers with regard to the constitutive elements of the universe. In the humoral pathology of the Hippocratics, two humors, bile and phlegm, play an essential role in several treatises. But the humoral theory that was to remain attached to the name of Hippocrates (no matter that it was actually the invention of his disciple Polybus) was that of the four humors: blood, phlegm, yellow bile, and black bile. In Hippocrates' time, it was only one theory among others.[99] However, the clearness with which it was stated, and the coherence of a system in which these four humors were related not only to the four elementary qualities (hot, cold, dry, wet) but also to the four seasons (winter, spring, summer, fall), no doubt help account for its widespread diffusion during the succeeding centuries, considering, too, Galen's role as an intermediary.[100]

These various theories, devised to account for what went on inside the body, were impressed upon the minds of certain Hippocratic physicians with such force that these authors sometimes sought to explain what was perfectly visible by appeal to the invisible. To take just one example from among many, the author of the *Haemorrhoids*, though he had actually examined hemorrhoids with his speculum and described clever methods for treating them, begins his treatise with this decisive phrase regarding the cause of the affection:

> The condition of haemorrhoids arises as follows. When bile or phlegm becomes fixed in the vessels of the anus, it heats the blood in them so that, being heated, they attract blood from their nearest neighbors. As the vessels fill up, the interior of the anus becomes prominent and the heads of the vessels are raised above its surface, where they are partly abraded by the faeces passing out, and partly overcome by the blood collected inside them, and so spurt out blood, usually during defecation, but occasionally at other times as well.[101]

Despite accurate observation of the dilation of the anorectal veins, the humoral theory of bile and phlegm interposes itself, serving to explain the visible by the invisible.

The Analogical Method: The Visible as Model for the Reconstruction of the Invisible

Physicians were thus apt to arrive at a position that was the very opposite of the one they sought to establish. Since they were conscious of the difficulties involved in penetrating the obscure world inside the body, they generally attempted to guide and to justify their reconstruction of invisible internal phenomena by analogy with the visible phenomena of the outside world.

The author of *Ancient Medicine*, in proposing his theory of the function of the organs ("structures") according to their configuration, affirms that pear-shaped ones are best adapted to attracting humors, and then goes on to declare:

One should learn this thoroughly from *unenclosed objects that can be seen*. For example, if you open the mouth wide you will draw in no fluid; but if you protrude and contract it, compressing the lips, and then insert a tube, you can easily draw up any liquid you wish. Again, cupping instruments, which are broad and tapering, are so constructed on purpose to draw and attract blood from the flesh. There are many other instruments of a similar nature. Of the parts within the human frame, the bladder, the head, and the womb are of this structure.[102]

This is without question the most representative example that can be given of the analogical method as practiced by the Hippocratics: the law is clearly formulated and two external phenomena are cited for purposes of reference, one drawn from daily experience (the attraction of liquid by the mouth), the other from medical practice (the attraction of liquid by a cupping glass).

Such a method obviously was not peculiar to physicians. The pre-Socratic philosophers, to the extent that they were interested in man in the way that physicians were, found themselves confronted with the same difficulties and used the same analogical method. The visible was a criterion of the invisible. This method has remained associated with the name of Anaxagoras, who had a felicitous expression for it that Democritus liked and that subsequently became a proverb: "The visible is the eye of the invisible."[103] But a fine phrase does not necessarily imply authorship. Empedocles, whose work predates that of Anaxagoras though he was the younger of the two, had already applied this method in a celebrated passage of his poem *On Nature*, in which he explains the mechanism of breathing by analogy with the behavior of water and air in a clepsydra.[104] Moreover, it was applied not only to man but also to the unexplored parts of the earth. The historian Herodotus, Hippocrates' contemporary (and neighbor), applied it to these domains in a rather singular manner. In "arguing from what is seen to what is not known," to use his terms, he reconstructed the upper course of the Nile, which was unknown, by analogy with the (symmetrical) course of the Danube.[105] In the event, "what is seen" was scarcely that: the Danube, Herodotus tells us, had its source among the Celts in the city known in ancient times as Pyrene (Pyrenaeus to the Romans)—which lent its name to the mountains we call today the Pyrenees. Aristotle was to correct the error, saying that it was a mountain rather than a city, but he continued to locate the source of the Danube there. One can readily see that this kind of analogical reasoning was liable to lead to false conclusions, causing authors to leap from poorly established facts into the unknown, which they sought to reconstruct on the basis of implicit rational categories that better suited a geometrical mind than a geographical map.

Hippocratic physicians continued more or less consciously to employ the same method when they tried to reconstruct aspects of physiology and pathology. The ones who seem boldest to us today are the ones who saw man in the image of the universe. This amounted to explaining the invisible by the invisible. For the most part, however, external phenomena much nearer to hand served as points of reference, as was the case in the example just quoted from *Ancient Medicine*. Among all the Hippocratic physicians, one—the author of *Generation / Nature of the Child*—stands out for his constant use of this form of reasoning in appealing to everyday reality. He was truly a giant in the art of analogy.[106] Analogy manages even to creep into passages of his treatise dealing with physiology, where one least expects it. Consider, for example, these two analogies drawn from everyday life that are slipped into a learned argument comparing a woman's pleasure in sexual relations with that of a man:

Among women, I maintain, as the genital parts are rubbed and the womb made to move in the course of union, a sort of titilation arises in the womb that provokes pleasure and heat in the rest of the body. The woman also emits a seed coming from the body, either into the womb—the womb then becomes wet—or to the outside, if the womb is more gaping than is suitable. And the woman experiences pleasure from the moment she begins to couple, during the whole time, until the man releases her. In fact, if the woman passionately desires union, she emits the seed before the man and the rest of the time her pleasure is no longer so intense. Everything occurs as when one pours water into boiling water: the water ceases to boil; in the same way the man's seed falling into the womb extinguishes the heat and the pleasure of the woman. But the pleasure and the heat are intensified at the very moment when the seed falls into the womb; then they cease. It is like pouring wine on a flame: the flame intensifies at first and increases for a brief instant from contact with the wine that is poured [on it], then ceases; in the same way in the woman the heat intensifies on contact with the seed of the man, then ceases. The woman experiences a less intense pleasure than the man, but feels it longer than he does. Why does the man feel a more intense pleasure? Because the excretion coming from the wet occurs abruptly in him following a greater disturbance than in the woman.[107]

The seed of the man therefore has a double effect, apparently contradictory, upon the pleasure of the woman. It extinguishes her pleasure, but momentarily arouses it beforehand. Two analogies illuminate this effect: cold water poured into boiling water and wine poured over a flame. The first analogy refers to cooking; the second, which appears the more unusual of the two to the modern mind, probably refers to ritual libations where wine is spilled onto a fire. It will be recalled that, in Homer's *Iliad*, Achilles offers libations of wine to the pyre of Patrocles and orders it to be extinguished with the wine.[108] Such a reference to ritual practices should not seem shocking. Religion among the Greeks was part of everyday life. The same author does not hesitate to compare the normal discharge of the lochies (*lochia*) to that of the blood of a sacrificial victim.[109] Sacrificial practice even had an influence on technical medical vocabulary. The Greek noun signifying throat-cutting (*sphagè*) also designated the part of the neck that was cut, and the vessels that we call the carotids were called in Hippocrates' time the sphagitids; that is, the throat-cutting vessels.[110]

The fields from which Greek physicians drew visible evidence in order to deduce by analogy the internal functioning of the human body were quite varied, among them plants, animals, and arts; but cooking in the broad sense of the term remained the preferred field of reference. The pot of water that boils on the fire, whose use in explaining the woman's pleasure in sexual relations we have just noted, was explicitly or implicitly one of the privileged models of explanation for the internal functioning of the body, from the physiology of digestion to the pathology of fevers. We have seen that digestion was regarded as a sort of cooking.[111] One author accounts for the yawns that accompany fevers by the mass of air that passes out from the mouth, and justifies his explanation by comparison with the steam that rises from a pot when water boils; similarly, he holds that the sweats that accompany fevers arise from blood vaporized by the heat and condensed upon the blood vessel walls, just as steam rises from a pot of boiling water and condenses on the lid.[112] Along with the model of the pot used to account for internal vaporization and condensation, there is another having to do with the manufacture of cheese and butter that serves to explain coagulation and separation. The coagulation of cheese by a juice, with the whey separated out, was familiar to the Greeks; among the Hippocratics it was used by their great specialist in analogy, the author of *Generation / Nature of the Child*, to explain the coagulation and separation of internal humors during the cold of winter.[113] But this author refines the analogy by seasoning his demonstrations with a dash of exoticism. To explain the influence of the heat of summer on the internal humors, which thus find themselves heated and agitated, he transports his reader all the way to Scythia—a land renowned for its cold climate—for the analogy he seeks is to be located in a special cheese made there from mare's-milk, called "hippace":

What happens [in the body] is comparable to what the Scythians do with mare's milk. Pouring the milk into wooden vessels, they shake it. The shaken part foams and separates: the fatty part, which is called butter, remains at the surface, due to the fact that it is light; the heavy and thick part remains at the bottom—[this is the] part that they separate and dry; when it is coagulated and dried, it is called hippace—; the whey remains in the middle. In the same way too in man, all that is moist being shaken in the body, under the influence of the first causes of which I have spoken, all the humors in him are separated: bile remains at the surface, for it is the lightest humor; next, blood; after that, phlegm; the heaviest of all the humors is water.[114]

The humors inside the body, when they are heated and shaken, separate into layers, like the butter, cheese, and whey of faraway Scythia. Everything now becomes clear!

In all these examples, the analogical method consists in observing what goes on in external reality in order to illuminate what goes on internally. In the latter example, the author contents himself with describing the practice of the Scythians. But the method can be taken a step further by devising a rudimentary experiment involving external reality in such a way that it will cast light upon internal reality. One of the laws that ancient physicians and philosophers invoked to explain the differentiation of the parts of the embryo was that like tends toward like. Aristotle was to combat this notion.[115] But our great specialist in analogies invokes and justifies it by an experiment, or rather by an embryonic experiment:

If one attaches a tube to a goatskin, introducing by means of this tube some earth, sand, and fine shavings of lead, and after having poured in some water one blows through the tube, first these elements will be mixed with the water, then under the effect of prolonged breathing the lead will go towards the lead, the sand towards the sand, the earth towards the earth. And if one lets [the inside] dry and examines the bladder after having opened it up, one will discover that like has gone towards like. In the same way, the seed and the flesh are formed and each like part goes towards its own kind.[116]

This analogy is no more convincing than the preceding one. It is true in its way, but one cannot help but feel that it takes only the first halting steps in the direction of genuine experiment. The author is attempting to recreate in external reality what he imagines to be the conditions to which the embryo is subject in the womb. The tube stands for the umbilical cord; the goatskin is the outer membrane surrounding the foetus; the air breathed into the bladder replicates, according to the author, the breath that the embryo receives through the umbilical cord from its mother. As for the different ingredients introduced into the bladder, mixed together at first but then separated under the influence of the breathing, these correspond to the flesh of the embryo, which initially is undifferentiated but then becomes articulated to form the distinct parts of the body of the child. All this is very rudimentary. But the comparison, inherited by Ionian science from Homeric epic, is imperceptibly tranformed into a method of investigation for deciphering the invisible with the help of the visible.

Not all Hippocratic physicians allowed themselves to be carried away to the same degree by the temptation to reason by analogy. Let us conclude this section on the reconstruction of the internal world with the more prudent and more scientific position of the physician whom we cited at the outset in order to introduce the problem, the author of *The Art*. Like Anaxagoras, he had a feeling for words. Both of them toyed with paradox in searching for an eye with which to scrutinize the invisible. But while for Anaxagoras it was the visible itself that, by analogy, became the eye of the invisible, for this Hippocratic author the eye of the invisible was the understanding.

Are these simply different ways of stating the same thing? Not entirely. For the physician's method was no longer analogical; it was interpretive. It no longer amounted to reconstructing the invisible by analogical transposition of the visible; it was a way of deciphering the invisible through the interpretation of visible signs. Though the inside of the body is invisible, it allows visible signs to escape, such as the "clearness or roughness of the voice, rapidity or slowness of respiration, and for the customary discharges the ways through which they severally pass, sometimes smell, sometimes colour, sometimes thinness or thickness."[117] The physician takes this category of signs as an evaluative criterion for judging which places inside the body are affected and what ills are being suffered. He even knows how to induce these signs artificially when they do not naturally reveal themselves. Thus the physician makes a patient climb a hill, for example, or makes him run a certain distance so that his breathing will reveal what it is needed to reveal. This was an altogether original idea. To be sure, one finds elsewhere in the Hippocratic Collection the notion that evacuations of all sorts are indispensable signs for diagnosis and prognosis. But nowhere else is the point so clearly expressed that these signs, whether noted or induced, enable the physician to interpret the invisible. "The principle of this exploratory method," Charles Daremburg was to comment many centuries later, "has survived in the practice of medicine and surgery; only its application has been modified by the progress of medicine and of science."[118]

THIRTEEN

Health, Sickness, and Nature

Hippocratic Reflection on Health

Health is a notion that occurs often in the writings of the Hippocratic physicians. One counts more than seven hundred uses of the Greek terms designating health (*hygiès* and *hygieia*). Admittedly, these words express a concept that is not entirely comparable to our own. The Greek concept of health is both more restricted, to the extent that it has a positive value and denotes "good health,"[1] and broader, for it also takes in the idea of "healing."[2] Given, then, that the words designating health belong also to the vocabulary of healing, it is natural to encounter them in the writings of a physician. But the reason they appear as frequently as they do is that the Hippocratic physicians had reflected profoundly upon health and upon the relation between health and sickness.

Health was, in Hippocrates' time, the supreme value in both the eyes of the people and those of physicians. Popular sentiment was echoed by poetry. A drinking song attributed either to Simonides or to Epicharmus, both poets of the sixth to the fifth centuries to whom Plato refers several times, establishes a hierarchy among the goods that a human being may desire and places health first, before beauty and wealth: "[T]o enjoy good health is the best thing; second is to have turned out good looking; and third—so the writer of the song puts it—is to be honestly rich."[3]

Health was considered by the Greeks to be so great a good that they deified it. There existed in fact a goddess Hygieia, the hypostasis of health, whose cult developed from the fifth century alongside that of Asclepius. She was the most venerated of the daughters of the god of medicine. Poets composed hymns in her honor.[4] Sculptors represented her either next to Asclepius or alone, feeding the god's sacred serpent, which is wrapped around her. At the

Asclepieum of Cos in the third century B.C., she was pictured as part of a group, sculpted by the son of Praxiteles, representing Asclepius and his entire family: Hygieia was placed at her father's side, and Asclepius shown touching her with his right hand.[5]

Physicians did not challenge the privileged position accorded to health by general opinion. To the contrary, they were staunch defenders of it. When the Sophist Gorgias defined rhetoric as the science of discourses that concern the most important human affairs, Socrates gets him to say that physicians would not fail to contest his claim. Here is the brief fictive dialogue that Socrates reports in this connection: "First the doctor said: 'Socrates, Gorgias is telling you a lie. It isn't his craft that is concerned with the greatest good for humankind, but mine.' If I then asked him, 'What are you, to say that?' I suppose he'd say that he's a doctor. 'What's this you're saying? Is the product of your craft really the greatest good?' 'Of course, Socrates,' I suppose he'd say, 'seeing that its product is health. What greater good for humankind is there than health?' "[6]

Certain statements of the Hippocratic physicians corroborate the portrait of the physician sketched by Socrates. "[N]either wealth nor anything else is of any value without health," says one of them;[7] "health is of the utmost value to human beings," says another.[8] As for the goddess Hygieia, she is present among the healing divinities whom the disciple invokes at the outset of *The Oath*: "I swear by Apollo Physician, by Asclepius, by Hygieia, by Panacea and by all the gods and goddesses." Even if this reference to Hygieia has had no influence on medical practice, it confirms the importance that Hippocratic physicians accorded to health.

Hygienics and Sports Medicine

Being a precious good, health must first be preserved. According to Galen's long treatise *On Preserving Health*,[9] medicine comprises two parts, preserving health and reestablishing health. In Hippocrates' time, preventive medicine was certainly not yet well developed. There exists no treatise exclusively devoted to the regimen of people in health.[10] Nonetheless, certain passages in the Hippocratic Collection bear upon this subject. The last part of the *Nature of Man* describes the regimen that seems to its author to be best advised for remaining in good health; regimen, it will be recalled, was taken to involve not only diet but also exercises and baths. This broad regime, suitably adapted to the individual, varies according to the season: "So in fixing regimen pay attention to age, season, habit, land, and physique, and counteract the prevailing heat or cold. For in this way will the best health be enjoyed."[11]

The treatise *Regimen* also devotes a long chapter to the regimen to be followed by season when one is in good health. This section displays similarities with that of the *Nature of Man*, but it is more complex.[12] The same tradition was to be pursued in the fourth century by the physician Diocles of Carystus, nicknamed the young Hippocrates, from whom we possess a long fragment detailing the regimen to be followed during the course of the day from waking till sleeping—yet another regimen that varied according to the seasons.[13] In short, there existed already in classical Greece a form of hygienics.

There existed also a kind of sports medicine. The training of heavyweight athletes participating in various contests of the Pan-Hellenic Games necessitated a special regimen. In addition to sports training proper, which was the responsibility of professional trainers, such athletes were forced to follow a meat-based diet to develop their strength and weight. This diet was not without its dangers for the health of such athletes.[14] Therefore it is not surprising trainers should have been keenly interested in dietetics,[15] nor that, conversely, physicians did not totally neglect the regimen of athletes. In his description of the regimen of people in health, the author of *Nature of Man* explicitly makes reference to the enforced regimen of athletes.[16]

Despite the growing attention to hygienics and sports medicine, which corresponds more generally to the development of dietetics in Hippocrates' time, the essential purpose of medicine remained to eliminate illness. According to the author of *The Art*, its object "is to do away with the sufferings of the sick [and] to lessen the violence of their diseases."[17] Thus the concept of health was most often considered in close relation to that of illness. This is particularly true of the theoretical definitions of health contained in the Hippocratic Collection, which are inseparable from the definitions of illness.

Hippocratic Definitions of Health and Illness

"Who among us," the philosopher Epictetus has the common man ask, "did not use the terms 'healthy' and 'diseased' before Hippocrates was born?"[18] By that he meant to imply that every man has an intuitive notion of health and illness. But at the same time Epictetus stressed that it was only from the time of Hippocrates that a serious attempt was made to examine the reality underlying these preconceptions.

The two principal definitions of health and illness attributed to Hippocrates are found in the two treatises where philosophy is rejected and the inde-

pendence of medicine is affirmed. The author of *Ancient Medicine*, after having criticized those physicians who reduce the cause of diseases to one or two
principles such as the hot, the cold, the dry, or the moist, states his own
doctrine on the nature of man, the state of nonsickness, and the state of
sickness. Here is his definition: "[F]or there is in man salt and bitter, sweet and
acid, astringent and insipid, and a vast number of other things, possessing
properties of all sorts, both in number and in strength. These, when mixed
and compounded with one another are neither apparent nor do they hurt a
man; but when one of them is separated off, and stands alone, then it is
apparent and hurts a man."[19]

Health is defined both negatively, by the absence of suffering, and positively, by the balanced mixture of the constitutive elements of man. But insofar as
this mixture holds together, the elements do not manifest themselves. In its
negative aspect this definition was to inspire a certain number of modern
definitions of health. "When we are well," Diderot was later to observe, "no
part of the body tells us of its existence; if one informs us of it through pain,
this is a sure sign that we are ill."[20]

In a similar manner, the author of *Nature of Man*, after having criticized
those philosophers and physicians who maintain that man is formed from a
unique principle, states his own doctrine about the nature of man, health (this
time defined positively), and illness:

The body of man has in itself blood, phlegm, yellow bile and black bile; these
make up the nature of his body, and through these he feels pain or enjoys health. Now
he enjoys the most perfect health when these elements are duly proportioned [*métriôs*]
to one another in respect of compounding, power and bulk, and when they are
perfectly mingled. Pain is felt when one of these elements is in defect or excess, or is
isolated in the body without being compounded with all the others. For when an
element is isolated and stands by itself, not only must the place which it left become
diseased, but the place where it stands in a flood must, because of the excess, cause
pain and distress.[21]

Despite divergences on points of detail regarding the elements that make
up the nature of man, these two definitions are comparable. In each, health
and sickness are radically opposed states. Health is defined by the mixing, or
crasis, of all the constitutive elements of the human body, and sickness by the
contrary concepts of separation and isolation of one element in relation to the
others. To this notion of mixture the author of *Nature of Man* adds that of
"measure," which is to say due proportion, or balance, among the elements.

It is probably accidental that the two chief Hippocratic definitions of health and sickness should appear in the two treatises that challenge the validity of philosophical knowledge in medicine. For this idea of balance serves also to define health in a treatise of philosophical inspiration, the *Regimen.* The author of this treatise boasts of having made a discovery about the prognosis and diagnosis of illnesses. According to him, it is the proportion between exercise and diet that determines health or illness: "For it is from the overpowering [*krateisthai*] of one or the other that diseases arise, while from their being evenly balanced [*isazein*] comes good health."[22]

In this definition, the elements in question are not of the same nature as in the two preceding definitions; they are not constituents of man, but components of regimen, exercise and diet. Nonetheless, the relation between the concepts of health and illness, as well as the notions that serve to define them, are analogous: the pathological state is the contrary of the state of health; sickness is an imbalance whereas health is a balance. In this third definition, however, the idea of equilibrium or disequilibrium is made explicit. Health results from an equality between the two principles, illness from the domination of one by the other.

The Definition of Health according to Alcmaeon of Croton

One cannot insist too much on the historical importance of these definitions, of which the best known is that of the *Nature of Man.* They are the most ancient definitions of health that can be directly located in Greek thought, and consequently in Western thought as a whole. But contrary to what Epictetus implies, Hippocrates was not the first physician to have given a definition of health and sickness. Alcmaeon of Croton, a physician associated with the Pythagoreans whom we met in a previous chapter, had already expressed his opinion on the subject a century earlier. Unfortunately his thinking is known only indirectly through a late account: "Alcmaeon says that what maintains health is the isonomy [i.e., equality] of properties, wet, dry, cold, hot, bitter, sweet, etc., while monarchy [i.e., the domination of one alone] among them brings on illness."[23]

As with every doxography that reports an opinion without explicitly citing it, it is difficult to distinguish between the author's words and those of the doxographer. It is generally agreed, however, that the picturesque terms "isonomy" and "monarchy," borrowed from political vocabulary, may be traced back to Alcmaeon of Croton himself.

Alcmaeon's teaching contained the gist of what one finds later in the Hippocratic treatises. Before *Ancient Medicine* and *Nature of Man,* Alcmaeon had defined health on the basis of the constitutive elements of man. And in this regard, the author of *Ancient Medicine* is nearer to his precursor than that of *Nature of Man*, for like Alcmaeon he admits an infinite number of constitutive elements, whereas the author of *Nature of Man* retains only four principles—the four humors, blood, phlegm, yellow bile, and black bile. As far as the equilibrium or disequilibrium between these elements is concerned, use of this distinction was already made by Alcmaeon to explain the state of health and of illness. And to the extent that Alcmaeon spoke of isonomy and of monarchy, he foreshadowed the definition of the *Regimen*, which speaks of equality and predominance.[24]

By comparison with Alcmaeon, the originality of Hippocratic medicine resided in the idea of mixture, or *crasis*. This innovation goes together with the development of humoral physiology and pathology. If one were to look for an analogical model implicit in the new concept, it would be found in the banquet—the archetypal image of the wine mixed with water that was offered in libation to the gods before drinking.

In any case, the Hippocratic definition, in its positive aspect, was to remain the classical definition in Greek medicine. "Almost all my predecessors," says Galen, "defined health by the good mixture [*eucrasia*] and proportion [*summetria*] of the elements."[25] The philosophers did not define it differently. The Stoic Chrysippus defined health by the good mixture (*eucrasia*) and proportion (*summetria*) of the hot, cold, dry, and moist in the body.[26]

From Health to Sickness: Rupture or Difference of Degree?

These theoretical definitions did not exhaust the thinking of the Hippocratic physicians about health and illness. Far from it. For though such definitions stressed the opposition between the two, they did not account for the passage from one to the other. Additional reflection was required for this purpose.

We do not have space here to review in detail the various kinds of causes that were supposed to determine the transition from the normal to the pathological.[27] It suffices to recall that internal equilibrium also assumes a balanced relation between the body and what comes from the outside; that is to say, between the organism and diet, on the one hand, and, on the other, between the organism and its environment. But what needs to be noted here is the way in which the Hippocratic physicians pictured this transition.

Since they conceived health and illness as two antithetical states, the passage from one to the other seemed to them to be an important change. The notion of change (*métabolè*) is in fact the basis of Hippocratic pathology. It was used both to explain and to express the passage from the normal state to the pathological state. "One should be especially on one's guard against the most violent changes of the seasons," says the author of *Airs, Waters, Places*.[28] "[T]he chief causes of diseases are the most violent changes in what concerns our constitutions and habits," says the author of the *Regimen in Acute Diseases*.[29]

This theme was not confined to the technical literature of the physicians. Two historians who were contemporary with Hippocrates, Herodotus and Thucydides, also claimed that diseases were triggered by change.[30] According to Thucydides, the Athenian prisoners penned up in the "quarries" of Syracuse during the disastrous Sicilian expedition fell sick owing to a change (*métabolè*) in temperature, as the stifling heat of summer gave way to cool autumn nights.[31]

The physicians brought an unprecedented refinement to thinking about this subject, however. The least change in diet seemed to them harmful. In this connection they were able to cite a particularly striking example. The dietary habits of the ancient Greeks were not uniform. As in our own day, some people were accustomed to eat two meals a day, one taken at noon and the other in the evening, while others limited themselves to a single meal in the evening. What would happen if the diets of these two types of people were switched for a day? Here is the answer of the author of the *Regimen in Acute Diseases*:

[S]udden changes cause harm and weakness, both to those who take one, and to those who take two full meals a day. Those too who are not in the habit of lunching, if they have taken lunch, immediately become feeble, heavy in all the body, weak and sluggish. Should they also dine, they suffer from acid eructations. Diarrhoea too may occur in some cases, because the digestive organs have been loaded, contrary to habit, when they are accustomed to a period of dryness, and not to be twice distended with food and to digest food twice. . . . But, indeed, those too who have the habit of taking two meals a day, should they omit lunch, find themselves weak, feeble, averse to all exertion, and the victims of heart-burn. Their bowels seem to hang, the urine is hot and yellow, and the stools are parched. In some cases the mouth is bitter, the eyes are hollow, the temples throb, and the extremities are chilled; most men who have missed lunch cannot eat their dinner; and if they do dine their bowels are heavy, and they sleep much worse than if they had previously taken lunch.[32]

The author does not stop at describing the remarkable troubles due to an inhabitual surfeit or absence of food; he even prescribes a regimen designed to compensate for the effects of the change. In his desire to draw attention to the dangers of the least change of diet, the author unconsciously exaggerates the harmful consequences of a modification that affects only the rhythm of meals during a single day.

This distrust of change implied a corresponding faith in the power of habit. The author goes so far as to assert that many people find it easy to eat three quite large meals a day—because they are used to it. Accordingly, he maintains that a habitual diet, even if it is bad, is surer to preserve health than an abrupt change to a better diet.[33] Habit thus becomes one of the factors to be taken into account in the evaluation of the health of individuals; hence, the mention of "habits" in the long list of the various elements that the Hippocratic physician must consider in arriving at a judgment.[34]

Habit was to remain an important consideration in Hellenistic and Roman medicine. One of the two great physicians of the Hellenistic period, Erasistratus, wrote at length in praise of habit, extending the argument of the author of *Regimen in Acute Diseases* and enlarging upon it to the extent that he stresses the importance of habit not only for the body but for the mind. Just as the body of the athlete is accustomed to physical exercise, the mind of the researcher is used to intellectual effort:

Those who are altogether unfamiliar with [research] become blinded and bewildered as soon as their minds begin to work: they readily withdraw from the inquiry, in a state of mental fatigue and exhaustion, much like people who attempt to race without having been trained. He, on the other hand, who is accustomed to research, seeks and penetrates everywhere mentally, passing constantly from one topic to another; nor does he ever give up his investigation; he pursues it not merely for a matter of days, but throughout his whole life.[35]

Erasistratus's tribute was recorded by Galen, who himself devoted a brief work to reminding the physician of the necessity of taking habit into account in treatment.

On this view, since habit is associated with health and departure from habit triggers illness, the onset of illness clearly marks a rupture with health. There seems therefore to be a discontinuity between the normal and the pathological. One passes directly, in effect, from a state of peace to a state of civil war. The fate of the body is comparable to that of a city. Both the human body and the body politic remain peaceful so long as all the elements of which they are composed are united and well integrated, or mixed. By contrast, they are prey to dissension and illness when a part isolates itself from the rest in order to seize power, and in this way causes damage to the whole. Such a comparison is never explicit in Hippocrates; for this one must wait for Plato.[36] But the metaphor crops up in Hippocratic writings, all the more readily as the vocabulary of force and of war is regularly used to describe physiological and pathological processes.[37]

On closer examination, however, it becomes clear that the antithesis between the normal and the pathological was not always so settled in Hippocratic writings. In certain respects, health was seen as being closely related to sickness. This deeper analysis of the relation between the normal and the pathological laid emphasis on three points: first, excellent health may quickly turn into illness; second, good health is sometimes only apparent; finally, health itself is a relative condition.

The Fragility of Excessively Good Health

The first argument assumed that there is in fact such a thing as excessively good health, and consisted in showing that it represents a fragile equilibrium which, ultimately, is dangerous. This conclusion was suggested chiefly by the evidence of ancient sports medicine. Heavyweight athletes were obliged, as we have seen, not only to undergo strenuous training but also to follow a strict meat-based diet to maximize their strength. To enhance their performance, these athletes ate beef, oxen, goat, and antelope.[38] But such an unvarying regime carried with it obvious dangers, of which Hippocratic physicians were indeed well aware: "In athletes a perfect condition that is at its highest pitch is treacherous. Such conditions cannot remain the same or be at rest, and, change for the better being impossible, the only possible change is for the worse. For this reason it is an advantage to reduce the fine condition quickly, in order that the body may make a fresh beginning of growth."[39]

A physician does not ordinarily recommend putting an end to good health. The author's point here is that good health pushed to the extreme risked tipping over into illness. Here is one of the accidents to which athletes subjected to a compulsory diet were liable: "This kind of diarrhoea attacks mostly persons of close flesh, when a man of such a constitution is compelled to eat meat, for the veins when closely contracted cannot take in the food that enters. This kind of constitution is apt sharply to turn in either direction, to the good or to the bad, and in bodies of such a sort a good condition is at its best only for a while."[40] Good health therefore represents a precarious and fragile equilibrium; and excessively good health is dangerous because it derives from excess, and so upsets a delicate balance.

Although these reflections were inspired by actual medical practice, they were part of a larger cultural context in which moral and religious thought condemned excess and valued the happy medium. This is why already in the theater of Aeschylus, without any reference to the experience of athletes, one encounters the idea that overly robust health is dangerous and a sign that illness is near. The old people who make up the choir in Aeschylus's *Agamemnon*, dimly fearing for the fate of their king, triumphantly returned home but nearing his downfall, gives several examples of prosperity leading to unhappiness, among which good health is cited: "Yet it is true: the high strength of men knows no content with limitation. Sickness chambered beside it beats at the wall between."[41]

Stripped of its poetic and metaphorical language, the underlying idea resembles that of the Hippocratic physicians: the dividing line between health and sickness is very thin indeed. Of course, the idea meant rather different things in the two cases. In Aeschylus, to the mind of the choir, illness that followed from overly good health came under the category of the effects of the jealousy of the gods against any excessive human prosperity, while for the Hippocratic physicians the dangers of an excess of good health were rationally explainable without any reference to divine punishment. But the physicians' analysis, based on recent developments in professional athletics, gave new life to an old idea.

The Appearance of Good Health

The experience of athletes was regarded, however, as atypical. One physician went so far as to say that the athletic constitution was not natural.[42] But even among people who led a normal life, good health was apt to be deceptive. Indeed, sickness was usually preceded by a period of apparent health.

This is an idea to which the author of the *Regimen* attached great importance; for he looked to take advantage of the period of apparent health, during which the disease was latent, in order to forecast, diagnose, and prevent it. We have noted that, in his opinion, the cause of all sickness is an imbalance between the two components of regimen, food and exercise. Now this disequilibrium cannot, at the beginning, be perceived by nonspecialists since people "appear to be in health."[43] Only the trained eye of the physician can make a preventive diagnosis: "But I have discovered . . . the forecasting of an illness before the patient falls sick, based upon the direction in which is the excess. For diseases do not arise among men all at once; they gather themselves together gradually before appearing with a sudden spring. So I have discovered the symptoms shown in a patient before health is mastered by disease, and how these are to be replaced by a state of health."[44]

In the description of particular cases that illustrates his discovery, the author very carefully distinguishes those signs that are harbingers of illness during the period of apparent health from the symptoms of illness once it has manifested itself. Here is an excerpt from the beginning of the first case, in which the disequilibrium arises from a predominance of food over exercise:

> The nostrils without obvious cause become blocked after dinner and after sleep, and they seem to be full without there being need to blow the nose. But when these persons have begun to walk in the morning or to take exercise, then they blow the nose and spit; as time goes on the eyelids too are heavy, and as it were an itching seizes the forehead; they have less appetite for food and less capacity for drink; their complexion fades; and there come on either catarrhs or aguish fevers, according to the place occupied by the surfeit that was aroused. . . . In such a case food overpowers exercises, and the surfeit gathering together little by little brings on disease. One ought not, however, to let things drift to this point, but to realize, as soon as one has recognized the *first of the signs*, that exercises are overpowered by foods that gather together little by little, whereby comes surfeit.[45]

The symptoms of illness appear only "with time." They are preceded by the "first signs." The physician must not wait for the symptoms, but intervene from the moment that the first signs appear to correct the disequilibrium between foods and exercises. This desire to begin treatment from the period of apparent health, before the illness manifests itself in all its force, grows out of an intuition that is far from absurd.

Relative Health

It was not only in this marginal period between the end of health and the onset of illness that the Hippocratic physicians saw a close relationship between the normal and the pathological. They were the first to note that health is a relative state consisting of degrees.

The sight of the handicapped had indeed already suggested this idea. Referring to persons suffering from the dislocation outwards of both thighs, whether from birth or as the result of disease, the author of *On Joints* notes that they can enjoy reasonably good health (*ikanôs hugièroi*) if there are no complications. But their condition is far from perfect; in particular, the body as a whole—with the exception of the head—does not achieve its full development.[46] Here then was a case of relative health noted by the physician.

Under these circumstances, the line separating the healthy and the pathological is blurred. It sometimes becomes so vague that in one treatise we encounter the altogether singular combination of a term denoting good health with a term signifying sickness: "Those whose nostrils are naturally watery, and whose seed is watery, are below the average when in health [*hugiainousi nosèrotéron*]," it is said in the *Aphorisms*.[47] Nonetheless, this is an extreme case. More generally, the physician might seek to establish a hierarchy among the degrees of health by ranking the various categories of constitutions according to their greater or lesser capacity to dominate external influences and to resist change. Let us return to the example of a change in the daily rhythm of meals. While the author of *Regimen in Acute Diseases* considers that such change is harmful for all human beings without exception, the author of *Ancient Medicine* sees in the different effects produced by it the occasion to define a hierarchy both within the range of what is normal and between the normal and the pathological:

For the great majority of men can follow indifferently either the one habit or the other, and can take lunch or only one daily meal. Others again, if they were to do anything outside what is beneficial, would not get off easily, but if they change their respective ways for a single day, nay, for a part of a single day, they suffer excessive discomfort. . . . Such constitutions, I contend, that rapidly and severely feel the effects of errors, are weaker than the others. A weak man is but one step removed from a sickly man, but a sickly man is weaker still, and is more apt to suffer distress whenever he misses the due season.[48]

In the last lines, where he draws the lesson of this example, the author formulates definitions that were to have great importance for the analysis of the relation between health and sickness. He displays an acute sense of continuity and gradation. For him there is no difference in kind—only one of degree—between the normal and the pathological, since the sick are the weakest of those who are in good health. This principle of continuity between the normal and the pathological was to reappear in the nineteenth century in the work of Auguste Comte as Broussais's principle.

Appraisal of the Relationship between the Normal and the Pathological

From this sketch it becomes clear that, for the Hippocratic physicians, the relationship between health and sickness was more complex than it first appeared. Health and sickness were indeed understood as antithetical states: equality was opposed to domination, mixture to separation. But at the same time they held that there is only a difference of degree between the normal and the pathological, to the extent that the body, whether healthy or ill, may be defined by its greater or lesser capacity to overcome external influences and to resist change. These two types of relations between the normal and the pathological may seem incompatible to a modern mind; this was not the case in Hippocrates' time, for they coexist in a single treatise, *Ancient Medicine*.[49]

The Course of Disease: Disorder or Order?

With regard to the conception of the pathological state itself, apparently contradictory pictures could also coexist. Hippocratic metaphors imply that disease was conceived as a disorder, as a disruption of the normal state. But at the same time, physicians sought rules governing the progress of disease through the space of the body and, above all, through time.

One metaphor points toward the progress of disease, or rather to its course: "For if disease and treatment start together, the disease will not win the race, but it will if it start with an advantage."[50] Is treatment being likened here to a runner in a stadium who crosses the finish line before his rival? Or rather to a hunting dog set off in pursuit of a wild beast? Or, better still perhaps, to a warrior chasing an enemy who has come to attack one of his own? These metaphors in any case often converge in a picture of the disease as an animate being, rapid and powerful, who abruptly establishes his hold over the patient in the manner of a warrior over his adversary, or of a wild beast over his prey. Indeed, the disease "approaches," "attacks," "seizes" the patient and "holds" him.[51] A sort of struggle is entered into by the disease and the patient. The disease "dominates" the patient if he does not manage to "resist" the violence of it.[52] And "when the disease wins out over the body, such a thing is incurable."[53] The disease, being voracious, feeds at the expense of the patient. In fact, when the patient is too weak, "it is plain that what is taken proves nourishment and increase to the disease, but wears away and enfeebles the body."[54] The fever also has need of nourishment, like fire.[55] And when the disease no longer finds suitable nourishment, it devours little by little the healthy flesh of the patient and causes his death: "The disease begins at that place. When there is no more *nourishment* in sufficient quantity, it *devours* in advancing little by little; when it has gone everywhere, the *nourishment* is exhausted for the disease, and there is no longer a healthy part to take it away. If that happens, the patient dies."[56] In the best case, the disease releases the patient from its grip. Even when it seems to be going away, however, it may rush back again and attack, aroused to fury once more in a new fit of anger.[57]

All these metaphors preserve the trace of a prerational and pre-Hippocratic conception of disease as a demoniacal creature that assails the patient, causing the greatest chaos, operating in unforeseeable ways and for an unknown length of time. The disease is a sort of inner storm.[58] On this view, the pathological is the reign of the disordered, the wild, and the capricious.

But alongside these vivid metaphors, which hark back to an ancient and obscure conception of disease, physicians imagined its movements through the body in much more sober terms. It was conceived as departing from a specific place, going to another place, and settling there; later it could go elsewhere inside the body, or move outside.[59] These shifts in the location of the disease, which were perceptible in the form of pain, had their counterpart in humoral theory, corresponding to the movements of the peccant (or errant) humor as it separates itself from the other humors. Here is how the author of *Nature of Man* imagines the link between pain and the movement of the humors:

For when an element is isolated and stands by itself, not only must the place which it left become diseased, but the place where it stands in a flood must, because of the excess, cause pain and distress. In fact when more of an element flows out of the body than is necessary to get rid of superfluity, the emptying causes pain. If, on the other hand, it be to an inward part that there takes place the emptying, the shifting and the separation from other elements, the man certainly must, according to what has been said, suffer from a double pain, one in the place left, and another in the place flooded.[60]

It is therefore the lack or, even more than this, the surfeit of a humor produced by its flow either within or outside the body that triggers pain and sickness.

It is impossible to give a detailed picture of the many different routes followed by pathological fluxes. Nonetheless, the beginning of the treatise *Places in Man* provides a good synthesis of the movement of diseases and humors inside the body:

Now, in my opinion, there is no beginning point of the body, but rather every part is at the same time both beginning and end, in the same way that in the figure of a circle, no beginning point is to be found. Likewise, diseases arise from the whole body indifferently, although the drier component of the body is disposed to become ill and to suffer more, the moist component less. For whereas any disease that occupies a dry part is fixed and unremitting, one in a moist part flows somewhere else and generally occupies different parts of the body at different times; through constantly changing, it has interruptions and goes away sooner, and so it is not fixed.

Every part of the body, on becoming ill, immediately produces disease in some other part, the cavity in the head, the head in the muscles and the cavity, and so on in the same way [as the cavity in the head and the head in the muscles and the cavity]. The cavity, for instance, when material enters it and it does not make a corresponding evacuation downwards, floods the body with moisture from the ingested food. This moisture, being turned away from the cavity, moves away all at once to the head, and when it arrives in the head, not finding room in the vessels there, flows anywhere it can.[61]

As a rule, the fluxes that cause disease were supposed to depart from the head. Certain physicians who were strongly influenced by arithmology fixed the number of these fluxes at seven. This was the case, for example, with the author of *Places in Man*. There, the flows leaving the head are said to go forth into the rest of the body at random. But chance has arranged things well, for the places where these flows arrive are seven in number: nostrils, ears, eyes, chest (in the case of empyema or consumption), spinal cord (a sort of consumption), the flesh near the vertebrae (dropsy), and hips. The author of *Glands* also puts the number of fluxes originating in the head at seven. This agreement with regard to their number did not prevent him from asserting a distinct theory, however, for the places in the body where they were supposed to end up are not all the same.[62]

Duration and Crises of Disease

The progress of disease may also be understood in terms of its evolution over time, of its changing degree of intensity: thus a disease is born, grows, reaches its height, passes through decisive moments, and then, in the best case, diminishes and disappears; otherwise, it worsens and carries off the patient.[63] The Hippocratic physicians set out to identify the rhythms of this evolution.

The general duration of illness was sometimes related to the cycle of the seasons.[64] With regard to the actual evolution of the disease, these physicians were chiefly interested in determining and predicting decisive moments, or crises. Here is the definition that one of them gives of these: "To be judged in diseases is when they increase, diminish, change into another disease, or end."[65]

The notion of crisis therefore did not have the pejorative sense it has for us; it was a significant moment in the evolution of the disease, for better or for worse. When crises were interpreted in terms of humoral theory, they were associated not only with the movement of peccant humors (in the case either of their accumulation or evacuation) but also with their qualitative modification. For peccant humors to cease to be noxious, they needed to lose their rawness, to be "cooked" by means of a process that was entirely analogous to that of cooking in the culinary sense or of the maturation of a fruit by the sun. This is what the Hippocratic physicians called coction. The following text brings together all three of these notions, crisis, coction, and accumulation (or "abscession"): "In all dangerous cases you should be on the watch for all favourable coctions of the evacuations from all parts, or for fair and critical abscessions. Coctions signify nearness of crisis and sure recovery of health, but crude and unconcocted evacuations, which change into bad abscessions, denote absence of crisis, pain, prolonged illness, death, or a return of the same symptoms."[66]

Periodicity of Critical Days: The Temptations of Arithmology

Physicians did not limit themselves to watching for the signs that heralded these crises; they looked to determine their periodicity as well.

The observation of malarial fevers ("tertians" and "quartans") encouraged them in this ambition. But they went too far in refining the number of periods and in distinguishing various types of intermittent fevers, with the result that today their classification has been partially abandoned. While one still speaks of tertian, quartan, and sometimes quintan fevers, there is no longer any mention of semitertian, septan, or nonan fevers.[67]

Above all, the Hippocratics were guilty of unwarranted generalization, extending the notion of periodicity to cover all sorts of other diseases in the belief that they had established laws that were part of a larger anthropological, or even cosmological, context. To an even greater degree than in the numbering of humoral fluxes, septenary theory enjoyed a vogue in the reckoning of critical days. Here, for example, is the way in which the author of *Fleshes* builds the rhythm of diseases into the biological rhythm of man, taking as his basic unit the hebdomad, or seven-day period:

Diseases are also most acute in patients according to this same pattern, the days in which they come to a crisis and either die or recover being four (half a seven-day period), the second most acute occurring in a whole seven-day period, the third most acute in eleven days (one and a half seven-day periods), the fourth most acute in two seven-day periods, and the fifth most acute in eighteen days (two and a half seven-day periods). Other diseases have no means by which to reveal in how many days patients will recover.[68]

This septenary rhythm was, according to this author, a necessity of nature or, as we would say today, a natural law that regulates all human life. "The period of life of man," he declares, "is seven days." This author was hardly the only proponent of septenary theory in contemporary medical or philosophical circles, as we have seen, nor was he the fiercest.[69] This theory was mainly applied, in addition to the periodization of diseases, to embryology and the stages of human growth.[70] The author of *Fleshes* presents several arguments drawn from embryology to justify his own septenary theory of man. For example, the different parts of the body are formed in seven days in the embryo; and foetuses in the seventh month that have reached an exact number of hebdomads are viable. Still stranger is the claim that men die for the most part at the end of seven days if they go without eating and drinking.

Given that these passed for decisive arguments, one suspects that physicians did not hesitate to fiddle with the facts in their reckoning of critical days in order to make them fit their own theories. The comparison of *Fleshes* with another treatise, the *Prognostic*, is instructive in this regard. Here is the picture of the progress of fevers given in the *Prognostic*:

> Fevers come to a crisis on the same days, both those from which patients recover and those from which they die. The mildest fevers, with the most favourable symptoms, cease on the fourth day or earlier. The most malignant fevers, with the most dangerous symptoms, end fatally on the fourth day or earlier. The first assault of fevers ends at this time; the second lasts until the seventh day, the third until the eleventh, the fourth until the fourteenth, the fifth until the seventeenth, and the sixth until the twentieth day. . . . From the first day, however, you must pay attention, and consider the question at the end of every four days, and then the issue will not escape you.[71]

The counting up of critical days is identical in the two treatises with only one exception. With regard to the five comparable periods, the first four correspond exactly to the same number of days (4, 7, 11, 14); only the last period has a different number of days: eighteen for the author of the *Fleshes*, seventeen for the author of the *Prognostic*. This difference, minimal though it may be, conceals in fact an important difference in the manner of calculating. The unit of measurement for the author of the *Fleshes* is the hebdomad (associated with the number 7); for the author of the *Prognostic*, it is the tetrad (associated with the number 4). The eighteenth day corresponds to two and one-half hebdomads in the reckoning of the former;[72] the seventeenth day corresponds to the fifth tetrad in the reckoning of the latter.[73]

Other authors chose a different method of calculation, adopting as their base not periods of days, such as the hebdomad or the tetrad, but odd and even days. "[T]he odd-numbered, especially, must be observed, since on them patients tend to incline in one direction or the other," says one physician.[74] Another physician holds instead that certain affections have their crisis on even days and others on odd days.[75] On this view, then, the first critical day was sometimes the third, sometimes the fourth.

Despite these discrepancies in detail regarding the methods of calculating and their results, the main thing to be noted is that all these physicians, despite sometimes quite different orientations in their approach to medicine, tried to discover an order beyond the apparent disorder of pathological phenomena. The word *cosmos*, in the sense of "order," is rightly employed by the author of the *Prognostic* to describe this unfolding of disease.[76] The progress of disease therefore obeys, in the most favorable cases, a mathematical calculation. Number (*arithmos*) is seen to govern the succession of critical days in the unfolding of disease, as in the normal growth of the embryo and the child.[77] In this sense, too, it may be said that there is no difference in kind between the normal and the pathological.

Hippocratic Periodicity and the Hesiodic Calendar

When the Hippocratic physicians concerned themselves with the problem of determining the lucky or unlucky days in the progress of a disease, their thinking was rooted in a quite ancient belief according to which certain days were fortunate or fatal, while others were indifferent. Hesiod, who was roughly contemporary with Homer, closes his poem *Works and Days* with a statement of the days in each month that are favorable or unfavorable to human beings. Knowledge of this, for him, was the possession solely of an elite. "Different persons praise different days, but few really know."[78] The first significant days of the month, according to Hesiod, were the first, the fourth, and the seventh—which correspond to the first critical days of illness according to the author of the *Prognostic* and to that of the *Fleshes*.[79] Of course, the coincidence is only partial since the other days do not correspond; even so, it deserves to be noted. In any case, the significance of these two interpretations derived from different traditions of thought. For the poet, it was a matter of divine custom: critical days were those that were sacred to Zeus. The physicians, by contrast, made no reference to the divine, attempting instead to apprehend pathological phenomena in a rational way by appeal to a law of number.

Hippocratic Arithmology and Pythagorean Arithmology

The attempt at rationalization, even mathematization, of the sensible world in which the physicians played a part is most famously associated with the Pythagoreans. It is tempting, therefore, to see in the importance assigned to number by the Hippocratics a sign of Pythagorean influence upon medicine. The theory of the world that underlies the Hippocratic reckoning of critical days does, in fact, sometimes draw upon genuine mathematical (and musical) knowledge. One statement of critical days explicitly makes reference to a theory of harmony:

The physician who wishes to aim correctly at the recovery of patients must consider odd days in their entirety, and among the even days the fourteenth, the twenty-eighth, and the forty-second. The limit to the calculation of harmony is drawn there by some and it is the perfect even number; for which reason it would take too long to describe it in detail here. The physician must also reckon in accordance with triads and tetrads; with linked triads in their totality, and with tetrads linked two by two and disjoint two by two.[80]

The mathematical competence of this physician is clear. He alludes to a technical theory that he knows well but that he does not consider worth elaborating upon. Moreover, his statement of critical days constitutes an excellent example of the different ways of calculating, for it mixes the calculation of odd and even days with various periods, triads, tetrads, even, implicitly, hebdomads.[81]

Nonetheless this new theory, to the extent that it does not overlap with earlier ones, confirms that the arithmology of the Hippocratic physicians exhibited considerable variation both with respect to the modes of calculation and to results. It becomes difficult therefore to reduce all these variants to a common Pythagorean source. The hypothesis of Pythagorean origin is all the less probable as the period judged perfect by the Pythagoreans, the decade, plays no important role in the reckoning of critical days among the Hippocratic physicians.[82] Besides, the essential originality of the Pythagoreans consisted in extending arithmological calculations to the whole set of beings which they defined by numbers. This does not mean that all arithmological analysis was Pythagorean. The physicians, for example, were able to carry out calculations about critical days without believing on that account that everything was reducible to number. It is significant that the author of *Ancient Medicine* should have asserted that number is of great importance in the evolution of disease and yet at the same time challenged the existence of number as the criterion for evaluating the proper adaptation of regimen to man.[83] Arithmology did not penetrate as far as treatment. Health was not defined by number.[84]

From Illness to Recovery: Relative and Total Recovery

"What you should put first in all the practice of our art is how to make the patient well," says the author of *On Joints*.[85]

Ideally, medicine aimed at total recovery. But the Hippocratic physician was well aware that he could not always restore perfect health. Just as there existed a relative state of health, so there existed a relative state of recovery. It is owing to Hippocratism that this notion was to make its way into the history of science. It entered chiefly through surgery: while no "harm" to the shoulder results from the oblique fracture of the shoulder blade, for example, there may persist a "deformity" to the extent that the setting of the bones is less than perfect.[86] But the notion also figured in gynecology: certain treatments do not completely restore a woman's full health, because they are accompanied by sterility.[87] The concept of relative recovery is even built into the definition of medicine given by the author of *The Art*: the purpose of medicine, he says, "is to do away with the sufferings of the sick, to lessen the violence of their diseases."[88] Whether total or relative, the patient's recovery is the aim of medicine.

"Combating" Disease

How did Hippocratic physicians conceive of this act of recovery? Above all they pictured it as an operation that consisted in "combating" the disease and its cause.[89] The expression recurs in the three most famous definitions of treatment:

—*Epidemics I*:
   The [medical] art has three factors, the disease, the patient, the physician. The physician is the servant of the art. The patient must co-operate with the physician in *combating* [*hypenantiousthai*] the disease.[90]
—*Nature of Man*:
   Furthermore, one must know that diseases due to repletion are cured by evacuation, and those due to evacuation are cured by repletion; those due to exercise are cured by rest, and those due to idleness are cured by exercise. To know the whole matter, the physician must *set himself against* [*enantion histasthai*] the established character of diseases, of constitutions, of seasons and of ages; he must relax what is tense and make tense what is relaxed. For in this way the diseased part would rest most, and this, in my opinion, constitutes treatment.[91]

—Breaths:

> For knowledge of the cause of a disease will enable one to administer to the body what things are advantageous [by using opposites to *combat* (*ek tôn enantiôn epistamenos*) the disease]. Indeed this sort of medicine is quite natural. For example, hunger is a disease, as everything is called a disease which makes a man suffer. What then is the remedy for hunger? That which makes hunger to cease. This is eating; so that by eating must hunger be cured. Again, drink stays thirst; and again repletion is cured by depletion, depletion by repletion, fatigue by rest. To sum up in a single sentence, opposites are cures for opposites.[92]

Hippocratism is therefore founded on allopathy, or treatment by agents producing effects contrary to those of the disease. The Hippocratic Collection is nonetheless so varied that one also meets there with the first clear definition of homeopathy, or treatment by like agents.[93] Still, as a general rule, treatment is envisaged in the context of combat. The role of the physician is to "struggle" (*antagonisasthai*) against the disease thanks to his art.[94] Sometimes the metaphor of war is still more explicit. Disease is hostile to man.[95] It is necessary therefore to respond by means of a treatment that is hostile to the disease. This is what the author of *The Sacred Disease* declares: "For in this disease as in all others it is necessary, not to increase the illness, but to wear it down by applying to each what is most *hostile* [*polemiotaton*] to it, not that to which it is conformable. For what is conformity gives vigour and increase; what is *hostile* [*polemiou*] causes weakness and decay."[96]

The Need for Treatment to Counteract Change Appropriately by Means of Another Change

After having thus situated treatment in the context of combat, the author of *The Sacred Disease* goes on to say by way of conclusion: "Whoever knows how to cause in men by regimen moist or dry, hot or cold, he can cure this disease also, if he distinguish the seasons for useful [*kairous*] treatment, without having recourse to purifications and magic."[97] This passage contains two essential ideas: treatment must modify the state of the body; but this change must be appropriately carried out.

The conception of therapy as change is a recurrent theme in the Hippocratic Collection. "Everything that *changes* from the existing state benefits what is ill, for if you do not *change* what is ill, it increases," says the author of *Places in Man*.[98] Now, as the disease has itself effected a change,[99] treatment ought logically to effect a proportional change in the opposite direction. "Give to each disease according to its nature," this same author goes on to say; "in weak diseases give medications by nature weak, in strong diseases, medications by nature strong."[100] Such reasoning, though logically irrefutable, was vigorously disputed by the author of the *Regimen in Acute Diseases*:

I am convinced that the practice of physicians is the exact opposite of what it should be; for they all wish at the beginning of a disease to reduce the patient by starvation for two, three, or even more days before administering gruel and drink. Perhaps they consider it natural, when a violent *change* is taking place in the body, to *counteract it by another violent change.*

Now to bring about [another such] change is no small gain, but the change must be carried out correctly and surely.[101]

For the change to be carried out correctly and surely, it must be gradual; for every major change that is abrupt is harmful to man. As a result, treatment that may seem best in theory (administering a strong change in the case of a strong disease, for example) is in reality the most harmful; it risks doing as much harm, in fact, as the illness itself. As a consequence, the contest between the physician and the disease was never an even one. In seeking to combat the disease, the physician had to know how to measure the proper degree of change to be introduced into the body, and to seize upon the appropriate moment for introducing it, if he wished to restore health without causing damage. The notions of suitable quantity and apt timing were expressed in Greek by a single word, *kairos*; though this has traditionally been rendered as "opportunity," it denoted both the right measure and the opportune moment. It was necessary to administer to the body neither too much nor too little, neither too soon nor too late. Accordingly, to intervene in the right way and at the right time was seen as being unquestionably the most difficult aspect of the whole art of medicine—thus the beginning of the *Aphorisms*: "Life is short, the Art long, opportunity [*kairos*] fleeting, experiment treacherous, judgment difficult."

Two Criteria of Therapeutic Action: The Healthy and the Natural

The physician sought criteria to guide his action in so delicate an undertaking. The most important of these were "good health" and "nature."

The regimen of healthy people was not only of interest to the physician in the context of hygienics, as we have seen; it also offered a means of comparative investigation for judging the regimen of sick people. Immediately after denouncing his colleagues for making poor therapeutic use of the principle of change, the author of the *Regimen in Acute Diseases* stresses the need to take the regimen of people in good health as a point of reference in evaluating the regimen of people who are ill: "A physician's studies should include a consideration of what is beneficial in a patient's regimen while he is yet in health. For surely, if men in health find that one regimen produces very different results from another, especially when the regimen is changed, in disease too there will be great differences, and the greatest in acute diseases."[102]

This necessary reference to the state of health for the purpose of directing treatment is supported by an a fortiori argument: any error in regimen that can be noted during a state of health will be all the more damaging in the conduct of regimen during a state of illness, for the patient is less resistant than a healthy person. The same argument is applied by the author of *Ancient Medicine* when he declares: "That the discomforts a man feels after unseasonable abstinence are no less than those of unseasonable repletion, it were well to learn by a reference to men in health."[103]

There is no notable difference between the notion "good health" and certain uses of the concept "nature." By the latter term, the Hippocratic physicians understood "human nature." This was defined by normal patterns of bodily organization, whether at the elementary, anatomical, or physiological level, and a normal capacity for reacting to external influences, whether regimental or environmental. The natural state, like the state of good health, was the normal state. Thus the physician was able to take the body's natural and healthy condition as the model for his art. When a surgeon discoursed on how to reduce a fracture or a dislocation, for example, he adopted as his point of reference the position of the member when this was "in conformity with nature" (*kata phusin*).[104] More generally, the physician needed to know the natural organization of the different parts of the human body. It was in this sense that the author of *Places in Man* could say: "The nature of the body is the beginning point of medical reasoning."[105] This formula was to remain famous. Galen attributed it to Hippocrates himself and reproached his contemporaries for praising the precept without following it. He remarked ironically upon this situation in the following terms: "[T]hey devote themselves with such ardor to this task that they disregard in the case of each part of the body not only its substance, its texture, its shape, its size, and its connection with adjacent parts, but even its position."[106]

Not only was it important for the physician to know the natural organization of the body; it mattered, too, that he knew its natural capacity to react.

But this capacity was liable to vary from one individual to another; accordingly it constituted a variable that the physician had to take into account in his approach to treatment. The treatise *On Fractures* considered it as having the same relevance as a patient's age in forecasting the length of time it would take for a broken bone to heal: "It takes about thirty days altogether for the bone of the forearm to unite. But there is nothing exact about it, for both *constitutions* and ages differ greatly."[107] Generally speaking, physicians knew that individual natures (or "constitutions") reacted differently to the different influences—climate, places, age, regimen, diseases—that affected them: "The *constitutions* of men are well or ill adapted to the seasons, some to summer, some to winter; others again to districts, to periods of life, to modes of living, to the various constitutions of diseases."[108]

We may now better appreciate why the author of *Epidemics I* heads his long list of the factors that the physician must take into consideration in examining the patient by "the common nature of all," followed immediately by "the particular nature of the individual."[109]

Finally, Hippocratic reflection upon human nature led to an idea that was to have a glorious future in the history of Western medicine; namely, that nature cures itself (*natura medicatrix*). This idea is nicely expressed in aphoristic form in a passage from *Epidemics VI*: "The body's nature is the physician in disease. Nature finds the way for herself, not from thought. For example, blinking, and the tongue offers its assistance, and all similar things. Well trained, readily and without instruction, nature does what is needed."[110]

The reference here is to the existence of reflexes by which, unaided, nature protects itself against disease. The example of the reflex blinking of the eyelids was to be taken up again by Aristotle: "[I]ts object is to prevent things from getting into the eyes. All animals that have eyelids do it, but human beings blink most of all, because they have the thinnest and finest skin," he says, adding, "[This] movement . . . is a natural and instinctive one, not dependent on the will."[111] This picture of nature as the possessor of an instinctive knowledge is also expressed in two celebrated aphorisms of the treatise *Nutriment*:

> Nature suffices in everything for all.
>
> In everyone nature is instructed without being taught.[112]

Despite the fame of these passages, the teleological conception of nature they express is not representative of what one finds in the most ancient core of the Hippocratic Collection.[113] It was only with Aristotle that this conception came to be clearly stated: "[T]he Final Cause (purpose) and the Good (Beautiful) is more fully present in the works of Nature than in the works of Art," he says in *De partibus animalium*.[114] No assertion of this kind is to be encountered in Hippocrates' time. The Hippocratic physician was convinced that there existed laws of nature called "necessities of nature"; but these laws were understood as expressing a determinism rather than a teleology.[115] To be sure, the Hippocratic physician respected nature; and, to be sure, he took nature as the fundamental criterion of his art—thus the author of the *Breaths*, for instance, having defined medicine as therapy by means of opposites, adds that "this sort of medicine is quite natural."[116] But nature was not always cooperative.

The art of medicine therefore sometimes found itself in the position of having to force nature to cooperate. The best example is found in the treatise *The Art*. In the case of hidden illnesses, for example, when the signs furnished by nature are not sufficient to establish diagnosis and prognosis, the art exercises its constraint upon nature: "When this information is not afforded, and nature herself will yield nothing of her own accord, medicine has found means of compulsion, whereby nature is constrained, without being harmed, to give up her secrets; when these are given up she makes clear, to those who know about the art, what course ought to be pursued."[117]

The metaphor refers to a judicial inquiry. In Hippocrates' time, such compulsion took one of two forms: oaths, in the case of free men, or the "question" (i.e., torture), in the case of slaves. Confessions were extracted from nature by comparable means of compulsion. This notion was later to be echoed in the Renaissance by Francis Bacon: "Nature irritated and tormented by art surrenders [its secrets] more clearly than when she herself freely confides [them]."[118] But the Hippocratic physician added an important qualification: it was essential that the constraint exercised by art do no harm to nature. For the violence of the physician was not like that of the disease; it was, rather, a soft sort of violence. The ultimate aim of medicine was never lost sight of: "To help, or at least to do no harm."[119]

FOURTEEN

The Legacy of Hippocratism
in Antiquity

The extraordinary prestige of a physician who very shortly after his death was to become known as the Father of Medicine makes it effectively impossible even to sketch a brief history of the legacy of Hippocratism. Over the course of more than twenty centuries, Hippocrates has exercised an influence upon medical thought comparable to that exercised by Aristotle upon philosophical thought. Sometimes challenged, often admired, and still more often distorted, depending on what purpose it was being used to serve, the Hippocratic Collection remained a standard authority for Western medicine from antiquity until the nineteenth century.

The Prestige of Hippocrates in Antiquity Prior to Galen

Famous during his lifetime, when already he was renowned as the very model of the physician, as the testimony of Plato and Aristotle confirms,[1] Hippocrates did not cease to dominate medicine throughout antiquity, despite the decisive advances in anatomical knowledge made during the Hellenistic era in Alexandria owing to the practice of human dissection, even vivisection.

Hippocrates' works achieved the status of classics in the Hellenistic period. The third century B.C. witnessed the development of two types of scholarly activity that were to continue throughout the centuries that followed: commentaries on the treatises themselves, on the one hand, and glossaries explicating rare and difficult words, on the other. These scholarly labors were undertaken mainly at the Library in Alexandria, where the works of Hippocrates had been collected, especially by the circle of the greatest physician of the Hellenistic period, Herophilus.[2] But there was another center of medical study at Pergamum, where a great library rivaling that of Alexandria was founded in the second century B.C. Unfortunately, the results of these labors are known only indirectly, with the exception of the commentary on the treatise *On Joints* by Apollonius of Citium, a physician of the empirical school who dates from the first century B.C. Indeed, in the introduction to this commentary, which was dedicated to a Ptolemy, we find Hippocrates styled "the very divine." Hippocrates' reputation did not weaken over time, not even during the Roman period. Cicero, whose work cites Hippocrates three times, did not call him divine, but he did regard Hippocrates as an authority and compared his achievements to those of the god Aesculapius.[3]

Scholarship during the first century of the Christian era also contributed to the survival of Hippocrates' works. The most ancient Hippocratic glossary that we have (albeit in altered form) is that of Erotian, who we know was a contemporary of Nero, for he dedicated his work to Andromachus, the emperor's personal physician.[4] From this period date also the first two editions of Hippocrates whose authors are known: Artemidorus, nicknamed Capiton, and his contemporary Dioscurides. Unlike Erotian's glossary, these two editions have been lost; but they are indirectly known through Galen, who used them a century later and criticized them for not preserving the ancient readings.[5]

Also dating from the first century A.D. are the oldest essays that have come down to us on the history of medicine. Hippocrates occupies a prominent place in these works, which were written in Latin. Particularly significant is the judgment of the encyclopedist Celsus, a contemporary of Tiberius, recorded in the preface to his *De medicina*. Here is how he describes the development of medicine in Greece:

This Art, however, has been cultivated among the Greeks much more than in other nations—not, however, even among them from their first beginnings, but only for a few generations before ours. Hence Aesculapius is celebrated as the most ancient authority, and because he cultivated this science, as yet rude and vulgar, with a little more than common refinement, he was numbered among the gods. After him his two sons, Podalirius and Machaon, who followed Agamemnon as leader to the Trojan War, gave no inconsiderable help to their comrades. . . . Therefore even after these I have mentioned, no distinguished men practised the Art of Medicine until literary studies began to be pursued with more attention, which more than anything else are a necessity for the spirit, but at the same time are bad for the body. At first the science of healing was held to be part of philosophy, so that treatment of disease and contemplation of the nature of things began through the same authorities; clearly because healing was needed especially by those whose bodily strength had been weakened by restless thinking and night-watching. Hence we find that many who professed philosophy became expert in medicine, the most celebrated being Pythagoras, Empedocles and Democritus. But it was, as some believe, a pupil of the last, Hippocrates of Cos, a man first and foremost worthy to be remembered, notable both for professional skill and for eloquence, who separated this branch of learning from the study of philosophy. After him Diocles of Carystus, next Praxagoras and Chrysippus, then Herophilus and Erasistratus, so practised this art that they made advances even towards various methods of treatment.[6]

This picture of the beginnings of Greek medicine is surely not a model of historical reconstruction. Its interest resides rather in the fact that it indicates the place accorded to Hippocrates by a Roman scholar of the first century A.D. in what later was to be an influential account of the birth of medicine. Hippocrates seemed to Celsus to be the first figure to come after Homeric times and the intervening dark ages whose name was worthy of being passed on to posterity, both by reason of his medical ability and of his talent as a writer. What is more, he recognized Hippocrates as the true founder of medicine to the extent that he had succeeded in detaching this art from philosophy. Elsewhere in the same work, Celsus says that Hippocrates is "the most ancient authority."[7] This judgment was shared by his contemporary, the Roman physician Scribonius Largus, who remarked in the preface to his *Compositiones* that "Hippocrates is the founder of our profession."[8] Also in the first century A.D., Pliny the Elder, who died during the eruption of Vesuvius in 79, gave an outline of the history of medicine in which he, too, assigned a privileged place to Hippocrates:

To its pioneers medicine assigned a place among the gods and a home in heaven. . . . [It was already] famous in Trojan times, in which its renown was more assured, but only for the treatment of wounds.

The subsequent story of medicine, strange to say, lay hidden in the darkest night down to the Peloponnesian War, when it was restored to the light by Hippocrates, who was born in the very famous and powerful island of Cos, sacred to Aesculapius.[9]

The chief stages in the history of medicine are the same as in Celsus: first comes the discovery of medicine by Aesculapius, who was deified, followed by the development of surgery during the Homeric era; then the centuries of darkness; and finally a period of renaissance during which Hippocrates played an essential role. Unlike Celsus, Pliny does not speak of philosophical medicine as preceding Hippocrates. On Pliny's account, Hippocrates drew his inspiration not from philosophical medicine but from religious medicine.

Hippocrates' stature as an authority in the various schools of medicine that developed in the Hellenistic and Roman eras (dogmatism, empiricism, methodism, pneumatism) was great, but varied among them. Some physicians referred to themselves as "Hippocrateans."[10] The diversity of his work accounts for the fact that partisans of opposed schools, dogmatists and empiricists alike, could claim him as their patron. Hippocratic scholarship remained a tradition of the empirical school. In the third century B.C. its founder, a dissident Herophilean named Philinus of Cos, had composed a glossary of Hippocrates in which he criticized the interpretations of the Herophilean Bacchius of Tanagra. A whole series of glossators and commentators on Hippocrates followed in his steps.[11] The methodists, by contrast, made a point of criticizing Hippocrates. One member of this school, Soranus of Ephesus (first to second century A.D.), denounced his errors in gynecology. We may note, in particular, Soranus's judgment of Hippocrates' claim to be able to predict the sex of a child before birth:

Hippocrates says[12] that the signs indicating that a woman is carrying a boy are the following: she has better color, she is more alert, her right breast is larger, ampler, and fuller, and above all the nipple stands up; the signs indicating that she is carrying a girl are the following: besides pallor, the left breast is more ample and above all the nipple [is sunken]. But it is as a result of a false supposition that he arrived at this conclusion; he imagined in fact that when the seed has been taken into the right parts of the womb a boy is formed, and into the left parts a girl. That this is not true we establish in our work on nature entitled *On the Generation of Living Beings*.[13]

Of all the physicians prior to Galen, the one who showed the most intelligence in his use of the works of Hippocrates was Aretaeus of Cappadocia, a member of the pneumatic school during the first century A.D., in his account of semiology and the treatment of acute and chronic diseases; Aretaeus went even so far as to write his own work in the Ionian dialect, in imitation of Hippocrates. But it was Galen in the second century A.D., far removed from the sectarianism of the schools, who was to restore Hippocrates to his former position and to help further extend his reputation by ceaselessly referring to the immense body of work that went under his name.

Before we discuss the golden age of Hippocratism in Galenic medicine, it is necessary to emphasize that the Hippocratic corpus had already by this point largely gone beyond the limited circle of specialists to which it was restricted previously, and that it now belonged to the cultural heritage of all educated men.[14] Plutarch, the sage of Chaeronea, who lived in the second half of the first century A.D., may serve as an example in this regard. Not only did he know the anecdotes about the life of Hippocrates that are once alluded to in his *Parallel Lives*;[15] he mentions the physician of Cos eleven times in his

Moralia. Nine out of these eleven times he cites a specific passage in Hippocrates, or refers to one.[16] The *Aphorisms* comes first with four citations, unsurprisingly since the *Aphorisms* were to be the most frequently cited work throughout the history of Hippocratism. Plutarch also cites the *Prognostic*, the *Epidemics*, and the treatise *Breaths*. Certain citations recall celebrated passages: for example, the beginning of the *Breaths* on the condition of the physician ("For the medical man sees terrible sights, touches unpleasant things, and the misfortunes of others bring a harvest of sorrows that are peculiarly his"), though not quite accurately quoted in Plutarch's version, was to be famous throughout late antiquity.[17] Other texts cited by Plutarch are rather less well known. Twice he says that, according to Hippocrates, silence is a way to avoid thirst.[18] The Hippocratic passage to which he refers is so little known that the modern editors of Plutarch's work were unable to locate it. Plutarch was in fact referring to a passage in *Epidemics VI*: "When it is necessary to prevent thirst, keep the mouth closed, do not speak, inhale cold wind with drink."[19] More interesting is the use Plutarch makes of Hippocratic teaching. He adapts, for example, what Hippocrates says in the *Prognostic* about the signs of disease to his own observation of anger: "Hippocrates says that the severity of an illness is proportionate to the degree to which the patient's features become abnormal, and the first thing I noticed was a similar proportion between the degree of distraction by anger and the degree to which appearance, complexion, gait, and voice change. This impressed upon me a kind of image of the emotion."[20]

And when Montaigne says in his chapter "On Anger" in the *Essays*, "[A]ccording to Hippocrates the most dangerous distempers are those which contort the face,"[21] it is clear that he is citing this secondhand, quoting Plutarch. Once Plutarch even advises taking Hippocrates as a model for becoming more virtuous:

[B]ut Hippocrates, who wrote down and published the fact that he did not understand the skull's sutures, is a model for anyone who is genuinely [committed to] progressing, because [a person who is not] thinks it quite wrong for Hippocrates to help others avoid the situation he found himself in by publicizing his own failing, while [such a person]—[being by contrast] committed to immunity from error—does not dare to be castigated or to admit his fallibility and ignorance.[22]

The reference here is to the following passage of *Epidemics V*:

Autonomus in Omilus died on the sixteenth day from a head wound in midsummer. The stone, thrown by hand, hit him on the sutures in the middle of the *bregma* [front of the head]. I was unaware that I should trephine, because I did not notice that the sutures had the injury of the weapon right on them, since it became obvious only later.[23]

Hippocrates' honesty in admitting his mistakes also won the approval of the Latin writer Quintilian: "For Hippocrates, the great physician, in my opinion took the most honourable course in acknowledging some of his errors to prevent those who came after from being led astray," he says in his *Institutio Oratoria*.[24]

The Golden Age of Hippocratism: The Role of Galen in Hippocrates' Survival

By the second century A.D., Hippocrates' reputation extended to the furthest frontiers of the Greek world. The funerary inscription of a Greek physician from the Milesian colony of Tomis (today Constantsa in Romania), found in the nineteenth century by the French archeologist Ernest Desjardins and today preserved at the Archeological Institute of Bucharest, shows us how a physician in a remote corner of this world was accustomed to speak of Hippocrates: "If someone wishes to know, after my death, my life, who I was, what I did and the name of my country, the stone that is here will indicate it, message for posterity. My country is the metropolis of the Euxine [Sea], illustrious city of the hero Tomis of the strong javelin. My name was Claudaeus; I was instructed in the art of the divine master Hippocrates, message for posterity."[25]

Hippocrates is described by this physician as divine, just as he was by Apollonius of Citium. He was the divine master of medicine.[26] In another funerary epigram from the same period, also preserved in stone, a physician rather proudly compares his own reputation to that of "the ancient Hippocrates." This epigraph takes us back to one of the great centers of ancient medicine after Hippocrates' time, for it concerns a physician from Pergamum named Philadelphus.[27] But another physician from Pergamum was to do more than anyone else in the second century A.D. to spread the reputation of the "divine Hippocrates." This was, of course, Galen, who, as Charles Daremberg remarked, "did not distinguish himself less by his admiration for Hippocrates, whom he called his master, than by the considerable progress he himself brought about in the medical sciences."[28]

No physician in antiquity cited Hippocrates more frequently than Galen. Hippocrates' name occurs more than 2,500 times in his work (a record that is sure never to be broken). It is true, of course, that Galen's work is so vast that it accounts for one-eighth of extant Greek literature from Homer until the end of the second century A.D., running to some ten thousand pages in the standard edition of the nineteenth century.

Galen had the good fortune to be born in Pergamum, a capital of medicine not only on account of its library but also, and above all, because of its Asclepieum, which was both a place of worship and a renowned medical center that attracted a great many patients and physicians alike. Galen also knew all the other great medical centers of the ancient world, notably Alexandria, where he went to complete his medical education, and Rome, where he lived and practiced medicine for two extended periods (first from 162 to 166, and then from 168 for some thirty years). His work represents the sum of the medical knowledge of his time.

Galen complained that his contemporaries praised Hippocrates by their words but failed to imitate his example by their deeds. A long passage in one of his short treatises, *The Best Physician Is Also a Philosopher*, perfectly illustrates this theme:

What happens to the majority of athletes who, while wishing to become winners at the Olympic games, take care to do nothing to obtain [this result], occurs also for the majority of physicians. Indeed they praise Hippocrates and consider him above all others, but in order to resemble him they do everything except that which needs to be done. [Hippocrates], in fact, declares that astronomy contributes not a small share to medicine and obviously [it is] geometry that is the necessary guide to it. But they not only practise personally neither of these two sciences, but even criticize those who do practice them. Moreover, concerning the nature of the body, [Hippocrates] thinks it right to know it with exactitude, declaring that it is the beginning of all reasoning in medicine. But they devote themselves with such ardor to this task that they disregard in the case of each part of the body not only its substance, its texture, its shape, its size, and its connection with adjacent parts, but even its position. Moreover, not knowing how to divide diseases by kinds and types leads physicians into error in the aims of therapy; Hippocrates [says] this when he invites us to follow the rational method; but physicians today are so far from conforming themselves to it that they denounce those who do follow it as concerning themselves with useless things. Moreover still, in connection with the prognosis of present, past, and future in a patient, Hippocrates says that great attention must be paid to it. But they, equally in this part of the art, show such ardor that, if someone predicts a hemorrhage or a sweat, they treat him with contempt as a soothsayer or as a teller of tales; still less will they tolerate other predictions; still less will they adapt the form of regimen to the period when the illness is to reach its height. In what domain, then, do they compete with this man? It is certainly not by skill of expression; in him this, too, is perfectly correct; in them it is the opposite, to the point that one may see many of them making two mistakes in the space of a single word, which is not easily explained.[29]

The contrast Galen draws in this passage between Hippocrates and the medicine of his own time could not be more complete. Unreserved praise for the ancient physician is used as the basis for an uncompromising critique of Galen's contemporaries. This does not mean that Hippocrates has been made into an idealized figure here. For the qualities that Galen attributes to Hippocratic medicine are based for the most part on specific references to Hippocratic treatises.[30] In the rest of this opuscule, Galen presents the contrast between the ancient physician and his contemporaries in moral terms. The moderns are not naturally inferior to the ancients, he holds, but they are corrupted by two vices, greed and sensuality. The physician who wishes to be a disciple of Hippocrates is therefore enjoined to be a philosopher.

Galen did not restrict himself to holding up Hippocrates as a model for his contemporaries. Proclaiming himself a true disciple, Galen also responded to criticisms that certain of his colleagues had dared to address to the venerable physician; for all this, however, he was not a slave to his master in the way that those who styled themselves "Hippocrateans" were.[31] Most importantly of all, he wrote extensive commentaries on many of the Hippocratic treatises as well as a glossary of rare words attested by the collection. We are perfectly informed with regard to the various works that Galen composed about the physician of Cos, because toward the end of his life he drew up a catalog of his own writings, organized by category. One of these categories unites all of his writings about Hippocrates:

On my Hippocratic commentaries. None of the works in general that I have dedicated to friends ought in my opinion get into the hands of a wide audience; this is the case in particular with my exegetical writings on the Hippocratic treatises. At first, it was not for publication but to train myself that I wrote commentaries on these treatises, just as I did for each of the parts of the whole of medical theory, working out for myself what makes it possible to take in all the passages of Hippocrates on the medical art that provide instruction [which is] both clear and fully worked out. It is in fact for private use that I wrote *On Critical Days* according to the opinion of Hippocrates; it is for private use that I wrote *On Crises*; it is for private use that I wrote *On Dyspnea*, and on each of the other parts; and in this same spirit I composed the whole *Therapeutic Method* in fourteen books. As I knew that explications bearing upon each of the sentences of Hippocrates had already been written by many of my predecessors in a way that was not bad, I thought it superfluous to criticize all that did not seem to me to have been well said. I manifested this sentiment in the commentaries that I used to dedicate to those who requested them of me, rarely uttering a criticism against those who proposed these explications. At the beginning I did not even have their commentaries with me in Rome; for all the books that I possessed were still in Asia. If on occasion I remembered that one of them had said something quite wrong, liable to cause great harm in the exercise of the art to those who credited it, I pointed it out; but all the rest I expounded according to my own point of view, without mentioning those who had given a different explication. It is thus that I composed the commentaries on the *Aphorisms, Fractures, Joints*, and moreover the *Prognostic, Regimen in Acute Diseases, Ulcers, Wounds in the Head*, and the first book of the *Epidemics*. After that, as I understood that someone had praised a bad explication of an aphorism, I composed all the commentaries that I subsequently dedicated, having in mind a public edition and not [their] private possession by the addressees alone. These were the commentaries written on the second, third, and sixth books of the *Epidemics*; beyond these, on the *Humours, Nutriment, Prorrhetic, Nature of Man, In the Surgery*, as well as the treatise on *Airs, Waters, Places*, which in my view should be called *On Dwellings, Waters, Seasons, and Countries*. . . . Concerning Hippocrates also the following books: *On Regimen according to Hippocrates in Acute Diseases*, as well as the *Explication of Rare Words* that are found in his work [the *Glossary*], the *Against Lycus* on an aphorism that begins: "Growing creatures have the most innate heat" [*Aphorisms* 1.14], just as *Against Julian* [gives] the method for defending against what he reproached in the Hippocratic *Aphorisms*. Also concerning Hippocrates is another small book in which I show that the excellent physician must in every respect also be a philosopher.[32]

The balance sheet is impressive: some twenty-five works, to which more could be added since other treatises by Galen bear the name of Hippocrates in their title. Among these are a brief treatise entitled *On the Elements According to Hippocrates and Plato*, and an important work in nine books entitled *On the Doctrines of Hippocrates and Plato* that is notable for its doctrine locating the "guiding principle" of the human organism in the brain.

But it is the *Commentaries*, a group of some fifteen treatises, that stand out from the list as a whole. Galen wrote these toward the end of his career, during his second stay in Rome. Initially, he intended them for the private use of his friends, without indicating in any systematic way the interpretations of his predecessors; later, he revised them for publication, including a scholarly apparatus in the form of a running commentary on the text that derived from Alexandrian philology. It consisted of recopying Hippocrates' text, section by section, and commenting in turn upon each section (or *lemma*) by explicating rare words or difficult passages and expounding doctrine. Thus, each treatise was presented as a succession of excerpts containing a part of the Hippocratic text together with Galen's commentary on it.

In composing the *Commentaries*, Galen was conscious of his place in an already long tradition of exegesis. He provides us with details about his predecessors in this tradition in a second work concerning his own books entitled *On the Order of My Books*:

To know which explications of Hippocrates are correct and which are not is possible for one who has begun to practice with my essays. He will also have, for certain treatises of Hippocrates, my commentaries; and since now these commentaries are written, I shall attempt to add the rest. This will be done if I remain alive; if I die before having explicated the most important treatises of Hippocrates, those who desire to know his thought will have first my essays, as I have said, along with the commentaries I have already finished and then the commentaries of the exegetes of Hippocrates: those of my teacher Pelops and, occasionally, such commentaries [as remain] of Numisianus—few are preserved; beyond these, the ones of Sabinus and Rufus of Ephesus. Quintus and the disciples of Quintus have not understood the thought of Hippocrates with precision; this is why in many places their explications are not correct. Lycus sometimes criticises Hippocrates and claims that he is mistaken; this is because he does not understand his doctrines. . . . My teacher Satyrus—he is the one [whose classes] I attended first before following the instruction of Pelops—did not give the same explications as Lycus for the Hippocratic treatises. Satyrus claimed instead to follow with the most extreme exactitude the opinions of Quintus, without adding or subtracting anything. Aephicianus, certainly, introduced some modification to them in the direction of stoicism. I, therefore, who heard first in a way the explications of Quintus from the mouth of Satyrus and who later read one of the works of Lycus, condemned them both for not having understood exactly the thought of Hippocrates. One finds a better understanding in Sabinus and Rufus. One who has begun to practice with my essays is capable also of judging the commentaries of these interpreters and of detecting what they have said well and, occasionally, the errors that they have committed.[33]

Galen gives here the names of the eight physicians who were his immediate predecessors as commentators on Hippocrates. The only one of these authors whose name can really be said to have survived in the history of medicine is Rufus of Ephesus (first to second century A.D.). Several of Rufus's treatises have come down to us in which Hippocrates is cited as an authority,[34] but his actual commentaries on Hippocrates have been lost. Galen's reference to his predecessors nonetheless gives some idea of the profusion of commentaries on Hippocrates that followed one after another during the Hellenistic period, of the liveliness of the polemics among the various interpreters, and finally of the rapidity with which such commentaries could disappear. This makes the survival of Galen's own *Commentaries* all the more stunning. Through these works, the majority of which were to be preserved either in Greek or in Arabic, Galen powerfully contributed to the diffusion of Hippocratism. But since Galen constructed his image of Hippocrates to suit his own views, Hippocratism in the succeeding centuries was often to be dependent upon Galen's reading of it: "Hippocrates sewed, Galen cultivated," as one commentator of the sixth century A.D. very nicely stated the matter.[35]

The Legacy of Hippocrates in Late Antiquity

After Galen, the works of medicine preserved in Greek were mainly encyclopedias. It is chiefly through these that the survival of Hippocratism is to be traced. Henceforth, however, Galen was to be regarded as a classic reference along with Hippocrates, sometimes overshadowing him; even so, outside the medical world, Hippocrates was to continue to represent the ideal physician. His influence surreptitiously crept even into Christian literature, where we find Saint Jerome using the phrase "spiritual Hippocrates"[36]—not (as too often has been wrongly assumed) to describe Christ, but rather a priest, Isidorus, who served as a mediator in a theological quarrel. Saint Jerome even awarded this Isidorus the title "Hippocrates of the Christians."[37] Much later, Dante was to make Saint Luke, who was himself a physician, a disciple of "the very great Hippocrates."[38]

The oldest and most important encyclopedia after Galen is that of Oribasius, physician to the Emperor Julian (fourth century A.D.). When Oribasius, at the demand of the emperor, set about bringing together the texts of the best physicians, his criterion for selection remained Hippocratism. But Galen, by virtue of his stature as the most eminent representative of this tradition,[39] was to occupy the largest place in this vast compilation, seventy books in all, of which only one-third has come down to us.

The second encyclopedia is due to Aëtius, a physician originally from Amida in Mesopotamia who lived under the Emperor Justinian (sixth century A.D.). This encyclopedia, though less voluminous than that of Oribasius, containing only sixteen books, is distinguished by its manner of presentation. While Oribasius limited himself to collecting excerpts from the work of the greatest physicians, Aëtius stated his own views, drawing upon sources that occasionally he thought to identify. Galen remains, as in Oribasius, the principal source; his name is cited some two hundred times. Hippocrates occupies a more modest place, being mentioned only thirty-six times. But Aëtius nonetheless had a detailed knowledge of the Hippocratic works, and he makes reference to several treatises, in particular the *Aphorisms* and the *Prognostic*. He even reproduces in Greek a passage from the Hippocratic treatise *Sevens*, which otherwise has come down to us only in Latin.[40]

Hippocrates was not merely a venerable authority, however; the tradition of medicine associated with his name continued to be relevant to current practice. As evidence of this we may cite the following passage from Aëtius: "It is necessary that the physician be trained in conformity with the *Prognostic* of Hippocrates and with other works and that he know the workings of nature, for 'natures are the physicians of living beings.' He must aid nature, which fights in favor of health against disease. Thus, nature, if it receives as allies the physician doing his duty and the patient himself obeying and not committing mistakes in his regimen, will triumph over disease."[41]

Everything about this excerpt is Hippocratic in its inspiration. Not only is it necessary for the physician to take the *Prognostic* as his model, but the formula "natures are the physicians of living beings" is a (corrupt) reference to *Epidemics VI*.[42] The metaphor of battle against disease is also Hippocratic. However, the reading given by Aëtius conceals a shift in meaning, because nature assumes a place here that it did not have in the oldest treatises. While in the *Epidemics* the physician had to ally himself with the patient in order to combat the disease, in Aëtius the physician allies himself with nature to combat the disease. A new actor has entered into the fray, and now plays a leading role: nature.[43]

From the time of Justinian also dates a satiric epigram by the poet Agathias that further attests to Hippocrates' prestige during this period. A physician of Cos follows the letter of his predecessor's teachings without, unfortunately, respecting their spirit:

Alcimenes lay in bed sore sick of a fever and giving vent to hoarse wheezings from his wind-pipe, his side pricking him as if he had been pierced by a sword, and his breath coming short in ill-sounding gasps. Then came Callignotus of Cos, with his never-ending jaw, full of the wisdom of the healing art, whose prognosis of pains was complete, and he never foretold anything but what came to pass. He inspected Alcimenes' position in bed and drew conclusions from his face, and felt his pulse scientifically. Then he reckoned up from the treatise on critical days, calculating everything not without his Hippocrates, and finally he gave utterance to Alcimenes of his prognosis, making his face very solemn and looking most serious: "If your throat stops roaring and the fierce attacks of pain in your side cease, and your breathing is no longer made thick by the fever, you will not die in that case of pleurisy, for this is to us a sign of coming freedom from pain. Cheer up, and summoning your lawyer, dispose well of your property and depart from this life, the mother of care, leaving to me, your doctor, in return for my good prognostic, the third part of your inheritance."[44]

This Coan physician knew Hippocrates' *Prognostic* by heart, just like Aëtius; but he had totally forgotten *The Oath*!

Let us come back to the subject of encyclopedias for a moment. The encyclopedias of Oribasius and Aëtius were both compiled at Constantinople and signal the new role played by the capital of the Eastern Empire in the history of medicine, a role that was to reach its height during the Byzantine Renaissance. Nonetheless, the ancient centers, particularly that of Alexandria, continued to flourish and to perpetuate the Hippocratic tradition. Oribasius and Aëtius, for their part, had both pursued their medical studies at Alexandria. A number of Hippocrates' works continued to be part of the curriculum at the school there, though not as many as those of Galen. They were the subject of commentaries whose method adopted the same schemas that the philosophers of Alexandria were then applying to Aristotelian exegesis. Some of these, from the sixth and seventh centuries, have been preserved: Palladius commented in the sixth century on book VI of the *Epidemics* and the surgical treatise *On Fractures*; in the following century, the treatise *Nature of the Child* was commented on by John of Alexandria, and, also in the seventh century, the *Aphorisms*, *Prognostic*, and *On Fractures* were commented on by Stephanus (sometimes said to be of Alexandria, sometimes of Athens).[45] We know from his commentaries that treatises of Hippocrates were studied at Alexandria and the order in which they were read.[46] Finally, it is to a physician of the seventh century, Paul of Aegina, who was trained at Alexandria and who practiced there, that we owe the third great medical encyclopedia of antiquity.

The work of Paul of Aegina is far less vast than that of Oribasius, or even that of Aëtius, comprising only seven books. Mention of Hippocrates is also less frequent here than in Galen, although the share of references to him is greater than in Aëtius.[47] Paul of Aegina was a practicing physician as well as a theoretician, and particularly valued everything in the Hippocratic treatises concerning surgery. Although he very rarely quotes long passages, he makes an exception in the case of Hippocrates' description of the dislocation of the jaw and his procedure for reducing it.[48] "With regard to the complete dislocation of the lower jaw," Paul writes, "it will be sufficient to deliver Hippocrates' account, being, at the same time, brief, complete, and clear." There follows a very long citation to chapters 30 and 31 of the treatise *On Joints*, after which the encyclopedist concludes, "This mode of reduction we have often practised."[49] Such unqualified praise for the technique of his illustrious predecessor comes from a practitioner who recognized that it had not been improved upon since Hippocrates' time. Moderns recognized this as well. "The procedure most generally employed in France," noted the surgeon Auguste Nélaton (1807–1873), "is that which has been most anciently used, since it is described by Hippocrates."[50]

Though the school of Alexandria was to die out after the Arab conquest in 642, the Greek tradition of Hippocratism seems not to have been extinguished in this city. It is significant that an Arab physician of the eleventh century living in Cairo received a list of fifty-five writings of Hippocrates from a Christian colleague who possessed a Greek version of the list and translated it into Arabic for the occasion.[51] This late Alexandrian heritage was to be transmitted to the West in the form of both Arabic and Latin translations.

The Role of Latin and Arabic Translations in the Survival of Hippocratism

Since the Hippocratic literature was used by practitioners, its diffusion in the West required it to be translated into Latin for those who had no Greek, above all from the time when knowledge of the Greek language began to decline. It was thus in the fifth or sixth century that Latin translations of a number of Hippocratic treatises were undertaken in Italy, particularly at Ravenna, seat of the Byzantine exarchate from 568 to 752.[52] They date from the time when Cassiodorus, in the monastery of Vivarium in southern Italy, recommended that the monks there who did not know Greek read Hippocrates and Galen in Latin.[53] These ancient Latin translations have come down to us in manuscripts that go back to the tenth century. While they scrupulously respect the Greek source manuscripts, they contain a great many copying mistakes—so many, in fact, that the result is rather disappointing; the Latin is in any case barbarous, and sometimes obscure. Nonetheless, one of these translations remains extremely precious since it is our only source of one of the Hippocratic treatises of which the Greek original has been lost, the treatise *Sevens*.

In the East, the Hippocratic treatises continued to be read in Greek at Alexandria, Pergamum, and Constantinople, and were also translated into Syriac and Arabic. Here we must mention the name of the great translator of the Greek physicians in the ninth century, Ḥunayn ibn Isḥāq. Ḥunayn was a Nestorian physician and director of the House of Wisdom, founded at Baghdad by an Abbasid caliph. Assisted by his disciples, his habit was to translate the Greek into Syriac, and then the Syriac into Arabic. Only one Arabic translation made directly from a Hippocratic treatise has been preserved.[54] But Ḥunayn contributed indirectly to the diffusion of the Hippocratic Collection, for he translated Galen's *Commentaries* on Hippocrates.[55] Indeed, he was responsible for a rather curious circumstance. It will be recalled that these commentaries consisted of alternating sections, the "words of Hippocrates" (to use Ḥunayn's terminology) being followed by Galen's commentary on these words. In the Arab tradition, however, the Hippocratic treatises were recomposed by removing the "words of Hippocrates" from Galen's commentaries. As a result of this remarkable surgery, Hippocrates was reborn, now springing forth fully armed from the head of Galen. Both Galen and Hippocrates were to exercise a profound influence on Arab medicine through these translations, but it was chiefly in the form of what might be called Galenic Hippocratism that Arab commentators came to know the Hippocratic Collection. This in turn gave rise to a Galeno-Arab Hippocratism.

Translators did not quit while the going was good, however. The Arab translations of Galen were themselves translated into Latin, beginning in the eleventh century, and in this new form enjoyed a broad diffusion in the West through the Renaissance. But this meant that henceforth Hippocrates was to be known only very indirectly indeed. Thus, for example, the medical school at Salerno in southern Italy knew Hippocrates via Galen's commentaries on the *Aphorisms*, *Prognostic*, and *Regimen in Acute Diseases*, which in turn had been translated from Arabic into Latin by Constantine the African in the second half of the eleventh century. From the twelfth century, there were Latin translations made directly from the Greek, notably by Burgundio of Pisa and later by Bartholomew of Messina, translator at the court of King Manfred (1258–66), and, in the following century, by Niccolò da Reggio of Calabria (between 1308 and 1345). But the later Latin translations of Hippocrates made directly from the Greek were much rarer than those of Galen. In the first great universities where medicine was taught in Europe from the thirteenth century, at Montpellier, Bologna, and Paris, it was mainly Galeno-Arabic Hippocratism that was taught; and despite the new translations that began to appear in the twelfth century, which to a limited degree revitalized the Hippocratic tradition toward the end of the thirteenth and the beginning of the fourteenth centuries, the corpus of texts forming the basis of teaching remained fundamentally that of the school of Salerno, known as the *Articella*. Hippocrates was represented in this collection only by the three treatises commented by Galen and translated from the Arabic by Constantine the African. Of the three, the *Aphorisms* was the main object of commentary and discussion; and of these, it was the first one ("Life is short, the Art long, opportunity fleeting, experiment treacherous, judgment difficult") that particularly stimulated reflection about medical method; that is to say, about the respective roles of experiment and reason.

For the Hippocratic Collection to become known once again, directly and in its full range and scope, it was necessary to wait for the Renaissance and the advent of the printed book. In 1525, Marcus Fabius Calvus published at Rome an integral Latin translation based directly on the Greek. One year later, Franciscus Asulanus published at Venice, through the Aldine Press, the first complete Greek edition. This was based on a manuscript that was subsequently offered to François I of France and is to be found today at the Bibliothèque Nationale in Paris.[56] But prior to this return to original textual sources, the printed book had already permitted the medieval tradition to become widespread. The *Articella*, published in 1473 at Padua, was to be reprinted fifteen times before the appearance of the first Greek edition of the whole Hippocratic Collection.

To trace the fate of Hippocrates in modern times would take us beyond the limits of this study—and the competence of its author. A synthetic history of Hippocratism from the Renaissance through the present day remains to be written, despite the existence of a number of excellent monographs. A satisfactory history would need to follow several paths.

One of these paths is the search for the authentic Hippocratic tradition through a return to the Greek text, stripped of its commentaries. This search, inaugurated by the edition of Franciscus Asulanus, was long the work of Hellenist physicians, editors, translators, and interpreters who from the sixteenth to the nineteenth century attempted to restore the Hippocratic text to a form that seemed to them the nearest to the original, whether on the basis of conjecture or through comparison of manuscripts. A dramatic start was made in the sixteenth century. The best known of all Renaissance editors was Rabelais, an advocate of the new "humanistic medicine" that insisted on going back to the Greek text or, failing that, to a precise Latin translation. But his partial edition of Hippocrates and Galen (1532), despite the success to which its many reprintings testify,[57] did not enjoy the same influence as the complete editions produced by two physicians who today are far more obscure, but in fact far more deserving of fame, Janus Cornarius of Zwickau (1538) and Anuce Foës [also Anutius Foësius] of Metz (1595). Their editions were still used in the eighteenth century, even by scholars.

It was necessary to wait for a second renaissance in Hippocratic studies in the nineteenth century for the appearance of Émile Littré's great ten-volume edition,[58] which finally supplanted those of the sixteenth; so great was the prestige of the "Littré edition" that it overshadowed the one published shortly afterwards by the Dutch physician F. Z. Ermerins. With these two great editions, the heroic enterprise of the Hellenist physicians came to an end; and with them also came to an end the type of monumental edition containing the entire work of Hippocrates edited by a single man. The editorial work of the Hellenist physicians was—and continues to be—carried on by trained philologists with the help of historians of science. But none of the three great projects undertaken in England, France, and Germany with the aim of revising the whole *Corpus Hippocraticum* has yet succeeded in providing a complete modern edition, even though they have all disposed of the resources of teams of scholars. No doubt the art of publishing has become too long, for the progress of medicine has not done anything to shorten the life of editors.

Another path to be followed has to do with the impact that Hippocratism has had on the modern history of ideas. A treatise such as *Airs, Waters, Places*, with its medical climatology and its climatological and political anthropology, exercised an incontestable and quite special fascination upon the thinkers of the sixteenth and seventeenth centuries. The Italian physician Girolamo Cardano (better known as Jerome Cardan, the inventor of the universal joint as well as a great mathematician) published a long commentary on it in 1570.[59] The English physician John Arbuthnot gave a detailed summary of the treatise in his *Essay Concerning the Effects of Air on Human Bodies* (1733). The French physician Pierre Barthez, of the school of Montpellier, made firsthand use of what this treatise had to say about the influence of climate and laws on peoples in his *New Elements of the Science of Man* (1778). And Georges Cabanis, in *On the Relations between the Physical and Moral Aspects of Man* (1802), also relied very heavily on *Airs, Waters, Places* in his section concerning the influence of climates on moral habits.[60] The most famous modern work that can be linked with the treatise is Montesquieu's *On the Spirit of the Laws* (1748). One scholarly commentator has pointed out that among Montesquieu's papers at La Brède there is a summary of *Airs, Waters, Places*.[61] Montesquieu says nothing, however, about Hippocrates. One wishes that he had. The Greek physician Adamantios Coray, in the preface to his celebrated edition of *Airs, Waters, Places* that appeared in 1800, after citing the laudatory judgment of one of his predecessors regarding the treatise, adds: "This judgment has been justified in our own time by another work of genius, the *Spirit of the Laws*, whose author would have taken nothing away from his own glory if he had had the noble courage to honor the Greek physician whose fertile principle gave him the idea for his work and was the basis of it."[62]

But the most important path to be followed involves the various faces of Hippocrates that have appeared in the course of modern medical progress and the "biological revolutions" associated with it, to use the expression of a contemporary historian of medicine.[63] More than anything else, this would amount to writing the history of a dual corruption of the Hippocratic corpus. On the one hand, the authority of the master of Cos, transmitted mainly in the distorted form of exegeses by Galen and the Arabs, acted as a brake upon science. Thus, for example, the discovery in the seventeenth century of the circulation of the blood by Harvey was combated by some in the name of

Hippocrates. At the same time, however, others sought to save the grand old man's reputation by transforming him into a precursor—after all, it was hardly a problem to find mention of a "circular motion" in his writings. By this means, it became possible for Harvey's discovery to acquire an illustrious pedigree and for Hippocrates' statue to remain untoppled. Faced with this double distortion, neo-Hippocratism went back to the actual text in order to try to draw useful teachings from it. Thus it was that later in the seventeenth century the "English Hippocrates," Thomas Sydenham, found in certain Hippocratic treatises, particularly the *Epidemics*, the model not only for a new kind of climatological epidemiology, but also for a style of clinical observation free of theoretical bias and of therapeutic restraint.[64] His admiration for Hippocrates was such that when he discovered smallpox, he concluded that it could not have existed in Hippocrates' time as it did in his own; otherwise, he noted, "[i]t would not have escaped him, he who understood the history of diseases more clearly and described diseases more precisely than any of his successors."[65] In France, neo-Hippocratism was traditionally associated with the school of Montpellier, as opposed to the Galenism of the Faculty of Paris. This school claimed to stand in succession to that of Cos, as the inscription painted at the end of the eighteenth century in the *salle des Actes* at Montpellier testifies: "Olim Cous, nunc Monspelliensis Hippocrates."[66] Hippocrates' teaching survived there longer than that of Galen.[67] In the nineteenth century, Hippocratic empiricism was brilliantly represented by Laënnec,[68] who reacted against the "physiological" medicine of Broussais and his followers. But in this moment of crisis, Hippocratism had become the object of passionate battles that largely ignored Hippocrates' own words.[69] The adversaries of the "Hippocratic sect" resorted to caricature in denouncing Hippocrates' fatalism and cautiousness in letting nature have its way; and whenever Hippocrates was shown to have had the bad taste to say that it was necessary to act with haste, they got around it by learnedly demonstrating that the passage in question was not authentic.

Since then, scholarly quarrels upholding or castigating Hippocratism have died out in the medical world. Hippocrates' scepter has been shattered. Yet Hippocrates himself has survived all his detractors and all his admirers. Although the work transmitted under his name may now be outmoded from a scientific standpoint, its human dimension remains a model for physicians. The Hippocratic Collection in any case constitutes—and will go on constituting—one of the richest and most impressive monuments of the awakening of the scientific spirit in Greece and in the Western world.

With regard to abbreviations of classical works and journal titles used in the notes and bibliography, the reader is referred to the list of authors and books given in *The Oxford Classical Dictionary*, 3rd ed. (Oxford, 1996), xxix–liv. Additional information may be found in the third edition of the THESAURUS LINGUAE GRAECAE *Canon of Greek Authors and Works* (Oxford, 1990).

Ant. Pal.	*Palatine Anthology* (referred to in this work as *Anthologia Graeca* [also, in the Loeb Classical Library, *The Greek Anthology*]).
Budé	*Hippocrate.* Collection des Universités de France (published under the aegis of L'Association Guillaume Budé). 8 vols. Paris, 1967–1996.
CMG	*Corpus medicorum Graecorum.* Leipzig and Berlin, 1908– ; Berlin, 1947– .
Diels-Kranz	*Die Fragmente der Vorsokratiker.* Edited by H. Diels and W. Kranz. 3 vols. 6th ed. Zürich, 1951–1952; reprint 1966–1967.
FGH	*Die Fragmente der griechischen Historiker.* Edited by F. Jacoby. 3 vols. in 15 vols. Leyden, 1923–1958; reprint 1954–1969.
Grene-Lattimore	*The Complete Greek Tragedies.* Edited by David Grene and Richmond Lattimore. 4 vols. Chicago and London, 1992.
Lattimore	*The Iliad of Homer.* Translated and with an introduction by Richmond Lattimore. Chicago and London, 1951.
Littré	*Oeuvres complètes d'Hippocrate.* Edited and translated by Émile Littré. 10 vols. Paris, 1839–1861.
Loeb	*Hippocrates.* The Loeb Classical Library. Edited by W. H. S. Jones et al. 8 vols. 1923–1995.
Tandy-Neale	*Hesiod's WORKS AND DAYS.* Translated with commentary by David W. Tandy and Walter C. Neale. Berkeley and Los Angeles, 1996.
Teubner	*Hippokrates.* Bibliotheca scriptorum Graecorum et Romanorum Teubneriana. 2 vols. Leipzig, 1894–1902.

The Oath

I swear by Apollo Physician, by Asclepius, by Health, by Panacea and by all the gods and goddesses, making them my witnesses, that I will carry out, according to my ability and judgment, this oath and this indenture. To hold my teacher in this art equal to my own parents; to make him partner in my livelihood; when he is in need of money to share mine with him; to consider his family as my own brothers, and to teach them this art, if they want to learn it, without fee or indenture; to impart precept, oral instruction, and all other instruction to my own sons, the sons of my teacher, and to indentured pupils who have taken the physician's oath, but to nobody else. I will use treatment to help the sick according to my ability and judgment, but never with a view to injury and wrong-doing. Neither will I administer a poison to anybody when asked to do so, nor will I suggest such a course. Similarly I will not give to a woman a pessary to cause abortion. But I will keep pure and holy both my life and my art. I will not use the knife, not even, verily, on sufferers from stone, but I will give place to such as are craftsmen therein. Into whatsoever houses I enter, I will enter to help the sick, and I will abstain from all intentional wrong-doing and harm, especially from abusing the bodies of man or woman, bond or free. And whatsoever I shall see or hear in the course of my profession, as well as outside my profession in my intercourse with men, if it be what should not be published abroad, I will never divulge, holding such things to be holy secrets. Now if I carry out this oath, and break it not, may I gain for ever reputation among all men for my life and for my art; but if I transgress it and forswear myself, may the opposite befall me.

Translated by W. H. S. Jones (Loeb I, 299–301)

An Honorary Decree in Praise of a
Physician of Cos

This decree does not concern Hippocrates, but a physician of Cos of the Hellenistic era (second century B.C.). However, it is useful to bring to the reader's attention this piece of epigraphic evidence, which was recently published for the first time (*Parola de Passato* 46 [1991]: 135–140; Greek text with commentary by R. Herzog in Latin; Italian translation by Pugliese Carratelli). The document is exceptional by reason of its length, its state of preservation, and the richness of the information it contains. Indeed, it gives very valuable information about the career of the honored physician Onasander, and also that of his teacher Antipater. The decree in honor of Onasander was voted by the popular assembly of Halasarna (the present-day Cardamina); that is, by the citizens of Cos belonging to this deme. The decree was proposed by the three magistrates of the deme, called *napoiai*. The decree is dated by reference to the eponymous magistrate of the city of Cos, who bore the title "monarch."

The inscription, found on a block of marble lodged in the absidal wall of the church *Agia Théotès* in Cardamina in 1907, and copied at that time by the German archaeologist R. Herzog, remained unpublished for almost a century. In the meantime, the stone, which had not been moved from antiquity until the beginning of the present century—since the *Agia Théotès* was built upon the ancient sanctuary of Apollo where the stone stood—disappeared.

Here is the translation of this decree:

Under the monarch Philiscus, the twenty-eighth day of Panamos, the *napoiai*, Nicarchus, son of Tisias, Ariston, son of Charmylus, [and] Philonidas, son of Didymarchus, proposed the following. Grounds: the physician Onasander, son of Onesimus, having learned the art from Antipater, son of Dioscuridas, at the moment when his teacher was public physician with us, displayed during his studies a courteous manner toward all and offered to those of the people who had need of it, without even being called, the succor of his art. Having become [Antipater's] assistant, during still many more years he showed to a [yet] higher degree his competence in the art and his good conduct in life, shrinking from no effort or expense without which the people would have been deprived of some advantage. And when his teacher was nominated to fulfill the functions [of public physician] in the city [of Cos], Onasander decided at once to aid him in his public responsibilities by remaining his assistant. As many of the inhabitants of the deme still went to him, having known from past experience his competence in the art and his conduct in life, he showed himself to all attentive and devoted, giving aid and contributing, so far as it was within his power, to their salvation, exactly as those who had had turned to him personally [in the past] had known him [to do]. Then, when he decided to open his own office and to practice as a private physician in the city [of Cos], while certain of those who used his services paid him fees, nonetheless he neither demanded payment nor accepted remuneration from any of the people who came to him for his competence in the art of medicine, though he could in this way have accumulated a considerable sum, given that many of the people who used his services had both grave illnesses and exceptional treatments. But always attaching a lesser importance to his [own] personal interest, he showed himself attentive and devoted to all in giving aid and, during the rest of his life, he remained courteous to all and worthy of being honored, not only on account of his practice of the art, but also on account of his benevolence toward the people. In order therefore that it be manifest that the people honor not only those among the citizens who are good and benevolent toward them, but also those among the *paroikoi* [residents] who behave attentively and enthusiastically in every circumstance toward the people, and in order that Onasander, distinguished by the honors that he deserves, shows himself [still] more devoted to the people, with the aid of good fortune it is decreed by the people of Halasarna that the physician Onasander, son of Onesimus, be commended for his behavior toward all the people and for his competence in the medical art; that he [be permitted to] participate in all the religious ceremonies in which the people participate; that the *napoiai* deduct the costs of the stele and of the inscription from the funds belonging to the gods and that they erect the stele in the sanctuary of Apollo next to the stele of his teacher Antipater. Votes ratifying the proposal of the *napoiai*. For: two hundred forty-eight. Against: zero.

* * *

Thanks to this inscription, it is possible to follow the various stages of the career of a physician, Onasander, that unfolded for a long while in the shadow of that of his teacher. This Onasander was a *paroikos* (a "resident"—either a foreigner or an emancipated slave or the son of an emancipated slave) who practiced at Halasarna and later in the city of Cos. When his teacher Antipator was public physician in the deme of Halasarna, Onasander was first his pupil and then his assistant. When his teacher became public physician of the city of Cos, Onasander followed him and remained his assistant for a certain time. He then decided to open his own office as a private physician in the city of Cos. When he left Halasarna, he nonetheless did not forget his former clientele in the deme. For all the services rendered by Onasander to the deme, a commendation was issued by the assembly of citizens along with the privilege of participating in the religious ceremonies of the deme. The stele publishing the decree was placed in the sanctuary of Apollo, next to that of his teacher. Antipater had therefore been honored previously, no doubt for his services as public physician of the deme, when he gave up this position in order to become public physician for the city of Cos as a whole.

There is not room here to bring out the exceptional importance of this inscription for the information it provides relating to the career of Greek physicians (public and private alike), to the title of assistant (known already from Plato *Laws* 720a–b), and to medical ethics (the question of fees). Let us simply emphasize that the close ties between teacher and pupil are not unworthy of those that we glimpsed earlier with *The Oath* of Hippocrates, reproduced in its entirety in appendix 1.

The Treatises of the Hippocratic Collection

The treatises are cited in the alphabetical order of their English titles. The principal editions given here are based on the Greek-French edition of Émile Littré (10 vols., 1839–1861). I have not bothered to mention the other complete nineteenth-century edition, F. Z. Ermerins's Greek-Latin version (3 vols., 1859–1864), since it is of use only to specialists.

1. *Address from the Altar (= Epibomios)*

Contents: Brief supplication by Hippocrates, who has taken refuge with his family, praying at an altar of Athena and addressing himself to the Thessalians. He asks them to come to the aid of his native island of Cos, . threatened with war by Athens.

Authorship and date: This biographical writing figures in Erotian's list; fourth century or Hellenistic period.

Editions: Littré IX, 402–404; Smith, 1990 (Greek-English).

2. *Affections*

Contents: The originality of this treatise derives from the fact that it was intended for lay readers rather than for specialists.

It consists of two parts, the first concerning diseases (chapters 2–35). The author, after having attributed all diseases to phlegm and to bile in the first chapter, goes on to treat particular diseases in terms of the care to be given in each case—though he also knows semiology, etiology, and prognosis. The order of exposition followed is roughly *a capite ad calcem*: first the affections of the head (2–5), then those of the cavities (6ff.). By "cavities" is understood the upper cavity or chest, whose affections include pleurisy and pneumonia (7–9), and the lower cavity or belly, whose affections include those of the spleen (20), ileus (21), dysentery (23), lientery (24), diarrhea (25), tenesmus (26), cholera and diarrhea (27); the author then goes on (31) to discuss a disease that affects the feet, podragra (or gout). Upon this first principle of classification is superimposed another, which takes into consideration the season when the disease typically appears. Thus he divides the beginning of his description of the diseases of the cavities into diseases that arise mainly in winter (6–12, comprising the acute diseases: pleurisy, pneumonia, phrenitis, and causus, as well as other fevers) and diseases that manifest themselves chiefly in summer (15–18, including tertian and quartan fevers).

The second part of the treatise (39–61) provides general advice regarding patients' diet (soups, foods, drinks). It is in this part that one encounters one of the two catalogs found in the collection of the properties of foods and drinks, the other being found in the treatise *Regimen*.

A final peculiarity of this treatise is that it refers the reader several times to a work called *Pharmakitis*, saying that it contains fuller information about remedies. This work is lost.

Authorship and date: The material of the first section, which exhibits similarities with certain passages of *Diseases II*, is probably Cnidian in origin. But the bihumoral etiology is quite systematic; and, moreover, neither the introduction nor the part on diet bears any relation to the Cnidian treatises. The date of the treatise may be put sometime in the 380s.

Editions: Littré VI, 208–271; Jouanna, 1974 [= Jouanna, *Hippocrate: Pour une archéologie de l'école de Cnide* (Paris, 1974)] (Greek-French; excerpts); Potter, 1983 (= Loeb V, 1–91).

3. *Airs, Waters, Places*

Contents: The treatise consists of two parts, one properly medical (1–11) and the other ethnographic (12–24). In the medical part, the author enumerates and analyzes the various external factors that the physician must consider for purposes of prognosis and in order to treat the general or particular diseases liable to occur in the course of a year. First are the local factors specific to a city: the orientation of the city with respect to winds and to the sun (3–6); also the quality of the waters drawn there (7–9). Next is a general factor that applies to all cities where the physician may happen to go: the climatic constitution of the year (10–11).

The second part offers a comparison of the peoples of Europe and of Asia, and attempts to explain the principal physical and mental differences between them. It discusses first the physique of the peoples of Asia (12–15) and their character (16); then the physique of the peoples of Europe, notably the Scythians (17–23), and their character (23). These differences have mainly to do with climate, and secondarily with the influence of customs and laws. In the last chapter (24), the author comes back to those external factors that influence the physique and character of peoples, adding to climate the influence of the land.

Authorship and date: The first part is intended for the specialist, and more particularly for the itinerant physician who arrives in a city unfamiliar to him, where he is to practice for a fixed period of time. The treatise is traditionally associated with the school of Cos. Galen wrote a commentary on it (preserved solely in an Arabic translation). The author is probably the same as that of *The Sacred Disease*. Second half of the fifth century.

Editions: Littré II, 1–93; Kühlewein, 1894 [= Teubner I] (Greek); Gundermann, 1911 (Greek-Latin); Jones, 1923 [= Loeb I, 65–137]; Heiberg, 1927 [= *CMG* I, 1] (Greek); Diller, 1970 [= *CMG* I, 1, 2] (Greek-German); Lipourlis, 1983 (ancient Greek-modern Greek); Jouanna, 1996 [= Budé II, 2] (Greek-French).

4. *Anatomy*

Contents: Very brief description of the trachea, lungs, heart, liver, kidneys, bladder, and digestive system.

Authorship and date: This work is not part of Erotian's list, but rather belongs to later treatises; Hellenistic or Roman period.

Editions: Littré VIII, 536–541.

5. *Ancient Medicine*

Contents: The treatise opens with a long polemical preamble (1–2) in which the author denounces the errors of innovators in the medical art who base their analysis on some simplifying postulate, such as the hot, the cold, the dry, or the moist, in order to explain the cause of diseases. To show that the art has no need of a new method, the author then retraces in a long passage what may be called the "archaeology" of medicine; that is, the birth of an art that has long been able to claim an origin and a method (3–12). The author returns next to his critique of those who follow the "novel fashion," demonstrating that their postulate is contrary to reality, and minimizes the role of the hot and the cold in the production of diseases. He later broadens his attack (20) to include physicians and philosophers, such as Empedocles, who hold that the philosophical knowledge of man is prior to medicine. According to the author, far from being prior to medicine, knowledge of man is possible only by means of medicine, properly understood; that is to say, through the study of causal relations between regimen (diet, baths, exercise) and man. The three final chapters (22–24) provide additional detail regarding the causes of diseases. They are due not only to the properties of the body, but also to the conformations of its parts.

Authorship and date: The treatise belongs to the category of discourses originally meant to be delivered before a mixed audience of specialists and laymen. The mention of Empedocles in chapter 20 indicates that the treatise comes after him. End of the fifth century.

Editions: Littré I, 570–637; Kühlewein, 1894 [= Teubner I] (Greek); Jones, 1923 [= Loeb I, 1–64]; Heiberg, 1927 [= *CMG* I, 1] (Greek); Jones, 1946 (Greek-English); Festugière, 1948 (Greek-French); Conrado Eggers Lan, 1987 (Greek-Spanish); Jouanna, 1990 [= Budé II, 1] (Greek-French).

6. *Aphorisms*

Contents: The most widely read, commented, and cited treatise of the entire collection. It was the bible of physicians until the eighteenth century. The beginning of the first aphorism is known to all: "Life is short, the Art long."
   It is impossible to convey briefly the richness of this treatise, which is made up of a group of often unrelated propositions that bear upon the various aspects of the medical art (mainly prognosis and etiology, but also regimen and medication). Certain subgroups may nonetheless be identified among this mass of aphorisms, which traditionally is divided into seven sections. The first section contains numerous aphorisms on regimen in diseases (the regimen varying with the evolution of the disease) and on evacuations (warning against evacuating humors prior to coction). The aphorisms of the second section concerning prognosis and therapy are quite varied. Some of the fundamental notions of Hippocratic medicine are found in this section: treatment by contraries (2.22), the importance of habit (2.49, 2.50), the unnatural character of all excess (2.51).

The third section is more unified: a large part is devoted to the influence of the seasons upon disease (3.1–23), the rest to the influence of age (3.24–31). The fourth part begins with a discussion of upward and downward purges (4.1–20); the remainder of the section is devoted to prognostic signs in various diseases, particularly in fevers (stools, humoral evacuations, sweats, chills, spasms, urines, etc.). The fifth section opens with aphorisms on prognosis (5.1–15), continues with aphorisms on heat and cold (5.16–26), and concludes with aphorisms on women (5.28–62). The sixth and seventh sections collect aphorisms on prognostic signs in a number of diseases.

Authorship and date: The *Aphorisms* was regarded in antiquity as the work of Hippocrates par excellence. The treatise was commented on by Galen. In reality it is a compilation whose wording is similar in rather many places to that of other treatises in the collection, particularly ones attributed to the school of Cos such as *Nature of Man, Airs, Waters, Places*, the middle group of *Epidemics* (*II, IV, VI*), and *Humours*. Several aphorisms are also found in another edited work, the *Coan Prenotions*.

Even though the treatise may preserve ancient material, it was not composed prior to the fourth century.

Editions: Littré IV, 458–609; Jones, 1931 [= Loeb IV, 97–221]; C. Magdelaine, 1994 (Greek-French; Paris doctoral thesis).

7. The Art

Contents: The author proposes to show, in response to detractors of the medical art, that medicine is indeed an art and that it has the power, within certain limits, to cure or lessen illnesses. After a polemical preamble against those "who have made an art of vilifying the arts" (1), the author begins by giving a general argument valid for every art that makes reference to the philosophical debates of the period on being and non-being and on the relationship between language and reality (2). Then he demonstrates the existence of the medical art by refuting the various allegations brought by its adversaries (4–8). Finally, he shows the powers of medicine to combat disease (9–12) [= 9–13 in the Loeb edition], distinguishing two broad groups of diseases: those that can be seen (9) and those that cannot be seen (10–12) [= 10–13]. In an epilogue (13) [= 14], medicine is asserted to be an art of great resources within the limits of what it can and cannot do.

Authorship and date: The treatise belongs to the category of discourses originally intended to be delivered before an audience. It is generally dated from the last quarter of the fifth century.

Editions: Littré VI, 1–27; Gomperz, 1910 [2nd ed.] (Greek-German); Jones, 1923 [= Loeb II, 185–217]; Heiberg, 1927 [= *CMG* I, 1] (Greek); Jouanna, 1988 [= Budé V, 1] (Greek-French).

Barrenness. See 20. *Diseases of Women I–II / Sterile Women*

8. *Breaths*

Contents: Medical discourse originally intended for oral delivery. A long exordium (1) concerns medicine, its difficulties, method, object, and definition; this chapter contains the celebrated passage defining treatment as allopathy: "opposites are cures for opposites." The author's purpose is to show that diseases, despite their diversity, are due to a single cause (2). After having stressed the power of air in the universe and in human beings (3–5), the author shows that it is the sole cause of diseases (6–14). He begins with fevers: epidemic fever due to air infected with miasmas (6); fevers caused by bad regimen (7–8); abdominal maladies (9); chest hemorrhages (10); lacerations (11); dropsy (12); paralyses (13); the sacred disease (14). The conclusion (15) is that air is the principal cause of disease, all the rest being secondary.

Authorship and date: Despite its polished style, the treatise is the work of a physician and not of a Sophist. Since the discovery of the *Anonymus Londinensis*, it has been the object of debate in relation to the Hippocratic question (see page 60). It dates from the last quarter of the fifth century.

Editions: Littré VI, 90–115; Nelson, 1909 (Greek-Latin); Jones, 1923 [= Loeb II, 219–253]; Heiberg, 1927 [= *CMG* I, 1] (Greek); Jouanna, 1988 [= Budé V, 1] (Greek-French).

9. *Coan Prenotions*

Contents: Like the *Aphorisms*, the *Coan Prenotions* is made up of a collection of propositions. But unlike the *Aphorisms*, the subject is restricted to prognosis and the organization is more systematic.

The propositions, which number 640 in all, are grouped according to signs, affected parts of the body, diseases, and evacuations. Four broad sections may be distinguished. The first (1–155) is the least homogeneous: the aphorisms are organized around chills and fevers. The second section (156–319) arranges the aphorisms according to the parts of the body affected by disease and obeys the *a capite ad calcem* order: head or part of the head (156–236); neck, throat, chest, back (256–272); hypochondria (273–296); loins (298–319). The third section (357–544) groups the aphorisms according to particular diseases, once again respecting the *a capite ad calcem* order: anginas (357–372); pleurisies, pneumonias, empyemas (373–425); consumptions (426–436); diseases of the liver, dropsies, diseases of the abdomen and bladder (437–465). This section concludes with wounds (488–500) followed by the diseases of women (503–544). The final section (545–640) brings together the signs furnished by evacuations: vomits, sweats, urines, and stools. Despite an obvious effort at organization, not everything is clear. Whereas one would expect the aphorisms on hemorrhages to be in the last section, for example, they appear at the end of the section on affected parts (320–340).

Similarities between the *Prognostic* and the *Coan Prenotions* have long been noted; certain scholars, Littré among them, have thought that the *Coan Prenotions* was the ancient source of the *Prognostic*. It is now unanimously recognized that the relationship is just the opposite; indeed, this was already Galen's opinion. The treatise is a compilation. The compiler made notable use of other works in the collection, in particular *Prorrhetic I* and the *Aphorisms*, more rarely *Epidemics II, IV, VI,* and *VII*, the nosological writings (*Diseases I, II,* and *III*), *Sevens*, and so forth.

Authorship and date: The compilation does not appear in Erotian's list, but it was known to Galen, who cites the treatise twice in his *Hippocratic Glossary*. It cannot be earlier than the end of the fourth century.

Editions: Littré V, 588–733; Langholf (forthcoming).

10. *Crisis*

Contents: This is a compilation on prognosis made up, for the most part, of excerpts from other treatises in the collection, notably *Prognostic, Aphorisms, Epidemics II, IV,* and *VI*. Some chapters contain otherwise unknown passages, the most important of which are chapter 11 on causus (or "ardent fever") and chapter 39 on recurrences of disease. These passages are probably taken from works that have been lost.

Authorship and date: The treatise does not appear in Erotian's list; it postdates the *Aphorisms*.

Editions: Littré IX, 274–295; Preiser, 1957 (Greek).

11. *Critical Days*

Contents: Brief compilation of excerpts from other works (*Epidemics III, Internal Affections, Diseases III*). The sole interest of this treatise is that the second chapter preserves the Greek version of a passage from the *Sevens* (46), a treatise that otherwise was transmitted only in Latin (and partially in Arabic). The title of the compilation seems to come from the last chapter, which gives a brief indication of which days in fevers are critical.

Authorship and date: Late compilation dating from after *Sevens*; it is not cited in Erotian's list.

Editions: Littré IX, 296–307; Preiser, 1957 (Greek).

12. *Decorum*

Contents: Short treatise that begins with a long preamble on wisdom (1–6) and gives advice to the physician on how to avoid all blame and to win credit (7–17). Certain themes are foreign to the oldest treatises of the collection: "For a physician who is a lover of wisdom is the equal of a god" (5); "[M]edicine is found mostly to be held in honour by the gods" (6). But the advice to the physician regarding "good manners" (hence the title of the treatise), on what he must do in his office or in visiting his patients, is not contrary to the Hippocratic spirit (absence of ostentation; competence and self-control; frequent visits and, if necessary, leaving a pupil behind to watch over the patient).

Authorship and date: The treatise is not part of the ancient core of the collection. It does not appear in the list of Erotian. It is to be dated from the first or second century A.D. (see U. Fleischer, *Untersuchungen zu den pseudohippokratischen Schriften* [Berlin, 1939]).

Editions: Littré IX, 222–245; Jones, 1923 [= Loeb II, 267–301]; Heiberg, 1927 [= *CMG* I, 1].

13. *Decree of the Athenians*

Contents: Text of a decree issued by Athens in honor of Hippocrates for his services rendered during a pestilence, for his works of medicine, and for his refusal to accept the offer of the king of Persia. For these things

Hippocrates was to be initiated into the great mysteries (of Eleusis), receive a crown of gold, and enjoy Athenian citizenship (including the right of dining at the *prytaneion*).

Authorship and date: The decree belongs to the group of biographical writings; it does not appear in the list of Erotian. The text that has come down to us is not authentic, but dates from after Hippocrates' time, from probably the Hellenistic period rather than the fourth century.

Editions: Littré IX, 400–402; Smith, 1990 (Greek-English).

14. Dentition

Contents: Brief collection of thirty-two aphorisms on small children and their diseases (in particular tonsillitis). The title is taken from several aphorisms on the period when teething occurs.

Authorship and date: The treatise is not part of Erotian's list. It is late; around the time of Jesus Christ.

Editions: Littré VIII, 542–549; Jones, 1923 [= Loeb II, 315–329]; Joly, 1978 [= Budé XIII] (Greek-French).

15. Diseases I

The treatises *Diseases I, II, III*, and *IV* do not form a series; they are composed by different authors and belong to different periods. They have been grouped in different ways depending on the era of the text's transmission.

Contents: Diseases I is a treatise intended to enable the physician to triumph over his colleagues in debate by showing himself to be a master of the art of dialogue and contradiction (1).

A first section takes up general questions: causes of diseases (2), prognosis (3–4), notions of opportunity (5), of correctness and incorrectness (6), of spontaneity (7), the role of chance (8), dexterity and clumsiness (10).

A second section is devoted to diseases: empyemas (11–17); erysipelas of the lungs; lung tumors (19); tumors in the side (20); fevers (23); chills (24); sweats (25); pleurisy and pneumonia (26–28 and 31–32), causus, or "ardent fever" (29 and 33); phrenitis (30 and 34).

Authorship and date: Although the nosology displays some similarities with the descriptions of the Cnidian treatises, the general reflections are foreign to Cnidian ways of thinking. As in the treatise *Affections*, the bihumoral theory (bile-phlegm) is preponderant in the etiology of diseases. *Diseases I* can likewise be dated to the 380s.

Editions: Littré VI, 138–205; Jouanna, 1974 [= *Hippocrates: Pour une archéologie de l'école de Cnide*] (Greek-French; excerpts); Wittern, 1974 (Greek-German); Potter, 1983 [= Loeb V, 93–183].

16. *Diseases II*

Contents: This is actually composed of two distinct treatises: a short treatise (1–11), the beginning of which is incomplete, and a long treatise (12–75); let us call the first *Diseases II* 1 and the second *Diseases II* 2. These two treatises consist of a series of case studies of individual diseases and contain no general discussions of a synthetic character—by contrast with the *Epidemics*, which, while its cases likewise treat of particular diseases, contains general discussions of just this sort. The order of exposition of the diseases is *a capite ad calcem*. *Diseases II* 1 deals exclusively with diseases of the head (1–8) and of the throat (9–11). *Diseases II* 2 describes successively diseases of the head (12–25), of the throat and nose (26–37), and then of the chest and back (44–62). Certain points remain obscure, however, concerning the details of the classification. Between the diseases of the nose and those of the chest there is inserted a series of six affections (38–43), at least some of which are caused by an excess of bile; and the treatise finishes with varied affections whose principle of classification is unclear.

Each case devoted to a disease or a variety of disease obeys a regular schema in *Diseases II* 2: identification of the disease in a conditional clause or a title, followed by semiology, treatment, and prognosis (the latter being given either between semiology and treatment or after treatment). In *Diseases II* 1 the schema is similar, except that treatment is absent and that moreover there is an etiological discussion referring to an elaborate humoral etiology. As each disease described in *Diseases II* 1 appears also in *Diseases II* 2, these treatises provide one example among others of the many parallel passages that, with rewriting, came to link together the various treatises on diseases (cf. above all *Internal Affections* and *Diseases III*).

Diseases II has an altogether special importance in the history of diagnosis by auscultation. For a very long time it was the fundamental text for the procedure known as "direct auscultation."

Authorship and date: *Disease II* 2 contains, in connection with a "livid disease," a long passage whose wording is similar to that of a passage by the physician Euryphon cited by Galen (*Commentary on Epidemics VI of Hippocrates* 1.9). And it displays other points of contact with what is known of Cnidian medicine: the use of evacuants, milk or whey depending on the season, is frequently recommended (66, 68, 70, 73; cf. the comment made by the author of *Regimen in Acute Diseases* in the first chapter about the *Cnidian Sentences*); also of "infusions" for evacuating pus from the lung (47, 50, 52; cf. [Galen] *On Sects* 10).

The Cnidian origin of the treatise is therefore likely. The parallelisms between *Diseases II* 1 and 2 testify to a common origin, probably the *Cnidian Sentences*. The material is ancient (middle of the fifth century?). But the various instances of rewriting are not necessarily contemporaneous with each other. The elaborate humoral etiology of *Diseases II* 1 is evidence of more recent rewriting than that of *Diseases II* 2, for example.

Editions: Littré VII, 1–115; Jouanna, 1974 [= *Hippocrate: Pour une archéologie de l'école de Cnide*] (Greek-French; excerpts); Potter, 1983 [= Loeb V, 185–333]; Jouanna, 1983 [= Budé X, 2] (Greek-French).

17. *Diseases III*

Contents: Like *Diseases II* (1 and 2), the treatise contains particular diseases without any general comments. The order of exposition seems, here again, to be *a capite ad calcem*, for the first diseases are those of the head (1–4); there follow a disease of the lungs (7) and a disease of the abdomen or belly, ileus (14). But this order is subsequently disturbed: a disease of the head (8) and a disease of the throat, angina (10), inexplicably appear after the disease of the lungs, and diseases of the "upper cavity" come after the diseases of the "lower cavity": pneumonia (15), pleurisy (16). Other diseases: lethargy (5), causus (6), phrenitis (9), jaundice (11), tetanus and opisthotonus (12–13). The treatise ends with a list of cooling preparations to drink in the case of causus (17).

Authorship and date: All the diseases described exhibit parallel readings with *Diseases II* and with *Internal Affections*. Cnidian origin.

Editions: Littré VII, 116–161; Jouanna, 1974 [= *Hippocrate: Pour une archéologie de l'école de Cnide*] (Greek-French; excerpts); Potter, 1980 [= *CMG* I, 2.3] (Greek-German); Potter, 1983 [= Loeb VI, 1–63].

18. *Diseases IV*

Contents: Like *Diseases I*, *Diseases II*, and *Diseases III*, *Diseases IV* forms an independent treatise (see section on authorship below). The nature of man is formed of four humors, phlegm, blood, bile, and water. It is from these humors that diseases arise, with the exception of those that are caused by violence (1) [= 32, Littré]. The author shows first how humors increase and decrease in the body: the belly is the source of the humors that stem from foods and drinks; each humor also has a particular source that communicates with the belly—the head for phlegm, the gall bladder for bile, the spleen for water, and the heart for blood. Four routes permit evacuation of these humors: the mouth, nostrils, anus, and urethra (2–10) [= 33–41, Littré]. Health obeys a cycle of foods that exit the second day and of humors that exit the third day. When the cycle is disturbed, there is disease. The fever due to a disequilibrium of the humors is decided on odd days; the same is true in the case of death and the inflammation of wounds (11–17) [= 42–48]. Overview of the diseases with a general conclusion to the treatise: there are three principles from which diseases arise (surfeit, violence, and bad weather that heats or cools excessively); explanation of fever by the settling of the morbid humor or its swirling motion (18–22) [= 49–53]. Appendices on the tapeworm (23) [= 54], lithiasis (24) [= 55], dropsy, with a lengthy refutation of the belief that liquids pass through the lungs (25–26) [= 56–57].

Authorship and date: Same author as *Generation / Nature of the Child* and of a treatise on diseases of women partially preserved in the gynecological treatises. In the editions based on Littré, this treatise is placed following *Generation / Nature of the Child* with consecutive numbering of the chapters. End of the fifth century or beginning of the fourth.

Editions: Littré VII, 542–615; Joly, 1970 [= Budé XI] (Greek-French). An English commentary by I. M. Lonie was published in Berlin in 1981.

19. *Diseases of Girls*

Contents: Very brief discussion on two pages. The title is misleading. The purpose of the author was not to treat particularly of the diseases of girls; he wished to discuss diseases. Short preamble on the necessity of knowing the original constitution of nature for understanding the nature of diseases. Then the author begins with a discussion of the disease called sacred (epilepsy) with attendant delirium and suicidal visions. Women are more liable to the condition than men. The author considers first the case of young girls—hence the title traditionally given to the treatise—and concludes the passage that has survived by noting that among married women the ones most affected by these illnesses are sterile. The way in which the author introduces his remarks about the sacred disease ("First of all . . . ") implies that what has come down to us is only the beginning of the work.

The interest of this fragment is twofold: first, as a physiological explanation of the sacred disease that is different than the one we have in the treatise *The Sacred Disease* (where the disease is said to be caused by a flux of phlegm descending from the head); second, as a sharp attack upon soothsayers, who are accused of "fooling" women.

Authorship and date: Despite its title, this treatise bears no relation to the gynecological treatises. It does not appear in Erotian's list. Fourth century.

Editions: Littré VIII, 464–471.

20. *Diseases of Women I–II / Sterile Women*

Contents, authorship, and date: These three books form a quite vast compendium on the diseases of women, which Littré published with the chapters continuously numbered (*Diseases of Women I*: 1–109; *Diseases of Women II*: 110–212; *Sterile Women*: 213–249). Erotian already knew the group in the same form as we know it from manuscript tradition; that is to say, in two treatises: *Diseases of Women* (in two books) and *Sterile Women*. Modern philological analysis (due to Grensemann) has shown that this group is heterogeneous despite a superficial unity:

A. The group contains the remnants of a treatise on the diseases of women written by the author of *Generation / Nature of the Child* and *Diseases IV* (layer C, Grensemann). This treatise, partially preserved, was broken up as a result of its insertion in the middle of a set of other treatises at an earlier period in the transmission of the collection. The essential part of what is preserved is in *Diseases of Women I*; a few remnants are found in *Diseases of Women II* (beginning at 145) and in *Sterile Women* (213). From what we can judge of these surviving parts, the treatise was composed in a rhetorical manner, began with diseases due to menstrual periods, continued with the diseases of pregnant women, then with accidents during birth and afterwards, and concluded with problems of sterility. From internal references made by the author from one treatise to another, it turns out that this work on the diseases of women was written after *Genera-tion / Nature of the Child* (cf. *Generation* 4, *Nature of the Child* 15, *Diseases of Women I* 1, 43, 73), but before *Diseases IV* (see *Diseases IV* 57). Its author was an independent physician whose attachment to any school cannot be proven. The fact that it became broken up within a larger group of trea-tises obviously does not prove that it originally belonged to this group.

B. The remainder is constituted for the most part by cases on diseases of women whose expository schema is similar to the one found earlier in *Diseases II* 2 (see entry above) and in *Nature of Women* (layer A, Gren-semann), as well as by lists of medicines. The account of diseases bears a good many parallels to other passages, both within this group and in *Na-ture of Women*, which attests the existence of a common source and of re-writing. The material is of Cnidian origin. Although it may be ancient (middle of the fifth century?), all or some of the rewriting may date to the fourth century. Special mention needs to be made of one instance of re-writing (layer B, Grensemann), which goes beyond the framework of the case studies of diseases by adding certain general comments (see, for ex-ample, 111, on the need to take account of environmental influences, sea-sons, places, and winds).

Editions: Littré VIII, 1–463; Grensemann (layer C), 1982 (Greek-German); Countouris (layer B), 1985 (Greek-German).

21. *Eight Months' Child* (containing *Seven Months' Child*)

Contents: These two opuscules, grouped separately in ancient editions, actually form a single treatise. The order of the two varies in ancient manuscripts, and modern scholars are divided over which is to be adopted.

A treatise of embryology explaining why the foetus is not viable at eight months but is viable at ten months and sometimes—what is more paradoxical—at seven months. The reason is that the foetus of eight months is subjected simultaneously to two shocks, the suffering of birth and another painful experience common to every child in the eighth month, whether it is inside the womb or outside. By contrast, these two shocks do not occur at the same time for those who are born at seven months, nine months, or ten months.

Authorship and date: The treatise was attributed to Polybus in ancient dox-ography (see Clement of Alexandria *Stromates* 6.16; cf. Pseudo-Plutarch

De placitis philosophorum 5.18). But it is improbable that *Nature of Man* and *Eight Months' Child* are by the same author. The latter can be dated from the end of the fifth century or the beginning of the fourth.

Editions: Littré VII, 432–461; Grensemann, 1968 [= *CMG* I, 2.1] (Greek-German); Joly, 1970 [= Budé XI] (Greek-French). There exists a late treatise on *Seven Months' Child* in an ancient manuscript (*Vaticanus gr.* 276); published in Grensemann, 1968 [= *CMG* I, 2.1] (Greek-German).

Embassy. See 58. *Speech of the Envoy*

Epibomios. See 1. *Address from the Altar*

22. *Epidemics I* and *III*

Contents: These two books form the first group of the seven books that make up the *Epidemics*.

Epidemics I: The first book is mainly taken up with three "constitutions"; that is, three descriptions of the climate in a given place (in this case Thasos) over the course of a year, noting the diseases that "stay" there in each season. General remarks have been added at the end of the last two constitutions.

The book concludes with fourteen cases of individual patients describing the day-by-day evolution of their illnesses. The names of the patients are generally given, and sometimes their address. Although their place of origin is indicated only in two cases (Thasos: 4 and 9), it is probable that all the patients are Thasian. In any event, this is certainly the case with two other patients, for their names also appear in the description of the third constitution, which is expressly concerned with Thasos: Philiscus (1) and Silenus (2).

Epidemics III: The book begins with a series of twelve case studies. Only in one case is the patient's native city indicated (the fourth patient is from Thasos), but it is believed that the other patients are Thasians as well. The book continues with a "constitution" on the island of Thasos. At the end of the constitution, the author adds some general remarks about the elements permitting a correct prognosis to be made. The book concludes with a new series of cases involving patients from different cities this time: Thasos, Abdera on the Thracian coast across from Thasos, Cyzicus on the Propontis, and also Larissa and Meliboea in Thessaly.

Authorship and date: These two books are written by the same author, an itinerant physician of the Hippocratic school if not Hippocrates himself. They were commented on by Galen. They are traditionally dated from about 410. For this scholars rely on one of the patients mentioned in the third constitution of *Epidemics I*, Antiphon, son of Critobulus, whose name also appears in two inscriptions of Thasos, one of which dates from the years 411–410 to 408–407 (see page 118 and note 29 on page 443). But while the inscriptions attest that Antiphon was theor (or magistrate of Thasos) at the time, they do not say whether he was sick during this period; given that he was lucky enough to pull through, he might have fallen ill either before or after assuming his duties as theor. Another piece of evidence: in *Epidemics III* 1.2, the "new wall" may refer to the wall reconstructed in 411 under the oligarchy; but it has been objected that this phrase may refer to an older wall.

Editions: Littré II, 598–717 and III, 24–149; Kühlewein, 1894 [= Teubner I]; Jones, 1923 [= Loeb I, 139–287]; Lichtenthaeler, 1994 (commentary on *Epidemics III*, 1–12).

23. *Epidemics II, IV, and VI*

Contents: Second group of the *Epidemics*. Unlike the first, it takes the form chiefly of notes. The unity among these three books is proven by the fact that some of the patients are the same from one book to another and by a certain amount of similar wording in each.

Epidemics II: It is impossible to give briefly an exact idea of the quite varied character of the notes composed by this author, a physician who practiced in Thessaly at Crannon (1.1), on the Thracian coast at Aenus (4.3), and above all along the Propontis at Perinthus, where physicians arrived as a group (3.1).

The three features noted about *Epidemics I* and *III* (i.e., "constitutions," general remarks, case studies) are found here in mixed and often fragmentary form. One recognizes passages relating to constitutions. General reflections occupy a much larger place than in *Epidemics I* and *III*: the relationship between the seasons and diseases, the development of diseases and the associated notions of "periods," "crises," "deposits," and so on. The best known of these reflections is a description of the veins (4.1). As for the case studies, these are mixed in with the other passages in no discernable order.

Epidemics IV: The sites of activity are the same here as in *Epidemics II*:

Crannon (14, 37); Aenus (48); Perinthus (21), where a group of physicians stayed. A series of villages is also mentioned: the villages of Hippolochus (31), of Boulagoras (35), of Amphilochus (45), and Medosades (45). Another place: Acanthus in the Chalcidice (20). The book contains fragments of constitutions that are not locally identifiable. The general remarks here are also mixed together with particular case studies.

Epidemics VI: Places where the physician practices that are identical to those of the two preceding books are Crannon (1.7), Aenus (4.11), and Perinthus (2.19, 7.10). Other places include ones already known from *Epidemics I* and *III*: Thasos and Abdera (8.29, 8.30); in addition to these, Pharsalus in Thessaly is mentioned (8.18). A remarkable passage in one constitution describes a cough that was prevalent in winter, with relapses and complications (7.1); although the place is not specified, comparison with other sections (cf. 7.10, for example) allows it to be identified as Perinthus. Otherwise general reflections alternate with descriptions of individual patients, as in the preceding books. It is in this book that one finds the criticism of the physician Herodicus, and the fine phrase "The body's nature is the physician in disease" (5.1). On similarities between this book and the *Humours*, see the entry for this treatise below.

Authorship and date: These three books are probably the work of a single writer. This author was an itinerant physician and belonged to a group of physicians drawn from Hippocrates' circle during the Thessalian period. Galen commented on the second book (preserved only in Arabic translation) and on the sixth.

The group is dated from the end of the fifth century or the beginning of the fourth. Mention of the appearance of a "large star" (*IV* 21) suggests one of two dates, 427–426 (see Aristotle *Meteorologica* 1.6.8) or 373–372 (see Aristotle *Meteorologica* 1.6.8, 6.10, 7.10); but neither of these is necessarily correct. Other reference points considered include Medosades (*IV* 45), one of the villages that the king of Thrace, Seuthes II, had awarded to his right-hand man Medosades (see Xenophon *Anabasis* 7.7.1); while the shift in control was an accomplished fact in 400, it can scarcely be dated earlier than this. More doubtful connections have been proposed: Cyniscus (who brought the author to see a patient in Perinthus: see *IV* 53 and *VI* 7.10) has been identified with the Cyniscus cited by Xenophon (*Anabasis* 7.1.13) as being in the Chersonesus, in Thrace, in 400 (Perinthus, however, is not in the Chersonesus: *obscurum per obscurius*); and Alcibiades ("The man who came from Alcibiades," *II* 2.7) with the great

Alcibiades who in 404 took refuge at Dascylium in the Propontis, across from Perinthus, and was assassinated the same year. In any case, the material was no doubt brought together by the author of this group over a number of years during the course of his travels as an itinerant physician.

Editions: Littré V, 43–197 and 260–357; *II* (partial), *IV* and *VI* (partial): Langholf, 1977 (Greek); *VI*: Manetti-Roselli, 1982 (Greek-Italian); Smith, 1994 [= Loeb VII, 18–151; 218–291).

24. *Epidemics V and VII*

Contents: Third group of the *Epidemics*.

Epidemics V: The fifth book, unlike the preceding ones, includes only a very few general comments (54, 57, 58) and pieces of descriptions of constitutions (73, 78, 94). It is mainly made up of case studies. Frequently the town where patients live (or where the physician practices) is specified: Elis (1–2), Oeniadae (3–8), Athens (9–10), Larissa (11, 13–15), Pherae (12), Omilus (27–31), Salamis (32), Acanthus (52), Delos (61), Cardia (100), Abdera (101), Olynthus (106), Malia (26). Taken together, the descriptions are remarkable and permit retrospective diagnoses to be made.

Epidemics VII: The seventh book is closely related to the fifth, for a whole series of cases given in *Epidemics V* (51–106, excepting 86) is also found in *Epidemics VII*. However, the order is not necessarily the same and the wording is not always as complete in the one book as in the other. While the two books have an important element in common, each also contains passages that are not found in the other. Among the passages unique to *Epidemics VII* are a good many descriptions of patients. Indications as to the place of origin of these new patients are fairly rare: the island of Syros (79), Olynthus (80) in Chalcidice, Abdera (112, 114, 115) in Thrace, Pella (118) and Baloea (17) in Macedonia.

Authorship and date: With regard to date, certain descriptions of patients are later than 358–357 (the date of the siege of Datum by Philip, mentioned in *Epidemics V* 95 and *VII* 121 in connection with a man injured by a catapult); others, by contrast, are prior to 348 (the date of Philip's destruction of Olynthus, a city mentioned in both *Epidemics V* and *VII*). This group belongs to the school of Hippocrates after the master's death.

Editions: Littré V, 198–259 and 358–469; Smith, 1994 [= Loeb VII, 152–217, 292–415].

25. *Excision of the Foetus*

Contents: Brief treatise on female affections; incomplete (see the reference at the end of the first chapter). The title is taken from the first sentence of the treatise and only takes into consideration the material of the first chapter: the extraction of the dead foetus, possibly by incision of the foetus. Chapters 1–4 deal with childbirth; the fourth contains the description of the manner in which the woman is to be shaken in the event that delivery is difficult. Chapter 5 treats of the collapse of the womb following delivery or owing to fatigue from incision of the womb. Notable here is the express prohibition against treatment if the collapse of the womb is not recent.

Authorship and date: Belongs to the group of gynecological treatises. The majority of the subjects treated in this treatise figure in other gynecological treatises; but the writing is original.

Editions: Littré VIII, 512–519.

26. *Fistulas*

Contents: Causes and various treatments of anal fistulas. The author uses a speculum in conducting examinations. Treatment of other anal affections, inflammation, prolapse, and so on.

Authorship and date: The treatise appears in Erotian's list. It is probably by the author of *Haemorrhoids*, and dates from the fourth century.

Editions: Littré VI, 446–461; Petrequin, 1877 (Greek-French); Joly, 1978 [= Budé XIII] (Greek-French); Potter, 1995 [= Loeb VIII, 390–407].

27. *Fleshes*

Contents: Despite its title, *Fleshes* is a work of medicine (see the opening chapter). After a short preamble in which he recalls the necessity of founding anthropology on cosmology (1), the author briefly reverts to the formation of the universe and proceeds to discuss the original formation of man (2–14). The pair "fat" and "gluey" is used to account for the formation of the various parts of the body: bones, tendons, vessels, digestive tract, spinal cord, heart, lungs, liver, kidneys, nails, teeth. Then he explains the functioning of the senses: hearing, smell, sight, speech (15–18). He concludes by offering a septenary theory (19): the number seven governs everything that concerns man (growth of the embryo, birth, formation of the teeth, diseases).

Authorship and date: A unique, entirely preserved example that gives some idea of what the Greeks of the fifth and sixth centuries meant by "inquiry into nature."

Editions: Littré VIII, 584–615; Deichgräber, 1935 (Greek-German); Joly, 1978 [= Budé XIII] (Greek-French); Potter, 1995 [= Loeb VIII, 127–165].

28. *Generation / Nature of the Child*

Contents: These two treatises, distinct in the manuscript tradition, actually form a single work on embryology.

Generation: The seed comes from all parts of the body, but descends from the brain via the spinal cord as far as the genitals (1–3). Account of coitus and conception (4–5). The seed comes from the man and the woman. Explanation of the birth of a girl and of a boy, of resemblances to parents, and of accidental or hereditary malformations (6–11).

Nature of the Child: Formation and development of the embryo. The seed is enveloped by a membrane, and both breathes and is nourished by the blood of the mother, which it receives through the umbilical cord; description of a seed of six days (12–16). Differentiation of the parts of the body by the breath in accordance with the làw of similars; it occurs more rapidly in the male foetus than in the female; the last parts to be formed are the nails and hair (17–20). First movements of the embryo and the formation of milk in the mother (21–22). Quite extended analogy with the growth of plants: "The natural growth of plants is similar to that of man" (22–27). Experiment with hen's eggs (29). Delivery at the end of ten months at the latest, for the mother no longer furnishes nourishment to the child, which then begins to stir and breaks the membranes (30). Explanation of the birth of twins (31).

Authorship and date: The author is the same as that of *Diseases IV* and of a treatise on the diseases of women that is mentioned in chapters 4 and 15 of *Generation / Nature of the Child* and partially preserved in the gynecological treatises (see *Diseases of Women I–II / Sterile Women* above). End of the fifth century or beginning of the fourth.

Editions: Littré VII, 470–542; Joly, 1970 [= Budé XI] (Greek-French); Lonie, 1981 (English commentary).

29. *Glands*

Contents: Anatomy, physiology, and pathology of the most important glands (the author makes no distinction between glands and ganglions). Their function is to attract the excess moisture of the body. The author treats the brain as a gland; rather long passage on the fluxes issuing from the brain, which are seven in number.

Authorship and date: The date is disputed. According to some, the treatise is not prior to the Hellenistic era; according to others, it belongs to an older period (end of the fifth or beginning of the fourth century). It does not appear in Erotian's list in any case.

Editions: Littré VIII, 550–575; Joly, 1978 [= Budé XIII] (Greek-French); Potter, 1995 [= Loeb VIII, 103–125).

30. *Haemorrhoids*

Contents: Brief treatise on this affection, its causes (bile and phlegm attaching themselves to the anus and attracting blood to it) and various treatments (cauterization, excision, medications either applied or inserted as suppositories). In examining patients, the author mentions using a speculum.

Authorship and date: It belongs to the list of Erotian. Probably the same author as that of the *Fistulas*; fourth century.

Editions: Littré VI, 434–445; Petrequin, 1877 (Greek-French); Joly, 1978 [= Budé XIII] (Greek-French); Potter, 1995 [= Loeb VIII, 377–389].

31. *The Heart*

Contents: A short treatise that offers what was to be the most precise description of this organ until the sixteenth century. Its author practiced dissection (7); this could only have been animal dissection (cf. 11). The physician has noted the pyramidal shape of the heart (1); knows that it is a muscle (4); has seen the pericardium and the liquid that it contains (1); knows the ventricles are separated by a partition (4); knows, too, the atriums (8) and describes with particular care the sigmoidal valves (10). If the anatomy is accurate, the physiology is far-fetched. The author has closely observed the beating of the heart, but he believes that part of what one drinks passes through the lungs and is lapped up by the heart (1–2).

The atriums play a role analogous to bellows and enable the heart to breathe. The inner fire is in the left ventricle. It is cooled by the air and also by the presence of the lungs, which are cold (5–6). The left ventricle is the seat of the intellect (10). The heart is the source of life for human nature (7). The author admires the work of nature, which he describes as that of a skillful artist (8 and 10).

Authorship and date: The treatise does not figure in Erotian's list. The anatomical knowledge is clearly superior to what was known in Hippocrates' time. The treatise dates from the Hellenistic era.

Editions: Littré IX, 76–93; Unger, 1923 (Greek-Latin); Bidez-Leboucq, 1944 (Greek-French); Manuli-Vegetti, 1977 (Greek with Italian commentary).

32. *Humours*

Contents: Despite its title, inspired by the opening sentence, the treatise does not confine itself to humors. It consists of general and varied pieces of advice in no very clear order. The enumerative style of the treatise links it with the genre of practitioners' notebooks. The advice given to the physician involves, among other things, the various signs to be observed in connection with disease (2–5), the progress of disease, and treatment; a final section (12–19) is devoted more particularly to the influence of the environment on disease: seasons, winds, places, waters. In chapter 11 one finds an interesting comparison of the earth to the stomach ("As the soil is to trees, so is the stomach to animals").

The treatise is undeniably related to the middle group of the *Epidemics* (*II, IV, VI*), for in chapter 7 there is a reference to those who suffered from coughing and angina at Perinthus (cf. *Epidemics VI* 7.1 and 7.10). Beyond this, the final chapter (20) is virtually the same as *Epidemics VI* 3.24–4.3, though the question remains whether it was added in the course of the text's transmission.

Authorship and date: Like the *Epidemics*, the treatise is associated with the school of Cos. It is contemporary with *Epidemics II, IV,* and *VI*; the author is believed to be the same.

Editions: Littré V, 470–503; Jones, 1931 [= Loeb IV, 61–95]. A study by Deichgräber was published in 1972.

Injuries of the Head. See 44. *On Wounds in the Head*

Instruments of Reduction. See 37. *Mochlicon*

33. *Internal Affections*

Contents: Treatise on diseases that lacks either preamble or conclusion; it is entirely devoted to particular diseases that are described in a succession of cases, one after another. These cases are arranged in roughly *a capite ad calcem* order, but they begin only with diseases of the chest. The principal diseases described are as follows: diseases of the lungs and trachea, and of the chest, back, and sides (1–9); three consumptions (10–12); four diseases of the kidneys (14–17); dropsies (23–26); diseases of the liver (27–29); diseases of the spleen (30–34); four jaundices (35–38); "typhus" (39–43); ileus (44–46); "thick" diseases (47–50); diseases of the hip (51); three tetanuses (52–54). Each case follows a more or less constant form of presentation: identification of the disease and causes of the disease; description of symptoms; prognosis; treatment.

Authorship and date: One of the characteristics of the treatise is the subdivision of certain diseases into a quite precise number of varieties. Now we know from Galen (*Commentary on the Regimen in Acute Diseases of Hippocrates* 1.7) that the physicians of Cnidus divided diseases into a number of specific varieties. Where comparison is possible, the Cnidian subdivisions and those of the *Affections* coincide perfectly: three consumptions, four jaundices, three tetanuses, four diseases of the kidneys. This is one of the chief reasons for linking it with the school of Cnidus. Moreover, the treatise contains wording similar to that of *Diseases II.* It may be dated to the decade 400–390.

Editions: Littré VII, 166–303; Jouanna, 1974 [= *Hippocrate: Pour une archéologie de l'école de Cnide*] (Greek-French; excerpts); Grmek-Wittern, 1977 [= *Archives Int. Hist. Sciences* 26 (1977): 3–32] (chapters 14–17); Potter, 1983 [= Loeb VI, 65–255].

34. *In the Surgery*

Contents: This is a manual concerning surgical operations in the physician's office. General advice on the examination of the patient (1). Advice regarding an operation: lighting; position of the surgeon, seated and standing; position of the hand that carries out the operation; instruments;

assistants (2–6). The remainder of the treatise is devoted mainly to the art of bandaging (7–25). Some remarks also on the use of affusions of water (13) and on "friction," or rubbing (17).

Authorship and date: This manual belongs to the group of surgical treatises; it is traditionally associated with the school of Cos. Galen commented on it.

Editions: Littré III, 262–337; Petrequin, 1878 (Greek-French); Kühlewein, 1902 [= Teubner II] (Greek); Withington, 1928 [= Loeb III, 53–81].

35. *Law*

Contents: The Oath makes reference to a "medical law." This opuscule on the "Law" was taken in antiquity to be the natural complement to *The Oath* (in Erotian's list, the *Law* comes just after *The Oath*). It is, in fact, more recent. It contains brief reflections on medicine, a noble art but one that is disparaged on account of bad physicians, these supernumeraries of tragedy (1). To be a good physician, it is necessary to combine natural talent with a sound training acquired from childhood in a good medical school, as well as a willingness to work hard (2). There follows a nice comparison between the physician's training and the cultivation of plants (3). Thus prepared, the disciple will be able to practice as a traveling physician (4). The last chapter likens the learning of science to a religious initiation into the mysteries (5). The prohibition against revealing what is holy to the profane recalls *The Oath*.

Authorship and date: Already part of the Hippocratic Collection in the time of Erotian, who classified the treatise among the works relating to the art, putting it just after *The Oath*. The opuscule cannot be earlier than the fourth century (note the use of *dogma* in chapter 3, a term that does not appear before Plato and Xenophon).

Editions: Littré IV, 638–643; Jones, 1923 [= Loeb II, 255–265]; Heiberg, 1927 [= *CMG* I, 1]; Jouanna, 1996 [= A. Garzya and J. Jouanna, eds., *Storia e ecdotica dei Testi medici greci* (Naples, 1996), 271ff.] (Greek).

36. *Letters*

Contents: The traditional corpus of the *Letters* comprises twenty-four letters supposed to have been written by Hippocrates, to Hippocrates, or about Hippocrates. They are divided into two broad groups.

The first group (1–9) relates to the invitation extended to Hippocrates by the Persian king Artaxerxes and Hippocrates' refusal despite the enticements of the barbarian: "Wisdom holds greater appeal for me than gold" (6). These letters are short, with the exception of the first two (in which figure a certain Paetus over whom much ink is spilled). The second letter contains biographical information about Hippocrates.

The second group (10–21 and 23) concerns Hippocrates and Democritus, the philosopher of Abdera. These are much longer and form a sort of novel in letters. The people of Abdera ask Hippocrates to come treat Democritus, who they think has gone mad because he laughs at everything, even at the misfortune of others. Arriving at Abdera from Cos, Hippocrates realizes that Democritus has not lost his mind, but is writing a book about madness and is laughing at the folly of men. Hippocrates and Democritus become friends, and exchange letters.

Two letters at the end of the collection (22 and 24) do not belong to these two main groups. In one Hippocrates recommends to his son Thessalus the study of geometry and arithmetic as sciences useful for the practice of medicine. In the other Hippocrates sends to Demetrius, the king of Macedonia (an anachronism: Demetrius Poliorcetes became king of Macedonia only at the beginning of the third century B.C.), precepts for remaining in good health.

Authorship and date: Obviously apocryphal, even if here and there they contain interesting details, these letters are not part of the list of Erotian, who, among biographical writings, knew only the *Address from the Altar* and the *Speech of the Envoy*. Nonetheless certain of them already existed in the first century A.D., because the oldest papyrus bearing a part of the corpus dates from this era (*POxy*. IX 1184v: letters 3 to 6 from the first group). Two other papyri, later by a century (*PBerl. Inv.* 7094v and *Inv.* 21137v and 6934v), give letter 11 from the second group as well.

Editions: Littré IX, 308–400; Putzger, 1914 (Greek); Sakalis, 1989 (Greek); Smith, 1990 (Greek-English).

N.B.: There exist other letters of Hippocrates that are not part of Littré's edition nor, curiously, any of the three editions that have appeared since; for these pseudo-Hippocratic texts see the entry below at no. 63. Two of these letters have been published separately: one by Ermerins as "Epistula ad Ptolemaeum regem de hominis fabrica" (in *Anecdota medica Graeca* [Lugduni Batavorum, 1840; reprint, Amsterdam, 1963], 278–297), the other by Boissonade as "Epistula ad Ptolemaeum regem" (in *Anecdota*

Graeca, vol. 3 [Paris, 1831], 422–428). The great number of manuscripts transmitting each of these two letters testifies to their fame.

37. *Mochlicon* [= *Instruments of Reduction*]

Contents: The title signifies that the treatise "relates to the lever." The lever (*mochlos*) is one of the instruments that serves for the reduction of fractures and dislocations (see chapters 25 and 38). Like the treatise *On Fractures / On Joints*, to which it bears a great similarity, the *Mochlicon* is a surgical work treating of the reduction of fractures and dislocations. After an introductory chapter on the disposition of the bones and joints (1), the author takes up in *a capite ad calcem* order fractures of the nose (2) and of the ear (3), and dislocation of the jaw (4); next, dislocations of the shoulder and of the upper limb (5–19), and of the lower limb (20–32); and, finally, deviations of the spinal column (36–37). The end of the treatise is taken up by general remarks on the means and methods of reduction (38 and 40), and on the treatment of complications (41).

Authorship and date: The treatise was known to Erotian and belongs to the group of surgical treatises; it is traditionally attributed to the school of Hippocrates. The work is presented as a guide to the teaching contained in *On Fractures / On Joints* with certain additions and modifications. The *Mochlicon* therefore cannot be earlier than *On Fractures / On Joints*.

Editions: Littré IV, 328–395; Petrequin, 1878 (Greek-French); Kühlewein, 1902 [= Teubner II] (Greek); Withington, 1928 [= Loeb III, 399–449].

38. *Nature of Bones*

Contents: The title was suggested by the beginning of the treatise, which quickly mentions the number of bones in different parts of the body; but it does not fit the treatise as a whole. The treatise consists in the main of descriptions taken from various sources of the blood vessels. Two of these descriptions were known to Aristotle and some even belong to other treatises in the collection (*Nature of Man* and *Epidemics II*); but the chief interest of the treatise is that it presents otherwise unknown descriptions (see 2–7 and 11–19).

Authorship and date: The treatise is not listed by Erotian. In Galen's time it was considered to be an appendix to the *Mochlichon*. It is in fact a recent compilation that contains ancient material.

Editions: Littré IX, 162–197.

39. *Nature of Man*

> *Contents*: In ancient manuscripts, the treatise includes not only the fifteen chapters edited by Littré (VI, 32–69) and Jones (Loeb IV, 1–41) but also the nine chapters edited by Littré under the title *Régime salutaire* (VI, 72–87) and by Jones under the title *Regimen in Health* (Loeb IV, 43–59).

In a first section (1–7), the author lays out his theory of human nature. In a polemical part he criticizes philosophers who hold that man is constituted by a single element, air, fire, water, or earth (1) and physicians who affirm that man is constituted by a single humor, blood, bile, or phlegm (2). In a positive part he asserts that generation occurs on the basis of several principles (3), and declares that the nature of man is constituted by four humors (blood, phlegm, yellow bile, and black bile), whose mixture explains health and whose separation brings on diseases (4). These humors, being distinct and always present in man so long as he is alive (5–6), grow or diminish according to the seasons (7).

After the statement regarding human nature, the author takes up pathology and therapy (8–15). In this part the argument hangs together more loosely. Diseases vary according to the seasons (8). They are particular or general: particular diseases are caused by regimen and must be treated by a modification of regimen; general diseases are due to the air, which contains miasmas, as a result of which it is necessary to move away from the infested region and to follow a slimming regimen in order to make the smallest possible demands on breathing (9). In the rest of this section, the best-known passages concern the description of the blood vessels (11), on the one hand, and fevers (15), on the other. One of the peculiarities of the treatise is the predilection for the number four: there are four fevers (continuous, quotidian, tertian, and quartan), just as there are four pairs of veins that descend from the head and four humors corresponding to the four seasons.

The last section treats of the regimen for preserving health (16–22 [= *Regimen in Health* 1–7]). The advice given there is directed first to those who lead a normal life. Regimen varies according to the season (16 [= 1]), and according to one's constitution and age (17 [= 2]). Regimen also includes walks and baths (18 [= 3]), as well as induced vomiting in winter to evacuate phlegm and clysters in summer to evacuate bile (20 [= 5]). The author concludes with advice about the regimen suitable to children and women (21 [= 6]) and on that of heavyweight athletes forced to observe a strict diet (22 [= 7]). The two last chapters (23–24 [= 8–9]) do not belong to the treatise; they are remnants of the beginning of *Diseases II* 2 (= chapter 12) and of *Affections* (chapter 1).

Authorship and date: This is the only treatise of the collection that can be attributed to an author known by name—Polybus, Hippocrates' pupil and son-in-law—if one admits the unity of the material as a whole (challenged by certain scholars); the description of veins is cited under the name of Polybus by Aristotle in the *Historia animalium* (3.3.512b–513a7) and the first section (3–4) is summarized by the *Anonymus Londinensis* (19.1–18), also under the name of Polybus. The treatise belongs therefore to the school of Cos. Galen, who commented on the treatise, attributes its first part containing the theory of the four humors to Hippocrates. The treatise is generally dated to the years 410–400.

Editions: Littré VI, 32–87; Villaret, 1911 (Greek); Jones, 1931 [= Loeb IV, 1–41]; Jouanna, 1975 [= *CMG* I, 1.3] (Greek-French).

Nature of the Child. See 28. *Generation / Nature of the Child*

40. *Nature of Women*

Contents: The title corresponds to the first words of the treatise but does not give an exact idea of what it contains. It is a treatise composed essentially of cases on the diseases of women to which an abridger later added a preamble inspired by a passage of the treatise *Diseases of Women II*, chapter 111 (= layer B, Grensemann), attaching to this a reflection upon the divine. The treatise consists of two parts: chapters 2–34 and 35–109. Each of these two parts is made up of a series of diseases that concludes with a long list of remedies. The most developed cases obey a schema similar to that of *Diseases II* 2 and of layer B of the gynecological treatises. Almost all of the diseases described have a counterpart description, indeed two such counterparts, in the other gynecological treatises (*Diseases of Women I–II / Sterile Women*). The diseases described in these cases are principally diseases of the womb, but there are others relating to the discontinuation of menstrual periods or to menstrual flows, to abortions, and to cases of sterility.

Authorship and date: The material is of the same origin as layer A of the gynecological treatises. It is not possible, however, to determine the affiliation of the abridger who composed the preamble. It is therefore a question of ancient material having been edited by a late epitomizer. The treatise is cited neither by Erotian nor by Galen.

Editions: Littré VII, 310–431; Trapp, 1967 (Greek).

41. *Nutriment*

Contents: Brief treatise presented in the form of intentionally enigmatic aphorisms, in which contraries are found side by side in the manner of Heraclitus. It concerns food in the broad sense of the term (air is also considered as a food; marrow as food for the bone; pus as food for the wound), so much so that unexpected subjects are broached (for example, periods for the formation of an embryo or for the healing of a broken bone). Several aphorisms on nature have remained famous: "Nature is sufficient in all for all" (15); "The natures of all are untaught" (39).

Authorship and date: The treatise was attributed by the ancients to Hippocrates; it is part of Erotian's list and Galen commented on it (the original commentary is lost). In reality, however, it is a post-Hippocratic treatise, as analysis of the vocabulary and the underlying medical and philosophical theories (knowledge of the pulse, for example; also the influence of Stoicism) indicates. It dates from the Hellenistic period. It was attributed to Hippocrates and commented on by Sabinus as early as 100 A.D. or so (see Aulus Gellius *Noctes Atticae* 3.16.8).

Editions: Littré IX, 94–121; Jones, 1923 [= Loeb I, 333–361]; Joly, 1972 [= Budé VI, 2] (Greek-French); Deichgräber, 1973 (Greek-German).

42. *The Oath*

Contents: See the text in appendix 1. An alternate rendering may be found, for example, in John Walton et al., eds., *The Oxford Medical Companion* (Oxford, 1994), 370–371.

Authorship and date: *The Oath* was always attributed by the ancients to Hippocrates. It is part of Erotian's list. The Arab tradition has preserved fragments of a commentary attributed to Galen. The authorship is disputed by the moderns. According to the most generally accepted interpretation, it is a document that gives information about the functioning of a medical school, probably the school of Cos. According to a more recent but not necessarily more correct interpretation, advanced by L. Edelstein, it is an oath issuing from Pythagorean circles. The date is also disputed. Fifth century according to some; fourth century according to others.

Editions: Littré IV, 628–633; Petrequin, 1877 (Greek-French); Jones, 1923 [= Loeb I, 289–301]; Jones, 1924; Heiberg, 1927 [= *CMG* I, 1] (Greek); Edelstein, 1969 (Greek-English, with commentary); Deichgräber, 1983; Lipourlis, 1983 (ancient Greek-modern Greek); Lichtenthaeler, 1984 (Greek-German, with a long commentary).

There exist also a Christian version of *The Oath* and another late version in verse. These two texts are given by Jones, 1924 and Heiberg, 1927 [⁻ *CMG* I, 1] (Greek); Jouanna, 1996 [= A. Garzya and J. Jouanna, *Storia e ecdotica dei Testi medici greci* (Naples, 1996), 269ff.] (Greek).

43. *On Fractures / On Joints*

Contents: These two treatises, written by the same author, form a single and indeed long work on surgery, treating of all manner of dislocations, diastases, and fractures, with the exception of those of the skull. Authority for the conventional order of reading (*On Fractures* before *On Joints*) is found in chapter 72 of *On Joints*, which refers to chapter 13 of *On Fractures*. As a technical treatise it is remarkable not only for the competence of the medical analysis and the quality of the writing, but also for the strong personality of the author. This physician was in every sense outstanding.

On Fractures: The author begins with simple fractures of the arm and the leg (1–23), then moves on to complicated fractures accompanied by a wound due to a protrusion of the bone (24–29); gives additional information in cases where the recommended modes of reduction are not suitable (30–36); and finally takes up dislocations and fractures of the elbow and of the knee (37–48).

On Joints: Dislocations of the humerus at the shoulder together with the various modes of reduction and treatment (1–12); dislocations and fractures of the clavicle (13–16). Chapters 17–29 do not belong to the treatise. Dislocations and fractures of the jaw (30–34); fractures of the nose (35–39), of the ear (40); deviations of the spinal column (41–48); fractures of the ribs and contusions to the chest (49–50); various types of dislocation of the thigh: signs indicating reduction and the consequences of nonreduction (51–61); procedures for reducing dislocations of the thigh (70–78) and of the fingers (80). The last chapters (82–87) do not belong to the treatise.

Authorship and date: The two treatises are mentioned by Erotian; but there is still more ancient evidence of them (see pages 52 and 61 regarding the attack brought against Hippocrates by Ctesias). Both were commented on by Galen. They are traditionally attributed to the school of Cos. End of the fifth century or beginning of the fourth.

Editions: Littré III, 338–563 and IV, 1–327; Petrequin, 1878 (Greek-French); Kühlewein, 1902 [= Teubner II] (Greek); Withington, 1928 [= Loeb III, 83–397].

On Sevens. See 56. *Sevens*

On Sterile Women. See 20. *Diseases of Women I–II / Sterile Women*

44. *On Wounds in the Head*

Contents: (False) description of the sutures of the skull and description of the nature of the bones of the head (1–2). Account of the different kinds of wounds, five in number: fracture, contusion, fracture with inward depression of the bone, hedra (or scratch fracture), and fracture by contrecoup (4–8). Modes of lesion to which the trephin is applied: fracture and contusion (9). Method for examining the injured person: by sight, touch, questioning, reasoning, and instruments (10). Various circumstances in which the different modes of lesion occur (11). Difficulty of diagnosis when the lesion occurs just at the sutures (12). Treatment and diagnosis of invisible bone lesions: applications, incision, trephining, scraping, "black drug" (13–14). Treatment of the flesh surrounding the wound (15). Removal of necrotic bone fragments (16–17). Differences presented by the skull of the child (18). Diagnosis of an incurably injured patient: description of traumatic meningitis (19). Further complication following a wound to the head: red erysipelatous edema of the face (20). The treatise concludes with advice on trephining: sawing trephine, perforating trephine (21). In chapter 14 it was said that the trephine should be used in the three days following the injury. Galen knew an appendix to the treatise not preserved in our medieval manuscripts.

Authorship and date: Belongs to the group of surgical treatises; traditionally attributed to the school of Cos. End of the fifth or beginning of the fourth century.

Editions: Littré III, 182–261; Petrequin, 1877 (Greek-French); Kühlewein, 1902 [= Teubner II]; Withington, 1928 [= Loeb III, 1–51].

45. *Physician*

Contents: The title, suggested by the first word of the treatise, corresponds
to the preamble, where the author draws a physical and moral portrait of
the ideal physician (1), rather than to the treatise as a whole, which is intended for beginners (see 2, 9, 13). The pupil must begin by practicing in
the office of the physician (cf. the treatise *In the Surgery*). An important
part of the treatise (2 9) is devoted to this topic: orientation of the office,
light for operating, seats for physician and patient, instruments (2); dressings and bandages (3–4); practicing incision; two types of lancets (5–6);
two types of cupping glasses (7); advice on bleeding a patient (8); conclusion about the instruments of the office (9). The author continues with a
section on ulcers and wounds (10–12). He leaves aside the question of
opportunity (*kairos*), for it is a subject for more advanced study (13). He
ends by advising the novice physician to apprentice himself to foreign ar-
mies in order to acquire experience of war wounds and to learn how to
extract shafts (14).

Authorship and date: The treatise entered the Hippocratic Collection late,
for it was known neither to Erotian nor Galen. It is of recent date
(Hellenistic era or beginning of the Christian era). However, its code of
ethics corresponds to that of the oldest treatises (refusal of theatricality,
concern for the interest of the patient). One ethical prescription is directly inspired by *The Oath* ("Patients in fact put themselves into the
hands of their physician, and at every moment he meets women,
maidens, and possessions very precious indeed. So towards all these self-
control must be used" [1]).

Editions: Littré IX, 198–221; Petrequin, 1877 (Greek-French); Jones,
1923 [= Loeb II, 303–313] (chapter 1 only); Bensel, 1923 [= *Philologus* 78
(1923): 88–130] (Greek); Heiberg, 1927 [= *CMG* I, 1] (Greek); Potter,
1995 [= Loeb VIII, 295–315].

46. *Places in Man*

Contents: After a preamble in which the author insists on the connected-
ness of all the parts of the body, which he compares to a circle (1), he describes the nature of the body (2–8): the head, veins, tendons, bones,

joints, stomach, and spleen. He next develops the theory of humoral fluxes at length (9–22): they are seven in number, originate in the head, and cause diseases in the places where they go—nostrils, ears, eyes, chest (empyema or consumption), spinal marrow (a sort of consumption), the tissues near the vertebrae (dropsy), joints, especially those of the hip. The order of topics in what follows is less clear. The author describes various other diseases with their treatment (23–40): among these affections are tumefaction of the spleen, "dry" pleurisy, fevers, jaundice, angina. General remarks on medicine (41–46): interesting remarks on allopathy and homeopathy, on the importance of opportunity (i.e., the aptness [*kairos*] of intervention) in medicine, and on the relationship between art and luck. The treatise concludes with a brief discussion of the diseases of women (47).

Authorship and date: Fourth century. The presence of the anatomical term "esophagus" (the only other attestation in the collection is in *Anatomy*) does not argue for an earlier date.

Editions: Littré VI, 273–349; Joly, 1978 [= Budé XIII] (Greek-French); Potter, 1995 [= Loeb VIII, 13–101].

47. *Precepts*

Contents: Throughout the treatise, the author draws a portrait of the ideal physician and castigates bad ones. The treatise begins with comments on method in medicine (1–3). One passage in this section displays a close relationship to Epicurus (cf. chapter 1 and Diogenes Laertius *Letter to Herodotus* 10.75). The treatise continues with recommendations regarding fees (4–7). The author discourses at length on the conduct to adopt with the patient (8–10); the physician must not hesitate to call upon colleagues in difficult cases; he must speak to the patient, encourage him, and try to please without charming him by ostentatious means. The author then criticizes physicians who have learned medicine late (13). The treatise ends with various aphorisms on particular points that bear no relation to what goes before (14).

Authorship and date: The treatise is not part of Erotian's list. It is later than Epicurus in view of the connection mentioned above. A gloss on the first chapter in a Vatican manuscript (*Urbinas gr.* 68), presented as an excerpt from Galen, says that the philosopher Chrysippus (third century B.C.) and the physician Archigenus (first to second century A.D.) had commented on the treatise. If this gloss is not false, the treatise would date from the Hellenistic and not the Roman period. It is, in any case, one of the late technical treatises of the Hippocratic Collection (see U. Fleischer, *Untersuchungen zu den pseudohippokratischen Schriften* [Berlin, 1939]).

Editions: Littré IX, 246–273; Jones, 1923 [= Loeb I, 303–333]; Heiberg, 1927 [= *CMG* I, 1] (Greek).

Presbeutikos. See 58. *Speech of the Envoy*

48. *Prognostic*

Contents: Preamble on the importance of prognosis (1); the author indicates he will treat of all the points that the physician must observe in the case of acute diseases in order to make the most accurate prognosis possible of the evolution and issue of the disease. In connection with each of these points he indicates the favorable and unfavorable signs: face, with the description of the Hippocratic facies (2); decubitus (3); hands, with carphology (4); breathing (5); sweats (6); hypochondrium (7); sleep (10); stools (11); urines (12); vomits (13); expectoration (14); suppurations (15–18); pains in the lumbar region and below (19); fevers (20); pains in the head (21); pains in the ears (22); pains in the throat (23); various prognoses to be made regarding recurrence, deposits (or "abscessions"), and more generally the evolution of the disease (24). Conclusion: a good prognosis must take into account the whole set of signs (25).

Authorship and date: This is a clinical work intended for the physician. It is traditionally attributed to Hippocrates by ancient critics, with not a single dissenting voice among them. It was commented on by Galen. It belongs to the school of Cos if not to Hippocrates himself. Second half of the fifth century.

Editions: Littré II, 110–191; Kühlewein, 1894 [= Teubner I]; Jones, 1923 [= Loeb II, 1–55]; Alexanderson, 1963 (Greek); Lipourlis, 1983 (ancient Greek–modern Greek).

49. *Prorrhetic I*

Contents: The treatise consists exclusively of observations relating to prognosis. It contains 170 aphorisms, arranged in no discernable order. The majority of these propositions were repeated, but reorganized, in the *Coan*

Prenotions. The interest of the treatise is that it shows that these aphorisms rest on clinical observation. Certain individual patients appear as examples. All but one are referred to by name. Their native city is indicated on two occasions: Cos and Odessa (the latter a city on the Black Sea, the present-day Varna in Bulgaria). These patients do not correspond to those of the *Epidemics*, despite two instances of homonymy. The treatise is the work of an itinerant physician who, having practiced in Cos, traveled all the way to the Milesian colony of Odessa. These names disappeared, with one exception, in the course of composing the *Coan Prenotions*.

Authorship and date: The treatise was known to Erotian, who challenges its association with Hippocrates. It was commented on by Galen. Although the examples of the patients refer to a sphere of activity different than that of the *Epidemics*, the treaty belongs by virtue both of its terminology and the notions it contains about the progress of disease to the same group of treatises. Middle of the fifth century.

Editions: Littré V, 510–573; Polack, 1954 (Greek; published in 1976); Potter, 1995 [= Loeb VIII, 167–211].

50. *Prorrhetic II*

Contents: Despite its title, this is not the continuation of *Prorrhetic I*. It is a treatise composed in its entirety by a physician whose personality shines through his writing. Following a polemic against overly bold prognoses (1–3) and an explanation of how to detect patients' faults in the observance of a prescribed regimen (4), the author studies prognosis in various diseases. Again, the exposition of these diseases follows no discernable order; the order is not, in any case, *a capite ad calcem*. Notably, the author considers dropsy (6), consumption (7), gout (8), the sacred disease (9), diseases of the eyes (18–20), diseases of the belly (22–23). One section is reserved for wounds and ulcers (11–16) and another for the diseases of women (24–28).

Authorship and date: The treatise has been rather neglected in Hippocratic studies, partly because neither Erotian nor Galen judged it worthy of Hippocrates, but also because Littré rejected it in volume IX of his edition. It needs to be rehabilitated and restored to the place it deserves alongside the *Prognostic*, from which it should never have been separated. On terminological grounds it is reasonable to suppose that these two treatises were written by one and the same author.

Editions: Littré IX, 1–75; Mondrain, 1984 (Greek-French; Paris doctoral thesis); Potter, 1995 [= Loeb VIII, 213–293].

51. *Regimen*

Contents: Long treatise, in four books in modern editions; in three books in Galen and in one of the two ancient manuscripts.

The first book is devoted to anthropology (1–36), for the author considers that it is not possible to treat of regimen without knowing the nature of man. Man, like other living beings, is constituted of two primordial substances, fire and water. These substances are indissociable and complementary. Fire, hot and dry, has the power of moving things; water, cold and humid, has the power of nourishing them, but exchanges may occur among these two elements as well as mixtures, which explains the diversity of living beings. Birth is only a reuniting of elements and death a separation of these elements (1–6). The author treats next of the formation of human nature in a long description of embryogenesis (7ff.). He explains in particular how fire organized the embryo in imitation of the universe by creating three circuits within the body that mirror the revolutions of the moon, the sun, and the stars (9–10). This organization of human nature is imitated by art (11–24). The author explains the formation of the male and female embryo (by the union of two seeds from the man and the woman respectively), and the development of twins as well as superfoetation (25–31). He describes the different types of bodily constitutions and of intelligence according to the different mixtures of water and fire (32–36).

The second book (37–66) is essentially a catalog of the natural and artificial properties of the elements of regimen (food, drink, exercise); it is the most elaborate such catalog in the entire Hippocratic Collection. Preceding it are two chapters on the influence of places and winds (37–38).

The third book (67–85 in modern editions; 67 to the end in Galen and one of the two ancient manuscripts) treats of regimen proper. The ideal, according to the author, is to achieve an exact balance between foods and exercises. But too many variables prevent this aim from being attained. The author distinguishes two classes of people: those who work and are unable to look after their health, and those who have the leisure to make health their first priority. For the first he describes an annual regimen varying as a function of each of the four seasons (68); but his main interest is in addressing himself to the elite that makes up the second class, revealing to them what he considers to be his own personal discovery. He thinks he has discovered a prognosis prior to illness, and a diagnosis of the cause of illness that always reduces to an imbalance in one sense or another between foods and exercises. He illustrates his discovery by a series of cases (70–85): six cases in which foods overpower exercises and eight cases in which the opposite occurs.

The fourth book (86–93 in modern editions; the subdivision does not exist in Galen or in one of the two ancient manuscripts) completes his exposition of prior prognosis by the use of dreams. The author distinguishes two categories of dreams: divine dreams that foretell good or evil and fall within the competence of interpreters of dreams; and dreams in which the soul reveals the state of the body, which come under the authority of physicians. With regard to the second category, the author establishes the prognostic and diagnostic signs of health and illness as a function of different visions. Various treatments may be indicated. It is in this context that the author recommends prayers to the gods.

Authorship and date: Although certain themes link up with those of the school of Cos (the influence of places and winds is comparable to what one finds, for example, in *Airs, Waters, Places*; the seasonal regimen is comparable to that of *Nature of Man*), the treatise occupies an original and independent place in the collection by virtue of its anthropology (the mixture of fire and water) and by its recourse to prayers to the gods. The treatise is put by scholars either at the end of the fifth century or in the first half of the fourth.

Editions: Littré VI, 466–663; Diels-Kranz VS 22C1 (Greek; excerpt); Jones, 1931 [= Loeb IV, 223–447]; Joly, 1967 [= Budé, unnumbered volume] (Greek-French); Joly, 1984 [= *CMG* I, 2.4] (Greek-French).

52. *Regimen in Acute Diseases*

Contents: The beginning of the treatise is famous for its polemic against the *Cnidian Sentences*, a work composed by several authors, then later reworked by several revisers. He reproaches the Cnidians for various inadequacies, notably in connection with their approach to medication (which consists essentially of evacuations based either on milk or whey) and with their conception of regimen; on the other hand, he also reproaches them for their excesses in determining the number of subdivisions of diseases (1) [= 1–3 in the Loeb edition]. The rest of the treatise concerns regimen in acute diseases (pleuritis, pneumonia, phrenitis, causus, etc.). According to the author, this is one of the most delicate questions in medicine, for the diseases are the most dangerous of all, excepting pestilential disease. However, physicians risk discrediting medicine by contradicting themselves on a matter of this importance, just as the contradictory assertions of soothsayers bring the art of divination into disrepute (2–3) [= 4–9]. The author considers successively the use of ptisane (or "gruel" made from barley) and the juice derived from it (4–7) [= 10–25], then of drinks. But before taking up the subject of drinks, he embarks on a long excursus on the effects of change in diet (8–13) [=26–49]. His account of drinks begins with wine (14) [= 50–52] and continues with hydromel (honey and water: 15) [= 53–57], oxymel (honey and vinegar: 16) [= 58–61], and water (17) [= 62–64]. He finishes his treatise with instructions on the use of baths.

Authorship and date: The treatise is traditionally attributed to the school of Cos. Galen, who commented on it, interprets it as an attack by Hippocrates against the Cnidians. The treatise dates from the end of the fifth century.

Editions: Littré II, 224–377; Kühlewein 1894 [= Teubner I] (Greek); Jones, 1923 [= Loeb II, 57–125]; Joly, 1972 [= Budé VI, 2] (Greek-French).

53. *Regimen in Acute Diseases (Appendix)*

Contents: Following the preceding treatise, the manuscripts contain additional material that is identified as a spurious (literally "bastard") part of *Regimen in Acute Diseases*. This appendix is partly concerned with acute diseases, but it is not clearly organized. It offers accounts (combining semiology, etiology, treatment, and prognosis) of several of the diseases considered acute by the preceding treatise (causus in chapter 1 [= 1–2 in the Loeb edition]; pneumonia and pleuritis in chapter 11 [= 31–34]) but not of all of them (phrenitis is omitted). By contrast, it treats of other diseases (anginas: 6 [= 9–10]; cholera: 19 [= 51]; dropsies: 20 [= 52]; and so on). In the course of his exposition, the author gives various pieces of advice on prognosis (the importance of odd days: 9 [= 21–22]) and on treatment (use of bleeding and purgation: 2 [= 3]). Certain of its themes (the danger of changing regimen, for example) link the *Appendix* to the *Regimen in Acute Diseases*.

Authorship and date: The main point of contention is whether the *Appendix* is due to the same author as the *Regimen in Acute Diseases*. Scholars are divided over this question, just as ancient physicians were divided over the treatment of acute diseases.

Editions: Littré II, 394–529; Kühlewein, 1894 [= Teubner I] (Greek); Joly, 1972 [= Budé VI, 2] (Greek-French); Potter, 1983 [= Loeb VI, 257–327].

Regimen in Health. See 39. *Nature of Man*

54. *Remedies*

Contents: Excerpt of a treatise on the use of evacuant medicines. The author advises the physician to use them with caution and not to forget that foods can serve the purpose of weaker evacuants. Before administering them, the physician should question the patient to determine if he or she is sensitive to evacuants. In the case of strong fevers, evacuants must not be given before the fever has subsided; better to give clysters that have a milder effect. "It is a shameful thing to kill a patient through the use of an evacuant." This maxim is not unworthy of the great Hippocratic treatises.

Authorship and date: The excerpt contains a passage that is parallel to one found in the treatise *Affections* (36), involving the distinction between four sorts of evacuants that eliminate four humors (bile, phlegm, water, and black bile). This similarity supports the dating of the extract to the first half of the fourth century as well. It is thought that the excerpt may belong to the book entitled *Remedies* that the author of the *Affections* cites on several occasions.

Editions: The excerpt was not published by Littré; H. I. Schöne, 1924 [= *Rheinisches Museum* 73 (1920–1924): 434–448] (Greek).

55. *The Sacred Disease*

Contents: Remarkable monograph devoted to a disease, "the disease called sacred"; that is to say, epilepsy. The treatise comprises a first polemical part (1) [= 1–4 in the Loeb edition] aimed against those who consider the disease to be due to the personal intervention of a deity, and who treat this disease by purifications, incantations, and dietary prohibitions. The author denounces their incompetence and their impiety; for him, the disease is not any more divine than others, and it is curable. In a second part (2–13) [= 5–16], the author proposes a rational explanation for the disease. It is hereditary and typically attacks persons of phlegmatic temperament (2) [= 5]. It is caused by the brain, which has not been sufficiently purged before or after birth. Fluxes of phlegm descend from the head and produce accidents according to the places where they end up (3–6) [= 6–9]. Epilepsy is caused by flows of phlegm descending from the head in two thick veins that come from the liver and the spleen: the cold phlegm coagulates the blood and blocks the passage of air. Description of the epileptic fit (7) [= 10]. The disease varies according to age: it is present above all in children and old people, or else in those who have had the disease since childhood (8–12) [= 11–15]. The chief precipitating cause is changes of the winds (13) [= 16]. The author then reverts to the role of the brain, the source of psychological life and of the intellect; its disturbance leads to madness; two sorts of madness: agitated madness due to bile, quiet madness due to phlegm; criticism of theories which hold that the diaphragm and the heart are the seat of intelligent thought (14–17) [= 17–20]. Conclusion: the disease is not more divine than others. Every disease is divine to the extent that it is caused by natural elements (cold, sun, winds); every disease is human to the extent that it is curable. Definition of treatment by contraries (18) [= 21].

Authorship and date: The author is probably the same as that of *Airs, Waters, Places*. The treatise is traditionally attributed to the school of Cos and dates from the second half of the fifth century.

Editions: Littré VI, 352–397; Jones, 1923 [= Loeb II, 127–183]; Grensemann, 1968 (Greek-German); Lipourlis, 1983 (ancient Greek–modern Greek).

56. *Sevens*

Contents: Long treatise lost in Greek (apart from a few passages), preserved in a bad Latin translation and, partially, in an Arabic translation. It is a classic example of philosophical medicine (establishing an analogy between man and the universe) and of arithmological medicine (insisting on the importance of the number seven). The treatise was used by scholars in the great debate over the influence of the Orient on Greek thought.

Authorship and date: The treatise does not appear in Erotian's list. Its date is highly controversial: between the sixth and fifth centuries B.C., according to Roscher; the first century A.D., according to Mansfeld. The rare passages preserved in Greek do not justify assigning an early date and associating it with the ancient core of the Hippocratic Collection.

Editions: Littré VIII, 634–673 and IX, 433–466; Roscher, 1913; West, 1971 (chapters 1–12); commentary on chapters 1–11 by J. Mansfeld, *The Pseudo-Hippocratic Tract Peri Hebdomadon, c. 1–11, and Greek Philosophy* (Assen, 1971).

57. *Sight*

Contents: Brief treatise relating to certain affections of the eye (pupils, eyelids) and their treatment. The author recommends delicate operations (scraping, cauterizing or excising the eyelid, and even trephining when sight is lost while the eyes are healthy). One chapter (3) treats cauterization on the back at length.

Authorship and date: The treatise does not appear in Erotian's list. Its date is debated. According to some, it is a late treatise; others locate it at the end of the fifth century or the beginning of the fourth.

Editions: Littré IX, 122–161 (ed. J. Sichel); Joly, 1978 [= Budé XIII] (Greek-French).

58. *Speech of the Envoy (= Presbeutikos)*

Contents: Long speech that Hippocrates' son Thessalus, sent by his father, is supposed to have delivered before the popular assembly in Athens on the occasion of a quarrel between Athens and Cos during the second part of the Peloponnesian War, pleading the cause of his native people. The main part of the speech recalls services rendered. These were four in number; the first two, the oldest of the four, were rendered by ancestors of Hippocrates and Thessalus.

The first service dates from the First Sacred War: aid furnished to the Amphyctions in the siege of Crisa by Nebros, physician of Cos, and his son Chrysos; privileges at Delphi accorded to the Asclepiads of Cos by way of thanks.

The second service dates from the First Persian War: Cos refused to participate in the expedition of the Persian king against Greece at a moment when Cadmus, Thessalus's ancestor on his mother's side, and Hippolochus, Thessalus's ancestor on his father's side, were leaders of the city. The island of Cos was then ravaged by the Persians and by their ally, Artemesia of Halicarnassus.

The third service was rendered by Hippocrates to the Greeks during the time of a pestilence that came from the north; he refused to aid the barbarians and with his sons and pupils brought help to Greece instead; on passing through Delphi, Hippocrates and Thessalus saw the privileges accorded to the Asclepiads renewed and inscribed on a stele.

The fourth service: Thessalus participated for three years as public physician in the Athenian expedition to Sicily.

After having reviewed these services, Thessalus asks the Athenians not to use force against Cos and to settle their differences by negotiation. He implies that other peoples were prepared to come to their aid, notably the Thessalians (see the *Address from the Altar*).

Authorship and date: This biographical writing was already known to Erotian. Even though the speech may not be authentic, it contains accurate information drawn from a reliable source. Certain details (particularly the reference to male descent in the family of the Asclepiads and to the relationship between the Asclepiads and Delphi) are confirmed by inscriptions; see pages 33–35. The text of this speech dates from the fourth or possibly the third century.

Editions: Littré IX, 404–428; Smith, 1990 (Greek-English).

59. *Superfoetation*

Contents: The title does not suit the treatise as a whole, only the first chapter. Like other physicians and scientists of his time, the author believes in superfoetation, which is to say the supplementary fertilization of a pregnant women obtained under special conditions through a second copulation. The first part of the treatise contemplates difficult situations in delivery (2–15); the end of the treatise (16–43) is centered instead on sterility, and gives tests and treatments with lists of remedies.

Authorship and date: The treatise does not appear on Erotian's list. Alongside original passages, it includes others that are parallel to ones in *Diseases of Women I–II / Sterile Women* (layer A, Grensemann). It belongs therefore to the group of gynecological treatises.

Editions: Littré VIII, 476–509; Lienau, 1973 [= *CMG* I, 2.2] (Greek-German).

60. *Testament of Hippocrates* [= *Qualem Oportet Esse Discipulum*]

Contents: Very brief ethical treatise enumerating the physical, moral, and intellectual qualities of the physician, his appearance (hair, nails, clothes), bearing, and attitude when he visits the patient. The physician must be free, naturally gifted, young, a decent person in every way, not covetous of wealth; he must be understanding in his relations with the patient and show evidence of his discretion and self-control.

Authorship and date: This treatise, while it does not figure in modern editions of Hippocrates, appears alongside *The Oath* and the *Law* at the head of the Hippocratic Collection in a part of the Greek tradition (at Alexandria in the eleventh century) and in the Arab tradition, where the treatise was well known as the *Testament* of Hippocrates and considered to be authentic. It does not belong to the ancient core of the collection, however; it may be dated to the first or second century A.D.

Editions: Deichgräber, 1970 (short version and long version in Greek; short version in the Arab tradition and long version in Latin).

61. *Ulcers*

Contents: The work describes what does and does not need to be done in the treatment of "ulcers." This term, which translates the Greek word *helkos*, is to be understood not only in its narrow pathological sense, but also in the more general sense of a wound; indeed, the treatise is known in French as *Plaies*, or "Wounds." It is impossible briefly to give a fair idea of the extremely varied and random advice contained in this treatise. One practice that seems peculiar, but which was shared by other Hippocratic physicians, consisted in administering evacuants of the "lower cavity" to patients suffering from injuries to the head or stomach (3). One of the original things about this treatise by comparison with the other works on surgery is that it gives, in the second part, a number of recipes for medicines to be used in treating wounds. The author sometimes notes the geographic provenance of these remedies or of their ingredients: this domain extends from Egypt (14, 17, 18) as far as Illyricum (13), passing through the islands (Cyprus, 13; Melos, 12), through Orchomenus (17), and through Caria, whence came the recipe for a particular medicine (16). It will be recalled that Caria is the family birthplace of the Asclepiads of Cos and Cnidus.

Authorship and date: The treatise is mentioned by Erotian. It can be dated from the fifth century or from the fourth.

Editions: Littré VI, 400–433; Petrequin, 1877 (Greek-French); Potter, 1995 [= Loeb VIII, 339–375].

62. *Use of Liquids*

Contents: Brief treatise on the external use of liquids (freshwater, saltwater, vinegar, wine) in the form of affusions, baths, or steambaths in various affections, and on the effects of hot and cold. Several passages are parallel to ones found in the *Aphorisms*. The author has a good medical background.

Authorship and date: The treatise is intended for specialists, as the reference at the beginning to the office of the physician indicates. It appears in Erotian's list under the title *On Waters*. It dates from the Hippocratic period, most likely the fourth century.

Editions: Littré VI, 119–137; Heiberg, 1927 [= *CMG* I, 1] (Greek); Joly, 1972 [= Budé VI, 2] (Greek-French); Potter, 1995 [= Loeb VIII, 317–337].

Wounds. See 61. *Ulcers*

Wounds in the Head. See 44. *On Wounds in the Head*

63. *Other Apocryphal Treatises*

There exist other manifestly late works that have been attributed to Hippocrates and have not been included in the so-called complete editions of Hippocrates. They are listed (along with the manuscripts that transmit them) in H. Diels, "Die Handschriften der antiken Ärzte. I. Teil: Hippokrates und Galenos," *Abhandl. der Königl. Preuss. Akad. der Wissenschaften* (Berlin, 1905): 39–57.

The Hippocratic treatises are collected in their entirety in É. Littré, *Oeuvres complètes d'Hippocrate,* 10 vols. (Paris: 1839–1861) (henceforth, "Littré"). For purposes of the present work, the vast majority of quoted passages in the Hippocratic Collection in English translation are taken from the incomplete, eight-volume Loeb Classical Library edition of the corpus (henceforth, "Loeb"). Reference is made in what follows first to the treatise in question and then to the corresponding volume and page number in either the Greek-French edition (e.g., "Littré IX, 418") or the Greek-English edition (e.g., "Loeb IV, 133"), or both. The publication history of the Loeb edition, together with the treatises contained in each volume, is as follows:

Vol. I: Translated by W. H. S. Jones. Cambridge, Mass.: Harvard University Press, 1923; reprinted 1984. *Ancient Medicine. Airs, Waters, Places. Epidemics I* and *II. The Oath. Precepts. Nutriment.*

Vol. II: Translated by W. H. S. Jones. Cambridge, Mass.: Harvard University Press, 1923; reprinted 1992. *Prognostic. Regimen in Acute Diseases. The Sacred Disease. The Art. Breaths. Law. Decorum. Physician* (ch. 1). *Dentition.*

Vol. III: Translated by E. T. Withington. Cambridge, Mass.: Harvard University Press, 1928; reprinted 1984. *On Wounds in the Head. In the Surgery. On Fractures. On Joints. Mochlicon.*

Vol. IV: Translated by W. H. S. Jones. Cambridge, Mass.: Harvard University Press, 1931; reprinted 1992. *Nature of Man. Regimen in Health. Humours. Aphorisms. Regimen I–III. Dreams.* (N.B.: this volume also contains the fragments of Heraclitus's *On the Universe.*)

Vol. V: Translated by Paul Potter. Cambridge, Mass.: Harvard University Press, 1988. *Affections. Diseases I* and *II.*

Vol. VI: Translated by Paul Potter. Cambridge, Mass.: Harvard University Press, 1988. *Diseases III. Internal Affections. Regimen in Acute Diseases (Appendix).*

Vol. VII: Translated by Wesley D. Smith. Cambridge, Mass.: Harvard University Press, 1994. *Epidemics II* and *IV–VII.*

Vol. VIII: Translated by Paul Potter. Cambridge, Mass.: Harvard University Press, 1995. *Places in Man. Glands. Fleshes. Prorrhetic I* and *II. Physician. Use of Liquids. Ulcers. Haemorrhoids. Fistulas.*

The same system has been followed in citing to the four-volume edition of *The Complete Greek Tragedies*, edited by David Grene and Richmond Lattimore (e.g., Grene-Lattimore III, 267). Where repeatedly cited works are referred to in abbreviated form by the names of their translators, as in the case of Richmond Lattimore's translation of the *Iliad*, this is indicated at their first instance in the notes. See the List of Abbreviations for a complete listing.

One. Hippocrates of Cos

1. On these coins, see page 38.

2. See Strabo 14.2.19; Diodorus of Sicily 15.76.2.

3. Cf. Tacitus *Annals* 12.61. The emperor Claudius, when he wished to grant immunity to the inhabitants of Cos, briefly recalled their history: " 'The earliest occupants of the island had,' he said, 'been Argives—or, possibly, Coeus, the father of Latona. Then the arrival of Aesculapius had introduced the art of healing, which attained the highest celebrity among his descendants' " (see the Loeb translation by J. Jackson [Cambridge, Mass., 1963], 405).

4. Plato *Protagoras* 311b–c; see the Hackett translation by S. Lombardo and K. Bell (Indianapolis, 1997), 749.

5. Plato *Phaedrus* 270c; translated by W. H. S. Jones in his introduction to the first volume of the Loeb edition of Hippocrates, xxxiii–xxxiv.

6. I leave to one side here the scholarly debates over what the Hippocratic method may actually have encompassed.

7. Aristotle *Politics* 7.4.1326a15–17; see the Loeb translation by H. Rackham (Cambridge, Mass., 1959), 555.

8. Aristophanes *Thesmophoriazusae* 272–274; see the Penguin translation by D. Barrett (Harmondsworth, 1964), 109–110, slightly modified here in accordance with Barrett's note. This play will be better known to some readers by its title in the Penguin edition, *The Women*.

9. Aristophanes' *Thesmophoriazusae* dates from 411 and Aristotle's *Politics* from the years 335–323.

10. Hippocrates *Letters* 15; see W. D. Smith, ed. and trans., *Hippocrates: Pseudepigraphic Writings* (New York, 1990), 71.

11. Hippocrates *Letters* 11; see Smith's translation in the *Pseudepigraphic Writings*, 59.

12. Hippocrates' *Speech of the Envoy* (or *Presbeutikos*) may be found in Littré IX, 404–428, among other editions; in English see Smith's translation in the *Pseudepigraphic Writings*, just cited, 110–125. See also the *Decree of the Athenians* (Littré IX, 400–403), and the *Address from the Altar* (or *Epibomios*) (Littré IX, 402–405).

13. See H. I. Shöne, "Bruchstücke einer neuen Hippokratesvita," *Rheinisches Museum* 58 (1903): 55–66.

14. This information is found in the *Life of Hippocrates* attributed to Soranus. The "monarch" referred to is to be associated with the old city of Astypalaea, located in the western part of the island, which was to become the deme of the Isthmus after the synoecismus of 366. According to G. Pugliese Carratelli ("Gli Asclepiadi e il Sinecismo di Cos," *La parola de Passato* 12 [1957]: 333–342 and "Il damos Coo di Isthmos," *Ann. Scuola Arch. di Atene*, n.s., 35–36 [1963–1964]: 150), who relies on the evidence of inscriptions, this monarch was a priest of Asclepius.

15. See Hippocrates *Speech of the Envoy* (Littré IX, 416.17). A copy of the decree of the *koinon* of the Asclepiads of Cos and Cnidus (fourth century B.C.) has been partially recovered at Delphi: see G. Rougemont, *Corpus des inscriptions de Delphes I: Lois sacrées et règlements religieux* (Paris, 1977), 122–124.

16. Plato *Symposium* 186e; see the Hackett translation by A. Nehamas and P. Woodruff (Indianapolis, 1997), 470. The term was probably already employed in the broad sense in Theognis (at line 432) and Euripides *Alcestis* 969ff. But it is in the narrow sense that "Hippocrates, he of the Asclepiads" is to be understood in Plato *Protagoras* 311b6 and *Phaedrus* 270c. The passage from the narrow to the broad sense is readily seen in the *Republic* 3.406a, where Plato opposes the old medicine of the time of Asclepius and his sons with modern medicine. "Asclepiads" is to be understood chiefly as designating the descendants of Asclepius and his sons, referred to in the immediately preceding lines; but as the Asclepiads were physicians par excellence, the term can also be broadened to designate physicians.

17. The term is employed in inscriptions of the classical period in the narrow rather than the broad sense. Several inscriptions about the Asclepiads have been found at Delphi. The restricted sense is clearly implied in the inscription about the Asclepiads of Cos and Cnidus, where reference is made to "descent by males" (see page 35). The most ancient inscription is the dedicatory inscription of an Asclepiad from Selinus in Sicily dating from the last quarter of the fifth century, the context of which does not suffice to decide which sense is intended (Delphi: Inv. no. 3522; see the most recent publication by L. Dubois, *Inscriptions grecques dialectales de Sicile* [1989], 83ff.). But one may compare it with the funereal epigram of the physician Pausanias, originally of Gela, also in Sicily, where the dual mention of physician and Asclepiad indicates that these two terms were not being confused: "His city Gela buried here Pausanias, son of Anchites, a physician of the race of Asclepius, bearing a name expressive of his calling, who turned aside from the chambers of Persephone many men wasted by chilling disease" (*Anthologia Graeca* 7.508; see the Loeb translation by W. R. Patton [Cambridge, Mass., 1960], 2:277). This Pausanias was a friend of Empedocles, who dedicated his treatise *On Nature* to him (Diels-Kranz 31B1). Even more recent inscriptions may use the term "Asclepiad" in the narrow sense; for example, a dedicatory inscription of an inhabitant of Iasus, a city in Asia Minor not far from Cos and Cnidus, dating from the second century B.C.: "Menes, son of Tyrtaeus,

of the city of Iasus, of the family of the Asclepiads, [offered this altar] to Asclepius Epibaterius, founder of the race" (see D. Levi and G. Pugliese Carratelli, "Nuove iscrizioni di Iasos," *Annuario Sc. At.* 39–40 [1961–1962]: 573–632; cf. L. Robert, "Nouvelles inscriptions d'Iasos," *Rev. Ét. Anc.* 65 [1963]: 314). Note also the inscription from Cos about a descendant of the Asclepiads and Heraclidae cited at page 17.

18. Tzetzes *Chiliades* 721ff.

19. See Homer *Iliad* 2.729–732; 4.204 and 219.

20. Ibid., 11.832–835; see the Richmond Lattimore translation [henceforth, "Lattimore"] (Chicago, 1951), 256. Before being wounded himself, Machaon had treated Menelaus (4.193–219).

21. Ibid., 11.514 (Lattimore, 248).

22. See *Little Iliad*, Frag. 30 Bernabé [= Pausanias 3.26.9]: "The author of the epic *The Little Iliad* says that Machaon was killed by Eurypylus, son of Telephus" (from the Loeb translation by W. H. S. Jones and H. A. Ormerod [Cambridge, Mass., 1926], 2:167). Cf. Hippocrates *Speech of the Envoy* (Littré IX, 426.3–5; Smith, trans., *Pseudepigraphic Writings*, 123): "Machaon laid down his life in the Troad when, as those who wrote of it say, he went into Priam's city out of the horse"; cf. also the *Life* of Brussels: "Machaon, as many sources report, died at the fall of Troy, without leaving descendants." But other traditions attribute sons to Machaon (see above all Pausanias 2.11.5, 23.4, and 38.6; 4.3.2 and 30.3) and some Asclepiads claimed to descend from him. In particular Aristotle, whose father Nicomachus was a doctor at Stagira, was said to belong to the family of Asclepiads descending from Machaon (Diogenes Laertius *Vitae philosophorum* 5.1).

23. See Pausanias 3.26.9.

24. Stephanus of Byzantium *Ethnica* s.v. Syrna. Certain witnesses call this Carian city Syrnos, like the island southwest of Cos: Pausanias 3.26.10, Theopompus (see note 26 below), and Aelius Aristides (see note 28 below). The city has recently been identified. Its ruins are those of Bayir, situated on the Asiatic continent across from Rhodes: see P. M. Frazer and G. E. Bear, *The Rhodian Perae and Islands* (London, 1954), 22ff.; cf. J. and L. Robert, *Bull. Epigr.* 212 (1955).

25. A variant explains Podalirius's settling in Caria with reference to the Delphic oracle (Apollodorus *Epitome* 6.18; scholium in Lychophron *Alexandra* 1047). A quite different tradition (ibid., 1050, with scholium; cf. Strabo *Geography* 6.3.9) has Podalirius dying in Daunia (Apulia). His tomb, next to a stream where the sick bathed together with their herds, was an oracular and healing hero-shrine (*héroon*).

26. See Theopompus, *FGH* 115F103 (14) Jacoby: "[C]oncerning the doctors of Cos and Cnidus, how they were Asclepiads, and how they came from Syrnos, the first offspring of Podalirius" (in G. S. Shrimpton, *Theopompus the historian* [Montreal, 1991], 232).

27. Galen *On the Therapeutic Method* 1.1.6; see R. J. Hankinson's translation of books I and II of this treatise (Oxford, 1991), 5.

28. See Aelius Aristides *Asclepiads* 11ff. Unlike Theopompus (see note 26 above), Aelius thought that both sons of Asclepius, Podalirius and Machaon, stopped off at Cos, then at Rhodes, and from there went on to Caria, Cnidus, and Syrnos (that is, Syrna), where they left heirs. On the Asclepiads of Rhodes, see *To the Rhodians on Concord* 45.

29. Nineteenth, according to the *Life* of Soranus; eighteenth according to *Letters* 2; seventeenth according to Tzetzes.

30. Tzetzes *Chiliades* 944–958. Compare Hippocrates *Letters* 2: "Hippocrates is Dorian by race, of the city of Cos. His father is Heraclides, son of Hippocrates, who is son of Gnosidicus, who is son of Nebros, who is son of Sostratus, who is son of Theodorus, who is son of Cleomyttades, who is son of Crisamis. . . . The divine Hippocrates is therefore the ninth from King Crisamis, the eighteenth from Asclepius, and the twentieth from Zeus" (Littré IX, 315). Yet a different accounting, based on a variant of the same text that gives Hippocrates' grandfather as Gnosdicus, omitting Hippocrates I, may be found in Smith, trans., *Pseudepigraphic Writings*, 47; according to this reckoning, Hippocrates is eighth from Crisamis, seventeenth from Asclepius, and nineteenth from Zeus.

31. There exist several versions of this "sacred war," the historical reality of which has been challenged recently. See Aeschines *Against Ctesiphon* 107ff.; Diodorus 9.16; Pausanias 10.37; Frontinus 3.7.6; Polyaenus 6.13.

32. Hippocrates *Speech of the Envoy* (Littré IX, 408.25–412.2); see Smith, trans., *Pseudepigraphic Writings*, 113–115.

33. Pausanias (10.37.7) mentions a similar ruse but attributes it to Solon. Other versions attribute authorship to Cleisthenes (Frontinus 3.7.6) and Eurylochus (Polyaenus 6.13).

34. Stephanus of Byzantium *Ethnica* s.v. Cos.

35. See Hippocrates *Speech of the Envoy* (Littré IX, 414.1–4). The hieromnemones were religious and administrative officials in many Greek states, delegates of the peoples belonging to the religious Confederation (or Amphictiony) who sat on the Amphictionic Council at Delphi; see Smith, trans., *Pseudepigraphic Writings*, 115 (n. 1).

36. Here, too, the *Speech of the Envoy* is our source, as for the fact that Cadmus may also have been known by Herodotus (7.163–164).

37. Hippocrates *Speech of the Envoy* (Littré IX, 414.13–416.18); see Smith, trans., *Pseudepigraphic Writings*, 115–117.

38. This is partially confirmed by Herodotus (7.164): Cadmus had succeeded his father as tyrant of the island of Cos.

39. See Herodotus 8.87–88.

40. Herodotus 9.76; see the translation by D. Grene, *The History* (Chicago, 1987), 646.

41. See Herodotus 7.99.

42. On Cadmus compare Hippocrates *Speech of the Envoy* (Littré IX, 416.18–24) and Herodotus 7.163–164.

43. Cape Mycale is on the tip of Asia Minor facing the island of Samos to the north of Cos.

44. See the *Life* of Brussels.

45. Hippocrates' mother is referred to as Phaenerete in both the Soranus and Brussels biographies, as well as in Tzetzes; but as "Praxithea daughter of Phaenerete" in *Letters* 2.

46. As sources regarding Hippocrates' origins, the *Life* according to Soranus cites the names of Eratosthenes, Pherecydes, Apollodorus, and Arius of Tarsus. Beginning with Eratosthenes of Cyrene, they extend back therefore from the third century B.C. as far as the Library of Alexandria.

47. The first of these two inscriptions dates from the first century A.D. (Maiuri, *N. Sill.* 461). The second—an inscription of the Museum of the Castle of Cos (EV 224)—is unpublished but a partial text can be found in G. Pugliese Carratelli, "Il damos Coo di Isthmos," 151; for the complete text, see Carratelli's contribution to the *festschrift* in honor of Marcello Gigante, noted in the bibliography at page 485.

48. Galen *Anatomical Procedures* 2.1; see Charles Singer, trans., *Galen: On Anatomical Procedures* (Oxford, 1956), 31.

49. Hippocrates *On Joints* 33 (Loeb III, 259).

50. This on the testimony of the *Suda*. Compare Galen *Regimen in Acute Diseases according to Hippocrates* 1.17: "Hippocrates' grandfather, the son of Gnosidicus, wrote absolutely nothing according to some, and, according to others, two writings only, the treatise on *Fractures* and the treatise on *Joints*"; cf. *Comm. Fractures* 1.1.

51. On Herodicus (of Selymbria) as Hippocrates' teacher, see the *Life* according to Soranus (where Herodicus's origin is not mentioned), *Suda*, Tzetzes, and scholium W at Plato *Republic* 3.406a: "He [Plato] speaks of Herodicus of Seylimbria. . . . This is the Herodicus with whom Hippocrates of Cos studied." In Pliny (*Natural History* 29.4) the reverse is claimed; namely, that Prodicus (read: Herodicus) was one of Hippocrates' disciples. It may be doubted whether this teacher of gymnastics and medicine, condemned by Plato as representative of the modern school of dietary medicine (see above all *Republic* 3.406a; but compare *Protagoras* 316e and *Phaedrus* 227d, as well as Aristotle, *Rhetoric* 1.5.1361b5) was Hippocrates' teacher, for a Herodicus (believed by scholars to be Herodicus of Selymbria) is harshly criticized in *Epidemics* 6.3.18 for his overly severe therapeutic method, which killed patients suffering from fever by a regime of running, repeated bouts of wrestling, and hot baths.

52. On Gorgias as Hippocrates' teacher, see the *Life* according to Soranus, *Suda*, Tzetzes. The influence of Gorgias's style on certain treatises of the Hippocratic probably gave rise to this belief. The papyrological record (*POxy.* 9.1184; see ¬, no. 36) contains a letter addressed by Hippocrates to Gorgias; this is a ¬ter contained in the manuscript record (*Letters* 6) but addressed there by ¬emetrius. Nothing can be concluded from the fact that the name ¬*nidemics* 5.11, where the wife of an inhabitant of Larissa named ¬ being sick: the name is too common. It should be noted, ¬rgias and Hippocrates lived in Larissa, where the Sophist's

instruction in rhetoric was valued by the Thessalian elite and particularly by the Aleuadae, the ruling family of the region (Plato *Meno* 70b).

53. On Democritus as Hippocrates' teacher, see Celsus *De medicina* Pref. 8 ("A disciple of Democritus, according to some, Hippocrates of Cos"), the *Life* by Soranus, *Suda*, Tzetzes. On the relations between Democritus and Hippocrates, see also the *Letters* 10–21 and 33. Modern scholars have also looked for traces of Democritus in the Hippocratic Collection. It should be added that according to one version, which survives in an ancient Latin translation of the corpus, Hippocrates studied physics with Melissus (*Ars medicina* in *Parisinus lat.* 7028, fol. 3v).

54. Strabo *Geography* 14.2.19; see the Loeb translation by H. L. Jones (Cambridge, Mass., 1950), 6:289.

55. Pliny *Natural History* 29.1–2; see the Loeb translation by W. H. S. Jones (Cambridge, Mass., 1963), 8:183–185.

56. See Pliny *Natural History* 20.264.

57. For further detail about these steles of Epidaurus, see chapter 8.

58. This is the thesis of F. Robert, "Hippocrate et le clergé d'Asclépios à Cos," *CR Acad. Inscr.* (1939): 91–99.

59. On this legend, see G. Huet, "La légende de la fille d'Hippocrate à Cos," *Bibl. de l'École des chartes* (Paris) 79 (1919): 45–59, and E. Wickersheimer, "Légendes hippocratiques du Moyen Age," *Archiv für Geschichte der Medizin* 45 (1961): 164–175.

60. See the *Life* according to Soranus. Other sources: the *Letters* and Athenodorus (cited in note 61 below). This encounter between Hippocrates and Democritus is also known in Arabic tradition: see, for example, Ali ibn Ridwan, *Sur la voie du bonheur par la profession médicale*, ed. A. Dietrich (Göttingen, 1982), 22: "The inhabitants of Abdera sent to Hippocrates ten *qintar* of gold for the treatment of Democritus, whom they believed had lost his reason. But Hippocrates returned the money and showed himself amicable to them. . . . When he visited Democritus, he recognized that he was sane and that the inhabitants believed that he had lost his reason because he had given up participating in the public affairs of the city in order to devote himself to science."

61. See Hippocrates *Letters* 10–21. Cf. also Athenodorus (first century A.D.), in Diogenes Laertius 9.42 (= Diels-Kranz 68A1) cited at page 41. See, too, Aelian *Varia Historia* 4.20.

62. See La Fontaine, *Fables* (VIII, 26); and Stendhal, *Vie de Henry Brulard* (chapter 3): "My grandfather adored the apochryphal correspondence of Hippocrates, which he read in Latin (although he knew some Greek) and Horace in the edition by Johannes Bond, printed in terribly small characters. He communicated to me these two passions."

63. See pages 29ff.

64. Sources: Hippocrates *Letters* 1–9 and *Decree of the Athenians*; Galen *Quod optimus medicus sit quoque philosophus* [henceforth, "*Med. Phil.*"] 3; *Life* according to Soranus; Stobaeus 3.13.51 (note that for Stobaeus the Great King is Xerxes); *Suda*. The anecdote is also known in the Arab tradition: see, for example, Ali ibn Ridwan, *Sur la voie du bonheur*, 22: "His renown was so great during his lifetime that the king of

Persia named Artaxerxes, the king of kings, offered him one hundred *qintar* of gold, a prominent position and splendid treasures if he came to him to be at his service as physician. But Hippocrates refused and gave no reply."

65. Hippocrates *Letters* 4; see Smith, trans., *Pseudepigraphic Writings*, 51.

66. Cyrus, father of Cambyzes, had brought from Egypt the best eye doctor (Herodotus 3.1).

67. See Homer *Odyssey* 4.231–232; cf. Isocrates *Busiris* 22.

68. See Herodotus 3.129–130.

69. Ibid., 3.130; see the Grene translation (cited above in note 40), 266.

70. See Herodotus 3.133–134.

71. Hippocrates *Oath* (Loeb I, 301).

72. See Xenophon *Anabasis* 1.8.26. He also treated the wife, mother, and children of Artaxerxes: see Plutarch *Life of Artaxerxes* 1.1.1012a. If Diodorus of Sicily (2.32.4) is to be believed, Ctesias was taken prisoner before being attached to the king's service by reason of his medical expertise. On this view, his career in Persia exhibits analogies with that of Democedes.

73. See Ctesias of Cnidus *Persica*, in *FGH* 3C688F14 Jacoby (34 and 44).

74. Hippocrates *Letters* 5; see Smith, trans., *Pseudepigraphic Writings*, 53.

75. Galen *Med. Phil.* 3.

76. Plutarch *Life of Cato the Elder* 23.3–4.350c; see Ian Scott-Kilvert, trans., *Makers of Rome: Nine Lives by Plutarch* (Harmondsworth, 1965), 146.

77. An entirely isolated version, mentioned by the Brussels *Life*, holds that Hippocrates went to the court of the king of the Medes Arfaxad (= Artaxerxes?) at Ecbatana.

78. Charles Baudelaire, *Le musée classique du Bazaar Bonne-Nouvelle* (Paris, 1846).

Two. Hippocrates the Thessalian

1. In the second part of this book we will examine the physical conditions faced by itinerant physicians of the period.

2. See pages 21ff.

3. Herodotus 3.131; see D. Grene, trans., *The History* (Chicago, 1987), 267. Other ancient accounts concerning Democedes may be found in Diels-Kranz 1:110–112; see, for example, the French edition of J.-P. Dumont et al., *Les Présocratiques* (Paris, 1988), 82–85.

4. See *Life of Hippocrates* according to Soranus.

5. Andreas was a student of Herophilus and later personal physician to the Egyptian king Ptolemy Philopater. He was killed in the king's very tent on the eve of the Battle of Raphia between Ptolemy and Antiochus III (217 B.C.): see Polybius 5.81.6. On Andreas's life and work see H. von Staden, *Herophilus: The Art of Medicine in Early Alexandria* (Cambridge, 1989), 472–477.

6. See page 18.

7. See Tzetzes *Chiliades* 963–965.

8. This information is contained in the *Life of Hippocrates* according to Soranus of Ephesus.

9. Galen *Med. Phil.* 3.

10. See chapter 3.

11. See Galen *Med. Phil.* 3. The distortion in Galen's account comes from his interest in denouncing the cupidity of certain of his colleagues, who were more "medicine peddlers than real doctors." On the clientele of the Hippocratics, see pages 114ff.

12. Hippocrates *Epidemics III* 17 (cases 5 and 12); *Epidemics V* 11 and 13–25 (i.e., sixteen cases in all).

13. On Meliboea, see Hippocrates *Epidemics III* 17 (case 16); on Crannon, see *Epidemics II* 1.1; *Epidemics VI* 14 and 37; *Epidemics VI* 1.7, 3.2 ("The woman I had first treated in Crannon"); for Pharsalus, see *Epidemics VI* 8.18; for Pherae, see *Epidemics V* 12.

14. The oldest group of the *Epidemics* (*I* and *III*) is traditionally dated from the years 419 to 410. For further details on the date of the *Epidemics*, see appendix 3, nos. 22–24.

15. See Tzetzes *Chiliades* 966.

16. See *Suda* s.v. "Hippocrates." On the relations between Hippocrates and Perdiccas, see pages 31ff.

17. On Thasos, see Hippocrates *Epidemics I* 1, 4, 7; 13.4, 13.9); *Epidemics III* 1.1, 1.4; 17.1–3, 17.11, 17.15. On Abdera, see *Epidemics III* 17.6–10, 17.13. On Cyzicus, see *Epidemics III* 17.14.

18. Abdera: Sacred Way (*Epidemics III* 17.7: "In Abdera the maiden who lay sick by the Sacred Way"); Thracian Gate (ibid., 17.8: "In Abdera Anaxion, who lay sick by the Thracian gate"). Thasos: ramparts (*Epidemics I*, case 1: "Philiscus lived by the wall"; *Epidemics III* 1.2: "Hermocrates, who lay sick by the new wall"); Heracleion (*Epidemics I*, case 6: "Cleanactides, who lay sick above the temple of Heracles"; *Epidemics III* 17.3: "Pythion, who lay sick above the shrine of Heracles"); Artemision (ibid., 17.1: "the Parian who lay beyond the temple of Artemis"); Heraion (*Epidemics I*, case 14: "Melidia, who lay sick by the temple of Hera"); temple of Earth (*Epidemics III* 1.1: "Pythion, who lived by the temple of Earth"); Liars' Market (ibid., 1.8: "The youth who lay sick by the Liars' Market"; 1.12: "A woman who lay sick by the Liars' Market"); fountain (ibid., 17.2: "the woman who lay sick by the Cold Water"); Platform (*Epidemics I*, case 2: "Silenus lived on Broadway"); Herdsmans' Gully (ibid., case 8: "Erasinus lived by the gully of Boötes").

19. On Thasos, see *Epidemics VI* 8.29, 8.32. On Abdera, see *Epidemics IV* 31, 56; *Epidemics VI* 8.30, 8.32. On Acanthus, see *Epidemics IV* 20c. On Perinthus, see *Epidemics II* 1.5, 3.1, 3.12; *Epidemics IV* 21; *Epidemics VI* 2.19, 7.10; cf. also *Humours* 8.

20. On Thasos, see *Epidemics VII* 112. On Abdera, see *Epidemics V* 101; *Epidemics VII* 112, 114–117. On Pella, see *Epidemics VII* 118.

21. This phrase, from *Epidemics II* 3.1, is also found in the other books of this group, *Epidemics IV* and *VI*, and indicates in all probability that several physicians of

the Hippocratic school came from Thessaly to Perinthus. The first person plural is also met with in the group of *Epidemics V* and *VII*.

22. Hippocrates *Prorrhetic I* 72.

23. Athens: Hippocrates *Epidemics V* 9, 10; Salamis: *Epidemics V* 32; Elis: *Epidemics V* 1, 2; Corinth: *Epidemics IV* 40; Syros: *Epidemics VII* 79; Delos: *Epidemics V* 61.

24. See Hippocrates *Prorrhetic I* 34. The patient from Cos mentioned is the son of Didymarchus.

25. Source of the story: *Life* according to Soranus; *Suda* s.v. "Hippocrates"; cf. also Tzetzes *Chiliades* 967, which notes only that Hippocrates was a contemporary of Perdiccas. See the earlier allusion in Galen *Med. Phil.* 3. Arab tradition follows Galen: see the version by Abî Usaib'a cited in F. Rosenthal, "An Ancient Commentary on the Hippocratic Oath," *Bull. Hist. Med.* 30 (1956): 79: "When he treated King Perdiccas for some disease he was suffering from, he did not stay with him all the time, but went away to treat the indigent and the poor in his own place." Not all sources are entirely in agreement on this point: according to Galen, Hippocrates treated Perdiccas reluctantly, while the *Suda* maintains that Hippocrates was a friend of Perdiccas and stayed in Macedonia for this reason.

26. See Pliny *Natural History* 29.5 and Plutarch *Life of Demetrius* 52–53; also Valerius Maximus 5.7.

27. See Hippocrates *Speech of the Envoy* (Littré IX, 418.20; Smith, trans., *Pseudepigraphic Writings*, 119), where Thessalus, son of Hippocrates, says: "We had an ancestral guest-friendship with the kings of the Heraclids."

28. F. Chamoux ("Perdiccas," in M. Renard, ed., *Hommages à Albert Grenier* [Brussels, 1962], 386–396) sees an illustration of the principal scene of this story, the diagnosis of Hippocrates, in the mosaic of Lambiridi held by the Gsell Museum in Algiers, which decorated the tomb of Cornelia Urbanilla (late third century A.D.). He also claims to see an illustration of the same episode from the life of Perdiccas in a very curious bronze statuette, currently in the collection at Dumbarton Oaks in Washington, D.C., but discovered more than a century ago in France, near Soissons. It represents a gaunt young man, holding out his left hand to another person. The inscription "Perdic" on the statue has long intrigued scholars. Chamoux believes it stands for Perdiccas, and that the person missing from the scene is Hippocrates. The quality of the sculpture, its realism, and the characters of the inscription permit it to be dated at least to the first century A.D.

29. Hippocrates *Speech of the Envoy* (Littré IX, 418–419); see Smith's translation in *Pseudepigraphic Writings*, 117–119. In addition to this speech, by Hippocrates' son, see the *Decree of the Athenians*; the *Life* according to Soranus; and Pliny *Natural History* 7.123: "Hippocrates, who foretold a plague that was coming from Illyria and dispatched his pupils round the cities to render assistance, in return for which service Greece voted him the honours that it gave to Hercules" (see the Loeb translation by H. Rackham [Cambridge, Mass., 1947], 2:589); cf. also Varro *De re rustica* 1.4.

30. See Thucydides 2.48.

31. Thessalus says that his trip to Athens during the pestilence took place eight years before the time when he is supposed to have delivered his speech. Since the speech was given after the end of the Athenian expedition to Sicily, occurring between the years 413–405—probably between the years 411–408—the years 419–416 represent the likeliest range of dates for the plague.

32. The (apocryphal) text of the decree is preserved in the Hippocratic Collection under the title *Decree of the Athenians* (see Smith, trans., *Pseudepigraphic Writings*, 107). Its apocryphal character is exposed by, among other things, the clause pertaining to the Athenian ephebia granted the children of Cos. The Athenian ephebia was extended to foreigners only from the second century A.D., and the Greek term used (*ephebeuein*) is not attested before the third century. The apocryphal character of the decree does not necessarily mean that everything in it was invented. It has been possible in this case, as in many others, to reconstruct a decree the historical existence of which is established, but whose exact text was lost.

The honors referred to by the *Decree* were later expanded upon. The phrase "It is decreed by the people to initiate [Hippocrates] into the great mysteries at public expense as was done with Heracles, the son of Zeus" assumed the form with Pliny the Elder (*Natural History* 7.123) already referred to: "[I]n return for [his] service [during the pest] Greece voted [Hippocrates] the honours that it gave to Hercules." Tradition became both vaguer and more general.

33. It no longer seems possible to identify this plague with the recurrence of the plague of Athens in 427–426 mentioned by Thucydides (3.87).

34. Thus in chapter 16 of [Galen] *De theriaca ad Pisonem* the plague treated by Hippocrates comes from Ethiopia, like the one described by Thucydides.

35. Aëtius of Amida, a physician of the sixth century A.D., and Pseudo-Galen attributed to Hippocrates and to Acron of Agrigentum (according to Aëtius 5.95), or to Hippocrates alone (according to [Galen] *De theriaca ad Pisonem* 16), the therapeutic method of lighting great fires throughout Athens; cf. Pliny *Natural History* 36.202. This method was in fact attributed to Acron of Agrigentum alone in other sources: Plutarch *De Iside et Osiride* 79.383d and Oribasius *Synopsis* 6.24.3–4. To these texts, Littré has the merit of adding a Latin manuscript preserved in Paris (vol. I, 40ff.): "A Latin manuscript of the royal library (no. 7028), still more detailed, asserts that Hippocrates, come from Athens, noticed that blacksmiths and all those who worked with fire were immune to the pestilential disease. He concluded from this that it was necessary to purify the air of the city by fire. In consequence, he caused great piles of wood to be burned; the air being purified, the sickness ceased, and the Athenians erected an iron statue to the doctor with this inscription: *To Hippocrates, Our Savior and Our Benefactor*. I do not know the source of these amplifications upon the [original] manuscript, whose writing is very old." One sees at once that Hippocrates, by reason of his greater fame, was substituted for Acron of Agrigentum in the development of the legend in order to intercede in a more famous plague.

36. See John Actuarius (Johannes Aktuarios) *Method. med.* 5.6.

37. Hippocrates *Speech of the Envoy* (Littré IX, 414.3ff.); see Smith, trans., *Pseud-epigraphic Writings*, 115.

38. Museum of Delphi, Inv. no. 225. The inscription was published by H. Pom-tow, "Hippokrates und die Asklepiaden in Delphi," *Klio* 15 (1918): 308. On the most reasonable restitutions, see R. Herzog, "Das delphische Orakel als ethischer Preis-richter," in T. Horneffer, ed., *Der junge Platon*, vol. 1 (Giessen, 1922), 164, as well as Herzog's complementary suggestions in "Die Grabschrift des Thessalos von Kos," *Quellen und Studien zur Geschichte der Naturwissenschaften und der Medizin* 3, no. 4 (1933): 57–58 [= 265–266].

39. This opinion is shared by R. Herzog in the two works cited in the previous note.

40. Pausanias *Periegesis* 10.2.6; see the Loeb translation by W. H. S. Jones (Cam-bridge, Mass., 1961), 4:379.

41. Museum of Delphi, Inv. no. 6687 A and B + no. 8131. The two most impor-tant parts of the inscription (no. 6687 A and B) were discovered in 1939 on the Sacred Way; the small fragment 8131 was discovered afterwards in 1956, in an area of the sanctuary very far from the place where the other two parts were found. Publication of no. 6687 A and B: Jean Bousquet, "Inscriptions de Delphes (7. Delphes et les Asclepiads)," *BCH* 80 (1956): 579–591. Publication of no. 6687 A and B + no. 8131: G. Rougemont, *Corpus des inscriptions de Delphes I: Lois sacrées et règlements religieux* (Paris, 1977), 122–124. From these one learns therefore that the Asclepiads, on arriving at Delphi, had to swear an oath that they were Asclepiad by male descent in order to be able to benefit from certain privileges, the exact nature of which is disputed in part.

42. Another inscription from Delphi (Inv. no. 2475 = G. Rougemont, *Corpus des inscriptions de Delphes*, vol. 1, no. 11, 119–121) also refers to privileges accorded by Delphi to certain Asclepiads: supply of victims for sacrifice at the expense of the city of Delphi; hospitality at the expense of the city; right to sit in the first row during competitions; exemption from civil taxes; enjoyment of the same rights as Delphians. Unfortunately, the inscription does not allow us to determine which Asclepiads were the beneficiaries of these privileges.

43. This difference can only be explained by the circumstances of Thessalus's speech. He sought to interest the Athenians in the fate of the island of Cos alone; because the fact that the privileges were said to have been accorded only to the Asclepiads of Cos in the *Speech of the Envoy* follows logically from the version of the legendary past presented there: Nebros was an Asclepiad of Cos.

44. The term *androgeneia* is not attested elsewhere in literary texts; it was suffi-ciently rare that Galen thought to include it in his *Glossary* of rare words in the works of Hippocrates. In the epigraphic record the term is attested only in two inscriptions from the same region, one from Cos, the other from Halicarnassus (see J. Bousquet, "Inscriptions de Delphes," 587, n. 1).

45. This dispute took place between 413 and 405, probably around 411–408.

46. Besides the *Speech of the Envoy*, see the *Address from the Altar* (*Epibomios*) and the *Life* according to Soranus.

47. Thucydides 8.41; see the Penguin translation by R. Warner, *History of the Peloponnesian War* (Harmondsworth, 1972), 560.

48. See Thucydides 8.44.

49. Ibid., 8.108; see the translation by Warner just cited, 604.

50. See Diodorus of Sicily 13.42.3 and 69.5.

51. See Hippocrates *Address from the Altar* (Littré IX, 402–404).

52. All these figures are found in the *Life* according to Soranus. According to the *Suda*, as well as Tzetzes, he died at the age of 104.

53. See the *Life* according to Soranus; Tzetzes 973.

54. *Anthologia Graeca* 7.135; see the Loeb translation by W. R. Paton (Cambridge, Mass., 1960), 2:77–79.

55. *Life* according to Soranus.

56. The source here is Soranus of Cos, who had conducted research in the local archives; the information is contained in the *Life* according to Soranus (of Ephesus).

57. On the coins representing Hippocrates, see page 38.

58. Inv. no. 1246, Cabinet des Médailles, Bibliothèque Nationale, Paris.

59. Hippocrates *Letters* 2; see Smith, trans., *Pseudepigraphic Writings*, 49–51.

60. See Lucian *Philopseudeis* 21.

61. The first to have identified the head as that of Hippocrates was G. Becatti, "Il Ritratto di Ippocrate," *Rend. Pont. Acc. XXI* (1944/1945): 123–141. Corroboratory evidence that this image of Hippocrates was part of the funerary repertoire of the period can probably be found in the Lambiridi mosaic in Algeria representing a physician taking the pulse of a patient, if one accepts with F. Chamoux that this mosaic indeed portrays Hippocrates examining Perdiccas.

62. See the *Life* according to Soranus.

63. A Hermes in the Uffizi Gallery, Florence (Inv. 1914, no. 353); a head in the Museum of Sculpture, Ny Carlsberg (I. N. 1975); a bust in the National Museum, Naples (no. 6131); a largely restored bust in the Chiaramonti Museum of the Vatican, Rome (Inv. 2219). Two others must be rejected: a head in the Prado, Madrid (Inv. no. 259 E) and a head in a private American collection (Frel, *Getty Greek Portraits*, no. 51). For illustrations, see G. M. A. Richter, *The Portraits of the Greeks* (London, 1965), I, 152ff., and M. V. Barrow, "Portraits of Hippocrates," *Medical History* 16 (1972): 85–88. On the bust of Hippocrates in the Faculty of Medicine at Montpellier, see note 66 on page 479.

64. Three types of coins are distinguished:

1. On the face, the head of Hippocrates turned to the right (inscription ΙΠ); on the reverse, the staff with coiled serpent (inscription ΚΩΙΩΝ): London, Berlin, and Paris (Cabinet des médailles, nos. 1273 and 1274).

2. On the face, the bust of Heracles with his club (inscription ΚΩΙΩΝ); on the reverse, Hippocrates seated, turned to the right (inscription ΙΠΠΟΚΡΑΤΗΣ): Paris (Cabinet des médailles, no. 1246).

3. On the face, the bust of Faustina II, the wife of Marcus Aurelius (inscription ΦΑΥΣΤΕΙΝΑ ΣΕΒΑΣΤΗ; on the reverse, Hippocrates seated, turned to the left (inscription ΙΠΠΟΚΡΑΤΗΣ ΚΩΙΩΝ): Berlin.

Illustrations in G. M. A. Richter, *The Portraits of the Greeks*, 153 and M. Putscher, "Das Bildnis des Hippokrates und das Kultbild des Asklepios in Kos," *Marburger Sitzungsberichte* 87, no. 1 (1966): 17ff.

65. In *Parisinus gr.* 2144: see the frontispiece to this book.

66. T. Meyer-Steineg, "Hippokrates-Erzählungen," *Archiv für Geschichte der Medizin* 6 (1912): 1–11.

67. Diogenes Laertius *Vitae philosophorum* 9.42 (= Diels-Kranz 68 A 1); see the Loeb translation by R. D. Hicks (Cambridge, Mass., 1958), 2:451–453. Let us close this survey of later legends by noting that, in the Arab tradition, the celebrated anecdote of Socrates and Zopyros was transposed to involve Hippocrates and Polemon: see the text of this anecdote in F. Rosenthal, *Das Fortleben der Antike im Islam* (Zurich, 1965), 342ff.

Three. Hippocrates and the School of Cos

1. The oldest account of Hippocrates' teaching is the *Protagoras* of Plato, cited at page 5.

2. See Homer *Iliad* 4.219.

3. See ibid., 11.839ff.

4. Pindar *Pythian Odes* 3.1–7; see F. J. Nisetich, *Pindar's Victory Songs* (Baltimore, 1980), 169.

5. See Dicaearchus frag. 60 (F. H.G. Miller).

6. See Herodotus 3.131.

7. See page 15.

8. Hippocrates *Speech of the Envoy* (Littré IX, 424).

9. Galen *Commentary on Hippocrates' Nature of Man* (preamble) and *Du foetus de sept mois* [= *Seven Months' Child*], translated from the Arabic by R. Walzer, *Riv. Stud. Orient.* 15 (1935): 345.

10. The inscription was published by R. Herzog, "Die Grabschrift des Thessalos von Kos," *Quellen und Studien zur Geschichte der Naturwissenschaft und der Medizin* 3, no. 4 (1933): 54–58 [= 262–268]. The phrase "son of Hippocrates" is Herzog's restitution.

11. See Hippocrates *Speech of the Envoy* (Littré IX, 418).

12. *Suda* s.v. Hippocrates (III and IV). They are both supposed to have written medical treatises.

13. Pliny *Natural History* 7.124. This Critobulus, whose place of origin Pliny does not mention, had to have been from Cos if one accepts that he is the same "Critobulus of Cos, son of Plato" who was named trierarch by Alexander during the Indian campaign (Arrian *Anabasis* 8.18.7).

14. Hippocrates *Epidemics V* 49 (Loeb VII, 189).

15. Arrian *Anabasis* 6.11; see the Loeb translation by P. A. Brunt (Cambridge, Mass., 1983), 2:131. This Critodemus is confused by Curtius Rufus (9.5.25.27) with the Critobulus who treated Philip.

16. Hippocrates *Speech of the Envoy* (Littré IX, 418.20); see W. D. Smith, ed. and trans., *Hippocrates: Pseudepigraphic Writings* (New York, 1990), 119.

17. *Suda* s.v. Hippocrates (IV).

18. Thymbraeus ("Timbreum") is mentioned in the list of Hippocrates' disciples given in the *Life* of Brussels.

19. *Suda* s.v. Hippocrates (V and VI).

20. Ibid. s.v. Hippocrates (VII). Nothing is known about him other than that he is supposed to have written medical works.

21. Galen *Anatomical Procedures* 2.1; see the translation by C. Singer (Oxford, 1956), 31.

22. See Hippocrates *Speech of the Envoy* (Littré IX, 412 and 414). Calydon is a city of Aetolia.

23. See Plato *Protagoras* 311b–c. The text is cited at page 5.

24. This commentary is known solely through the Arab tradition. Accounts of it have been brought together by F. Rosenthal, "An Ancient Commentary on the Hippocratic Oath," *Bulletin of the History of Medicine* 30 (1956): 52–87.

25. See Galen *On the Therapeutic Method* 1.1.

26. Galen indicates that Polybus remained at Cos, more precisely at Astypalaea, where he found himself entrusted with the instruction of the young; see *Commentary on the Nature of Man of Hippocrates* (preamble): "Polybus who was a disciple and received in turn [responsibility for] the teaching of the young"; "Thessalus son of Hippocrates who did not remain constantly in his native land [or, according to the variant reading in the Arab manuscript, "in the city Aithulija"; that is, Astypalaea; cf. the following citation] as Polybus, for he attended the king of Macedonia Archelaus"; and Galen *Du foetus de sept mois* 345 (Walzer edition): "Polybus was the disciple of Hippocrates and inherited after him the teaching of disciples, because he stayed in the city of Astypalaea. Thessalus, by contrast, was traveling most of the time, given that he was in the service of the king of Macedonia Archelaus." Compare Galen *Med. Phil.* 3. From these accounts it emerges that Polybus remained at Cos. A divergent source, the *Speech of the Envoy*, indicates that Polybus served at Hippocrates' side in Thessaly.

27. See pages 56–57.

28. See the *Life* of Brussels.

29. *Suda* s.v. Dexippus.

30. On the medical theories of Dexippus, see *Anonymus Londinensis* 12.8–36.

31. See Galen *De optima secta ad Thrasybulum* 13; *De venae sectione adversus Erasistratum* 9; *Commentary on Hippocrates' Regimen in Acute Diseases* 1.24; 3.42; 4.5.

32. See Aristotle *Historia animalium* 3.2.511b23ff. In the *Life* of Brussels, Syennesis is mentioned among the disciples native to Cos. Aristotle's far older account is more trustworthy.

33. See Aristotle *Historia animalium* 3.2.511b24–30 and Hippocrates *Nature of Bones* 8; also page 57.

34. Oribasius *Collectiones medicae* 8.8.

35. This Euryphon had to have been fairly famous in his time to be mentioned by the comic author Plato (not to be confused with the philosopher): thus we learn that Euryphon had treated the dithyrambic poet Cinesias (second half of the fifth century B.C.), who suffered from empyema following a bout of pleurisy, which left him with a great many bedsores over his body (Galen *Commentary on the Aphorisms of Hippocrates* 7.44). Euryphon was (wrongly) supposed in Galen's time to be the author of the *Cnidian Sentences* (see Galen *Commentary on Epidemics VI of Hippocrates* 1.29). On the causes of diseases according to Euryphon, see the (doubtful) account in the *Anonymus Londinensis* 4.31–40. Another Cnidian physician was known, Herodicus of Cnidus; his theories on the causes of diseases are reported in the same document (ibid., 4.40–5.34). This Herodicus is not to be confused with Herodicus of Selymbria.

36. The antiquity of the account in question, *Regimen in Acute Diseases*, is established by the fact that it is found in the Hippocratic Collection itself. The first chapter begins with the words, "The authors of the work entitled *Cnidian Sentences*." It goes on to add that the Cnidian work was also the object of collective revision, referring to "the later revisers" (Loeb II, 63–65).

37. See what was said earlier (page 30) regarding the significance of the use of the first person plural in the two most recent groups of *Epidemics* (*Epidemics II, IV, VI* and *Epidemics V, VII*). But the first person singular is frequently used there as well. It is not a question, then, strictly speaking, of collective works.

38. Some commentators have wished to see the *Coan Prenotions* as a collective work that was to the school of Cos what the *Cnidian Sentences* was to the school of Cnidus. This hypothesis is now abandoned. The *Coan Prenotions* is a relatively recent compilation, as it turns out.

39. See page 26.

40. Galen *Commentary on Hippocrates' On Joints* 4.40.

41. See Galen *On the Therapeutic Method* 1.1.6: "Even in the old days there was no shortage of dispute, as those in Cos and Cnidus strove with each other to make the greater number of discoveries; for there were still two schools of Asclepiads in Asia, even when the school of Rhodes had fallen into decline" (see R. J. Hankinson's translation of books I and II of this treatise [Oxford, 1991], 5). Galen opposes this good rivalry among the ancients to the bad rivalry among the moderns of his own day, singling out for blame the attacks on Hippocrates by the "methodist" physician Thessalus of Tralles.

42. See Galen *Regimen in Acute Diseases according to Hippocrates* 1.1.

43. See pages 33ff.

44. On this oath of the Asclepiads at Delphi, see pages 34–35.

45. Among these false Asclepiads must be counted those relatives by marriage who were not physicians.

46. This broad sense of the term "Asclepiads" is well attested in classical literature. Plato, for example, employs the term sometimes in its narrow sense (*Protagoras* 311b6 and *Phaedrus* 270c3), sometimes in the broad sense (*Republic* 3.406a6). On the two senses of the term, see the account of Tzetzes cited at page 10 (together with notes 16 and 17 elaborating on the discussion there).

47. On this polemic, see page 50.

48. See page 27.

49. On Praxagoras the Elder, disciple of Hippocrates, see the *Life* of Brussels ("Praxagorem seniorem"). The famous Praxagoras of Cos, who lived in the fourth century, was a "descendant of Asclepius" (Galen *On the Therapeutic Method* 1.3). He was son of Nicarchus (Galen *On the Natural Faculties* 2.9). Tzetzes (*Chiliades* 969) cites Praxagoras of Cos, without further qualification, as among Hippocrates' disciples: he must have confused the two Praxagorases. The accounts of Praxagoras the Younger are collected in F. Steckerl, *The Fragments of Praxagoras of Cos and his School* (Leiden, 1958).

50. The text of this inscription was published by J. Benedum, "Griechische Arztinschriften aus Kos," *ZPE* 25, no. 3 (1977): 272–274 and in *SEG* 27 (1977): 514.

51. The neighboring cities include:

—Calymna, island north of Cos: decree for the physician Praxilas of Cos from the third century B.C.; text in M. Segre *Tituli Calymnii* 14. Decree for the physician Antipater of Cos from the second century B.C.; texts in ibid., 78 and vol. 24.

—Samos, island north of Cos: decree for the physician Philistos of Cos from the third century B.C.; text in J. Benedum, *ZPE* 25 (1977): 265–270, no. 1 and in L. Robert, "Décret pour un médecin de Cos," *Revue de philologie* (1978): 242–251. The city awarding the decree is not mentioned in what remains of the inscription. From Herzog (1903) through Benedum (1977) it was thought to be Iasos. The attribution of the inscription to Samos was demonstrated by Robert.

—Halicarnassus, city on the continent across from Cos (today called Bodrum): decree in favor of the physician Hermias of Cos from the second century B.C.; text in L. Robert, "Hellenika," *Rev. philologie* 13 (1939): 163–165, no. 11, and in Paton and Hicks *Inscr. of Cos* 13.

—Theangela, city on the continent to the east of Halicarnassus (today called Etrim): decree in honor of a physician of Cos whose name is not preserved along with the response of the city of Cos, from the third century B.C.; text in J. Benedum, *ZPE* 27 (1977): 229–235, no. 1.

52. For the distant cities, the reader is referred to the list of inscriptions of public physicians given in L. Cohn-Haft, *The Public Physicians of Ancient Greece* (Northampton, Mass., 1956), 76–84. This list, though convenient, needs to be updated. Cities of Crete: Cnossus, no. 18 (physician Hermias of Cos: Guarducci *Insc. Creticae I* 8.7; Pouilloux *Choix d'inscr. gr.* 16); Gortyn, no. 19 (same physician: Guarducci *Inscr. Creticae IV* 168* [p. 230]; Pouilloux *Choix d'inscr. gr.* 15); Aptera, no. 46 (physician

Callipus of Cos: Guarducci *Inscr. Creticae II* 3.3*). See, too, Delos, nos. 28 and 31 (physician Philip of Cos: Laurenzi, *Clara Rhodos* 10, no. 4 (1941): 37–38; *IG* 11. 4.1078 and *Inscr. Delos* [4] 399 A.36–38); Delphi, no. 20 (physician Philistus of Cos: *Fouilles de Delphes* 3.4.362).

53. In principle, one copy of the decree was found in the city that honored the physician and another copy was displayed in the Asclepieum of Cos.

54. On the sixty-six inscriptions listed by L. Cohn-Haft, one counts sixteen physicians from Cos but not a single physician from Cnidus. Obviously, this is a list only of public physicians. From elsewhere, two important Cnidian physicians are known: Aristogenes, physician to the court of Antigonus Gonatas (277–239) in Macedonia (*Suda*), and Chrysippus, Erasistratus's teacher (Diogenes Laertius 7.186). See also two epigraphic attestations of physicians at Cnidus dating from the Hellenistic and Roman periods: *GIBM* 4.1.799 (Servius Sulpicius, son of Apollonius, Hecataeus, physician) and 838 (Cleitus, son of Cleitus, physician).

55. Tacitus *Annals* 12.61; see the Loeb translation by J. Jackson (Cambridge, Mass., 1963), 405.

56. Ibid., 12.67; see the translation by Jackson just cited, 415.

57. Xenophon obtained from the emperor, Claudius, fiscal immunity for the inhabitants of Cos. He financed new building at the Asclepieum of Cos and founded a library there, as local inscriptions testify. Unlike Hippocrates, Xenophon of Cos was both a physician and a priest of Asclepius. For the coins representing Xenophon, see *Greek Coins of British Museum, Caria* 215 (nos. 211–215).

58. Herophilus was a native of Chalcedon in Bythnia (opposite Byzantium); and Erasistratus was born at Iulis on the island of Ceos, not far from Attica.

59. On Herophilus, disciple of Praxagoras, see for example Galen *On the Therapeutic Method* 1.3: "Herophilus the dialectician, his fellow-pupil Phylotimus, their teacher Praxagoras the Asclepiad" (from R. J. Hankinson's translation [Oxford, 1991], 15). Accounts of Herophilus have been collected by H. von Staden, *Herophilus: The Art of Medicine in Early Alexandria*. Philinus of Cos, a physician of the third century B.C., began as a disciple of Herophilus before breaking away to found the empirical school; see for example Pseudo-Galen *Introductio sive medicus* 4: "Philinus of Cos was at the head of the empirical sect, having been the first to separate it from the logical sect, having initially been influenced by Herophilus, whose disciple he was also." Accounts of the empiricists have been collected by K. Deichgräber, *Die griechische Empirikirschule* (Berlin/Zurich, 2nd ed., 1965).

Four. Writings in Search of an Author

1. É. Littré, *Oeuvres complètes d'Hippocrate*, 10 vols. (Paris: 1839–1861).

2. See Aristotle *Historia animalium* 3.3.512b12–513a7.

3. See Hippocrates *Nature of Man* 11. This description appears also in *Nature of Bones* 9.

4. See Aristotle *Historia animalium* 3.2.511b23–30.

5. See Hippocrates *Nature of Bones* 8.

6. This according to the *Life* of Brussels; see pages 48–49.

7. See Herodotus 2.84: "About medicine, [the Egyptians] order it thus: each doctor is a doctor for one disease and no more. The whole land is full of doctors; there are some for the eyes, some for the head, and some for the teeth, and some for the belly, and there are some for the diseases that have no outward sign" (viz. D. Grene, trans., *The History* [Chicago, 1987], 165). The only trace of a division of labor in ancient Greek medicine is found in a lost poem of the Cycle entitled "The Sack of Troy" (*Iliu Persis*), which assigns specialties to the two physicians of the epic (see scholium to *Iliad* 11.515): the one, Machaon, is the surgeon; the other, Podalirius, is the expert on "invisible diseases" (compare the "diseases that have no outward sign," or "hidden diseases," of the Egyptians).

8. See Hippocrates *Diseases II* 1–11 and 12–75.

9. See Plato *Phaedrus* 270c. The passage is quoted at page 6.

10. Galen *Commentary on Hippocrates' Nature of Man* (preamble).

11. See Littré I, 295ff.

12. The first edition by H. Diels, which is still the best, appeared very shortly after the discovery: *Anonymi Londinensis ex Aristotelis Iatricis Menoniis et aliis medicis eclogae* (Berlin, 1893).

13. Col. 5.35–col. 6.18 and col. 6.31–43, translated in W. H. S. Jones, *The Medical Writings of Anonymus Londinensis* (Cambridge, 1947), 35–39. I leave aside the end of this doxography, due to a later author who contests the attribution to Aristotle (col. 6.43–45 and col. 7.1ff.).

14. See page 50. This polemic among partisans and opponents of the practice of setting a dislocated hip was to continue throughout the history of ancient medicine. See the account of the great physician of the empiricist school, Heraclides of Tarentum, cited by Galen (*Commentary on The Joints of Hippocrates* 4.40) and Celsus (*De medicina* 8.20.4).

15. See Hippocrates *On Joints* 70ff.

16. It should nonetheless be pointed out that this account of Ctesias's attack, like everything that touches indirectly upon the Hippocratic question, has aroused passionate scholarly debate since the beginning of the century, and that no conclusion, not even a conclusion as restrained as the one advanced here, would command unanimous assent.

17. Diocles is cited after Hippocrates on the list of those who performed the setting of a dislocated hip, along with Heraclides of Tarentum and Celsus.

18. See Galen *Commentary on the Joints according to Hippocrates* 3.23 (= Diocles frag. 187 Wellmann).

19. See Hippocrates *Nature of Man* 15. Plato, in *Timaeus* 86a, endorses a comparable systematization, making each of the four fevers correspond to each of the four elements (fire, air, water, earth).

20. See Hippocrates *Epidemics I* 11; also Galen *Commentary on Epidemics I* 3.2 (= Diocles frag. 97 Wellmann).

21. See Galen *Commentary on the Nature of Man according to Hippocrates* (preamble).

22. See *Anonymus Londinensis* 19.2ff.

23. See chapter 14.

24. See Caelius Aurelianus *Tardae passiones* 4.8.113 (= Herophilus frag. 261 von Staden); cf. Galen *Commentary on the Prognostic of Hippocrates* 1.4 (= Herophilus frag. 33 von Staden).

25. For accounts of Bacchius of Tanagra, see von Staden, *Herophilus*, 484–500. Bacchius's glossary was preceded by that of Xenocrites of Cos.

26. Bacchius edited *Epidemics III* (*Ba. 7* von Staden) and commented on treatises that were difficult to understand, among them *In the Surgery* (*Ba. 8* von Staden), the *Aphorisms* (*Ba. 9* von Staden), and *Epidemics VI* (*Ba. 10* von Staden).

27. Other treatises known to Bacchius: *Sacred Disease, On Fractures, On Joints, Mochlicon, Regimen in Acute Diseases, Epidemics I, II,* and *V, Prorrhetic I, In the Surgery, Places in Man, On Wounds in the Head, Diseases I, Use of Liquids.*

28. See *Erotiani vocum Hippocraticarum collectio cum fragmentis*, ed. E. Nachmanson (Göteborg, 1918), 9.

29. Other treatises transmitted in medieval manuscripts that were not glossed by Erotian: *Affections, Anatomy, Decorum, The Heart, Crises, Dentition, Excision of the Foetus, Eighth Months' Child, Generation* [?], *Critical Days, Diseases IV* [?], *Diseases of Girls, The Physician, Nature of Women, Precepts, Prenotions of Cos, Superfoetation, Sight*; and, among the biographical writings, *Decree of the Athenians* and *Letters*.

30. See Littré I, 434ff. It should be noted that Littré does not include the *Breaths* in his list. The London papyrus, discovered after the publication of Littré's edition, indicates that this treatise was considered authentic by the Aristotelian school. *Breaths* was included, by contrast, in Erotian's list.

31. It goes without saying that the date of composition of the treatises does not necessarily coincide with the date of their insertion in the Hippocratic Collection. While several of the treatises absent from Erotian's list are unanimously recognized as coming after Hippocrates (for example, *The Heart, Precepts, Decorum, Physician*), treatises such as *Fleshes* and *Regimen* are contemporaneous with Hippocrates.

32. This is not the place to describe each of the treatises that make up the Hippocratic Collection in detail. Appendix 3 lists all the treatises in alphabetical order and provides a succinct summary of each one, also indicating authorship and date.

33. See pages 28–29.

34. For the dates of these three groups, see note 14 on page 425 and appendix 3, nos. 22–24.

35. Besides *Humours*, see *Prognostic, Prorrhetic I, Prorrhetic II, Prenotions of Cos, Aphorisms, Regimen in Acute Diseases, Regimen in Acute Diseases (Appendix)*.

36. This is the title that the treatise bears in Erotian (see the list given at page 64) and also in one ancient manuscript (*Parisinus gr. 2253*).

37. See pages 46ff.

38. On the school of Cnidus, see the discussion at pages 49ff.

39. For these accounts see G. Grensemann, *Knidische Medizin*, vol. 1 (Berlin, 1975), 1ff., and J. Jouanna, ed. and trans., *Hippocrate: Maladies II* [= Budé X, 2] (Paris, 1983), 29ff.

40. See Hippocrates *Diseases II* (part 2) 66, 68, 70, 73; *Internal Affections* 3, 6, 13, 16, 48.

41. See Hippocrates *Internal Affections* 10 (three consumptions); 14 (four diseases of the kidneys); 35 (four jaundices); 52 (three tetanuses). The Cnidian subdivision of diseases is given by Galen in his *Commentary on Hippocrates' Regimen in Acute Diseases* (1.7): seven diseases of bile, twelve diseases of the bladder; four diseases of the kidneys; four kinds of strangury; three tetanuses; four jaundices; three consumptions.

42. For an analysis of this complex set of treatises, see appendix 3, no. 20.

43. Hippocrates *Regimen* 10 (Loeb IV, 247).

44. This treatise, almost entirely lost in Greek, has been preserved in an ancient Latin translation discovered by Littré. It is not possible to determine with certainty whether it was glossed by Erotian.

45. Hippocrates *Precepts* 6 (Loeb I, 319).

Five. The Physician and the Public

1. Hippocrates *Law* 1 (Loeb II, 263).

2. See pages 21ff. and 25ff.

3. Regarding some of these inscriptions, see the section on "The Medical Tradition at Cos after the Departure of Hippocrates" at 52–55.

4. Aristophanes *Acharnians* 1030ff.; see the Penguin translation by Alan H. Sommerstein (Harmondsworth, 1973), 96, here slightly modified. This is the first attestation of the verb *démosieuein* in the sense of "to be a public physician." The references to Pittalus below are found at line 1222 of the *Acharnians* and line 1432 of the *Wasps*, respectively.

5. See pages 32–33.

6. A physician was able to remain in the same city for up to twenty years: see *IG* 12.1.1032 (Hiller 1895) = Cohn-Haft 37.

7. Hippocrates *Epidemics V* 14 (Loeb VII, 165). Note the use of the plural (my italics).

8. See, for example, Hippocrates *Prorrhetic II* 1 (Loeb VIII, 219): "A person seems to be mortally ill both to the physician attending him and to others who see him, but a different physician comes in and says that the patient will not die, but go blind in both eyes."

9. Plutarch *Lives of the Ten Orators* 1.18; see the Loeb translation by H. N. Fowler in *Plutarch's Moralia* (Cambridge, Mass., 1960), 10:351.

10. See Diodorus of Sicily 1.82: in Egypt, "[P]hysicians draw their support from

public funds" (from the Loeb translation by C. H. Oldfather [Cambridge, Mass., 1960], 1:281).

11. See Aristotle *Politics* 3.15.1286a12–14, and Diodorus of Sicily 1.82.

12. See Hippocrates *Law* 1.

13. The most elaborate attack against medical charlatans is found in the treatise *The Sacred Disease*; see pages 184ff.

14. Xenophon *Cyropaedia* 1.6.15; see the Loeb translation by W. Miller (Cambridge, Mass., 1960), 1:101.

15. The figure traditionally given for the population of Athens during antiquity is twenty thousand citizens (see, for example, Demosthenes *Against Aristogiton* 1.51). This figure includes neither women nor children, still less slaves. But not everyone attended the assembly, except for great occasions. Absenteeism is denounced by Aristophanes in the *Acharnians*.

16. Plato *Gorgias* 514d; see the Hackett translation by D. J. Zeyl (Indianapolis, 1997), 858.

17. Xenophon *Memorabilia* 4.2.5; see the Loeb translation by E. C. Marchant (Cambridge, Mass., 1979), 4:271.

18. Plato *Gorgias* 456b–c; see the Hackett translation by Zeyl, 801 (slightly modified).

19. To the first group belong the treatises *Airs, Waters, Places, The Sacred Disease*, and the set formed by *Generation, Nature of the Child*, and *Diseases IV*. The only representatives of the second group in the strict sense are the treatises *The Art* and *Breaths*; to this list may be added, however, longer treatises such as *Ancient Medicine* and the beginning of *Nature of Man*, which were certainly delivered before an audience.

20. Hippocrates *Generation* 1.

21. Hippocrates *Breaths* 3 (Loeb II, 231). The immediately preceding quotation about the doctor's condition, from the first chapter of the same treatise, is found at page 227 of the Loeb edition.

22. See Lucretius *De rerum natura* 1.271ff.

23. See note 57 on page 478. The preceding quotation is from chapter 51 of the *Tiers Livre*; see D. M. Frame, trans. *The Complete Works of François Rabelais* (Berkeley and Los Angeles, 1991), 408.

24. See Diodorus of Sicily 12.53.3.

25. See page 18. It should be noted that the wife of a certain Gorgias residing at Larissa was treated by a Hippocratic author (see *Epidemics V* 11). But the name Gorgias is too frequently encountered to permit a connection to be made between this Gorgias and the Sophist.

26. Scholars thus make the mistake of applying to the classical era a term that appears in Greek only in a later one.

27. Hippocrates *Art* 1.

28. See Hippocrates *Nature of Man* 1.

29. See Hippocrates *Sacred Disease* I.

30. See Hippocrates *Art* 1. The treatise *Precepts*, in its twelfth chapter (Loeb I, 327), displays a more general reticence with regard to verbal jousting: "And if for the sake of a crowded audience you do wish to hold a lecture, your ambition is no laudable one, and at least avoid all citations from the poets, for to quote them argues feeble industry." But this is a late treatise (see appendix 3, no. 47); even so, its account has the merit at least of proving that this practice must have persisted through the Hellenistic and Roman periods, and that such speakers did not hesitate to adorn their speeches with references borrowed from the poets.

31. See Hippocrates *Art* 13.

32. Hippocrates *Nature of Man* 1 (Loeb IV, 3–5).

33. On gymnastic teachers and athletic trainers, see pages 166, 238, and 331.

34. On the criticisms leveled by Hippocratic physicians against these charlatans, see pages 184ff.

35. Hippocrates *Art* 1 (Loeb II, 191).

36. Hippocrates *Diseases I* 1 (Loeb V, 99–101).

37. See Plato *Republic* 3.405a.

38. It is cataloged in the Louvre as Inv. CA 2183; cf. J. D. Beazley, *Attic Red-Figure Vase-Painters* (Oxford, 2nd ed., 1963), 813 (no. 96).

39. Compare this with the very fine funerary stele from the same period, preserved in the collection of the Museum of Basel, representing a physician and a patient: two cupping glasses are hung on the wall (Antikenmuseum, Inv. no. BS 236; cf. E. Berger, *Das Basler Arztrelief* [Basel, 1970]).

40. See Hippocrates *Physician* 2.

41. Hippocrates *In the Surgery* 3 (Loeb III, 59–61); cf. *Physician* 2.

42. Physicians do not seem to have had a monopoly on the sale of medicines. According to the testimony of ancient authors, there also existed "pharmacopoles," or medicine vendors, who were closer to the snake-oil salesmen and fair hawkers of modern times than to true pharmacists. Aristotle (*Historia animalium* 8.4.594a21–24) refers to pharmacopoles who raised tarantulas and snakes.

43. See Plato *Laws* 1.646c.

44. Hippocrates *Decorum* 10 (Loeb II, 293).

45. See Hippocrates *Physician* 2–9.

46. See ibid., 2–3.

47. See Hippocrates *Mochlicon* 38.

48. Hippocrates *On Joints* 72 (Loeb III, 373–375).

49. A drawing of it is found in medieval manuscripts of Hippocrates; it was this drawing that the surgeons of the Renaissance relied upon.

50. See Rufus of Ephesus, quoted in Oribasius 49.27: "Hippocrates often gave the machine invented by him the name of beam, sometimes that of board. Later, it was named bench in adding feet to it." While Rufus attributes the invention of it to Hippocrates, the author of *On Joints* does not confirm this. Unto those that have shall more be given.

51. Cf. Hippocrates *On Fractures* 13.

52. See Hippocrates *In the Surgery* 5.

53. Ibid., 6 (Loeb III, 63). The emphasis is mine.

54. Hippocrates *On Fractures* 13 (Loeb III, 127–129).

55. Ibid., 15 (Loeb III, 133).

56. Hippocrates *On Joints* 76 (Loeb III, 379–381). Again, in this and the quoted passage immediately following, the emphasis is mine.

57. Ibid., 70 (Loeb III, 367–369).

58. Such an aide is also called "experienced" (*empeiros*) in *On Joints* 76.

59. The term is used in *In the Surgery* 2, when the various characters of the "drama" in the dispensary are enumerated: "the patient, the operator, assistants [*hyperetai*]." See also the new inscription from Cos reproduced in appendix 2.

60. Plato *Laws* 4.720a–b; see the Hackett translation by T. J. Saunders (Indianapolis, 1997), 1406.

61. The assistants could also be "residents"; that is, foreigners or emancipated slaves; see the new inscription from Cos cited in appendix 2. I leave to one side here the much debated question, raised by Plato's text, whether slaves could be physicians. The Athenian's assertion that doctors' aides were also called doctors is not supported by the evidence of the Hippocratic Collection, where the names are clearly distinguished. The distinction is clearly made as well in the new Coan inscription, but this inscription recounts the career of an "assistant" who later became a "physician."

62. See Hippocrates *Prorrhetic II* 4.

63. Hippocrates *Physician* 2 (Loeb VIII, 303).

64. Ibid., 9 (Loeb VIII, 311).

65. See Hippocrates *In the Surgery* 2.

66. See Plato *Gorgias* 514d; also pages 79ff.

67. Hippocrates *Physician* 1 (Loeb II, 311).

68. Aeschylus *Prometheus Bound* 473–475 (Grene-Lattimore I, 328).

69. Hippocrates *Decorum* 7 (Loeb II, 291).

70. Hippocrates *Physician* 1 (Loeb II, 313).

71. Hippocrates *In the Surgery* 3 (Loeb III, 61).

72. See page 86.

73. Hippocrates *In the Surgery* 3 (Loeb III, 61).

74. Ibid., 4 (Loeb III, 63).

75. See Hippocrates *Physician* 5.

76. Hippocrates *Diseases I* 10 (Loeb V, 121).

77. See page 86.

78. Attic cup, dating from 500/490 B.C., work of the painter Sosias. Antikenmuseum, Berlin, Inv. no. F. 2278.

79. See Homer *Iliad* 11.832.

80. See ibid., 833–836.

81. On the public physician, see pages 76ff. (citing the example of Thessalus, public physician at Athens during the Sicilian expedition, and the passage in Xenophon [*Cyropaedia* 1.6.15] on public physicians who accompanied military expedi-

tions). Later inscriptions praise the devotion of physicians in times of war as in times of peace; see, for example, the letter-decree sent by the city of Gortyn to Cos in 218 B.C. (M. Guarducci, *IC* 4.168, 230 = Cohn-Haft 19 = Pouilloux, *Choix d'inscr. gr.* 15): the physician of Cos Hermias, who was public physician at Gortyn in Crete, is praised for having saved many citizens and allies in the course of a (civil) war.

82. See page 22.

83. This is the treatise *Wounds and Traits*: see page 64.

84. See Hippocrates *Physician* 14.

85. Hippocrates *In the Surgery* 10 (Loeb III, 69).

86. Ibid., 7 (Loeb III, 65).

87. Hippocrates *On Joints* 35 (Loeb III, 265–267).

88. Hippocrates *Physician* 4 (Loeb VIII, 305).

89. Hippocrates *On Fractures* 2 (Loeb III, 99).

90. Ibid., 1 (Loeb III, 95).

91. Hippocrates *On Joints* 42 (Loeb III, 285).

92. Ibid., 44 (Loeb III, 289).

93. Hippocrates *On Fractures* 30 (Loeb III, 169).

94. Hippocrates *On Joints* 70 (Loeb III, 367). This procedure was mentioned earlier in connection with the physician's aides at page 90.

95. See Hippocrates *Decorum* 8.

96. Ibid., 11 (Loeb II, 295).

97. Ibid., 12 (Loeb II, 295).

98. Ibid., 11 (Loeb II, 295).

99. Hippocrates *Prognostic* 1 (Loeb II, 7–9).

100. Homer *Iliad* 1.68–70 (Lattimore, 61).

101. Hippocrates *Prorrhetic II* 42 (Loeb VIII, 291).

102. Hippocrates *Regimen in Acute Diseases* 1 (Loeb II, 63).

103. See pages 183ff.

104. See Aeschylus *Suppliants* 263; *Eumenides* 62; cf. *Agamemnon* 1623.

105. Hippocrates *Prorrhetic II* 1 (Loeb VIII, 219).

106. Ibid., 2 (Loeb VIII, 221).

107. Ibid. (Loeb VIII, 223).

108. Ibid.

109. See Plato *Gorgias* 456b.

110. Hippocrates *Epidemics V* 74 (Loeb VII, 203) [= *Epidemics VII* 36].

111. Ibid., 95 (Loeb VII, 213) [= *Epidemics VII* 121].

112. See Hippocrates *On Joints* 1.

113. Hippocrates *Regimen in Acute Diseases (Appendix)* 23 (Loeb VI, 287). Note that the last part of Potter's translation ("and it is good to predict this") has been modified since the concept underlying the Greek text is beauty (*kalos*) rather than the good; an ethical implication is, however, deducible from this concept, as the following comment makes clear.

114. See Hippocrates *Art* 11.

115. Hippocrates *On Wounds in the Head* 10 (Loeb III, 21). The emphasis is mine.

116. Hippocrates *Prognostic* 2 (Loeb II, 9).

117. Hippocrates *Diseases II* 48 (Loeb V, 277); translation very slightly modified.

118. Hippocrates *Diseases of Women I* 71; cf. *Sterile Women* 233.

119. See Hippocrates *Prorrhetic II* 12.

120. Hippocrates *Art* 8 (Loeb II, 203).

121. Ibid.

122. Ibid.

123. Ibid., 3 (Loeb II, 193).

124. Plato *Republic* 2.360e–361a; see the Hackett translation by G. M. A. Grube, rev. C. D. C. Reeve (Indianapolis, 1997), 1001.

125. Stobaeus *Ecl. IV* 38.9 (= Herophilus Frag. 51 von Staden); note that the title *Eclogae*, given to the work by Diels in his *Doxographi graeci*, corresponds to the *Anthologium* of the THESAURUS LINGUAE GRAECAE *Canon of Greek Authors and Works* (New York, 3rd ed., 1990), 371.

126. See Galen *Commentary on the Aphorisms of Hippocrates* 2.29.

127. Hippocrates *On Joints* 58 (Loeb III, 339).

128. This is true in the case of the author of *Ancient Medicine*; see page 238.

129. Hippocrates *Places in Man* 24 (Loeb VIII, 65).

130. Hippocrates *On Fractures* 36 (Loeb III, 183).

Six. The Physician and the Patient

1. Plato *Laws* 4.720a–d; see the Hackett translation by T. J. Saunders (Indianapolis, 1997), 1406, as well as the partial reference to this account at page 91.

2. See Hippocrates *Decorum* 17.

3. Hippocrates *Epidemics V* 41 (Loeb VII, 185).

4. See Hippocrates *Epidemics IV* 2.

5. See ibid., 38.

6. See Hippocrates *Epidemics II* 4.5.

7. Xenophon *Oeconomicus* 7.37; see the Loeb translation by E. C. Marchant (Cambridge, Mass., 1979), 4:425–427.

8. Xenophon *Memorabilia* 2.10.2; see the Loeb translation by E. C. Marchant (Cambridge, Mass., 1979), 4:163.

9. Hippocrates *Epidemics IV* 2 (Loeb VII, 93).

10. Hippocrates *Epidemics VI* 7.1 (Loeb VII, 271).

11. Hippocrates *Airs, Waters, Places* 21 (Loeb I, 127).

12. Inscription of the first century B.C. from Gytheum in Laconia: *IG* 5.1.1145 (Kolbe 1913) = Cohn-Haft 51.

13. See Hippocrates *Epidemics V* 74 [= *Epidemics VII* 36]. This case study has already been cited in connection with prognosis at pages 104–105.

14. See Hippocrates *Epidemics V* 45.

15. See Hippocrates *Epidemics II* 2.9.

16. See Hippocrates *Epidemics IV* 20.

17. See ibid., 50; cf. *Epidemics VI* 3.8.

18. It is not always the trade of the patient that is mentioned. In *Epidemics V*, for example, the first case study gives the trade of the husband of the patient, who is herself referred to as "the wife of the gardener" of Elis.

19. Fullers: *Epidemics IV* 36, *V* 59, *VII* 79; stonecutter: *Epidemics IV* 20c; miner: *Epidemics IV* 25; cook: *Epidemics V* 52; shopkeeper: *Epidemics VII* 13.

20. Vinedressers: *Epidemics IV* 25 and 50 (cf. *Epidemics VI* 3.8); gardener: *Epidemics V* 1; groom: *Epidemics V* 16.

21. Boxer: *Epidemics V* 71; wrestling master: *Epidemics VI* 8.30.

22. Schoolmaster: *Epidemics IV* 56.

23. Menander's vinedresser: *Epidemics IV* 25; Cleotimus's shoemaker: *Epidemics VII* 55; Palamedes' groom: *Epidemics V* 16.

24. See Hippocrates *Epidemics II* 2.17 (Loeb VII, 37).

25. Galen *Med. Phil.* 3.

26. Timenes' son: *Epidemics IV* 25; woman (probably slave) in the household of Timenes' sister: ibid.; Timenes' niece: *Epidemics II* 1.7 and *IV* 26; man (probably slave) in the household of Timenes' niece: *Epidemics VI* 2.19.

27. Apemantus: *Epidemics II* 2.9; Apemantus's wife: *Epidemics IV* 23; wife of Apemantus's brother: *Epidemics IV* 22; young slave of Apemantus's sister: *Epidemics IV* 27.

28. See Hippocrates *Epidemics I* 8.

29. *IG* 12.8.263: Antiphon, son of Critobulus, was one of the three theors under whom a decree was issued for the confiscation of the goods of the opponents of the oligarchs, who remained faithful to Athens, for the benefit of the temple of Apollo; this decree dates from the years 411/410 to 408/407. The same Antiphon, son of Critobulus, appears in the list of theors: *IG* 12.8.277.81.

30. Dyseris: *Epidemics V* 25 (compare Dyseris, the wife of the Thessalian prince Echecratidas, known to Simonides [schol. Theocritus 16.34] and Anacreon [*Anth. Pal.* 6.136 and 142]); Simus: *Epidemics V* 53 (compare Simus, the father of an Aleuas, grandfather of the family [schol. Theocritus, 16.34] and Simus, Aleuad, tyrant of Larissa, who called on Philip II to help him in 357 against the tyrants of Pherae [cf., for example, Demosthenes *On the Crown* 48]); Echecrates: *Epidemics VII* 57.

31. See Hippocrates *Epidemics II* 1.10.

32. See Hippocrates *Epidemics V* 16.

33. See pages 44ff.

34. Aristotle *Politics* 3.16.1287a.36ff.; see the Loeb translation by H. Rackham (Cambridge, Mass., 1959), 265.

35. Pindar *Pythian Odes* 3.54ff.; see F. J. Nisetich, *Pindar's Victory Songs* (Baltimore, 1980), 171.

36. See Plato *Republic* 3.408c.

37. Heraclitus frag. 58 Diels-Kranz; see J. Barnes, *Early Greek Philosophy* (Har-

mondsworth, 1987), 103. This paradox is stressed also by Xenophon in his *Memorabilia* (1.2.54): "[A man] lets the surgeon cut and cauterize him, and, aches and pains notwithstanding, feels bound to thank and fee him for it" (see the Loeb translation by E. C. Marchant cited in note 8 above, 4:39).

38. Euripides *Electra* 426–429 (Grene-Lattimore IV, 415).

39. Aristophanes *Plutus* 407–408.

40. See Plato *Republic* 3.406cff.

41. See Hippocrates *Regimen* 68–69.

42. Hippocrates *Precepts* 6 (Loeb I, 319). Compare the new inscription from Cos (appendix 2), where the physician Onasander is publicly thanked for having treated the people of Halasarna without charging a fee.

43. On the illnesses of women and their treatment, see pages 171ff.

44. Euripides *Hippolytus* 161–164 (Grene-Lattimore III, 174). The choir goes on in this passage to note "the torturing misery of helplessness, the helplessness of childbirth and its madness are linked to it forever."

45. Ibid., 293–296 (Grene-Lattimore III, 179).

46. See Herodotus 3.133.

47. Hippocrates *Diseases of Women I* 62 (layer C). The excerpt immediately following is taken from the same chapter.

48. Plato *Theaetetus* 149d; see the Hackett translation by M. J. Levett, rev. Myles F. Burnyeat (Indianapolis, 1997), 166. The passage on the special qualifications of older women occurs at 149bff. of the same treatise.

49. The first attestation of a female physician appears on the funerary stele of Phanostrate dating from the middle of the fourth century B.C. (National Museum, Athens, Inv. no. 993). This woman is described both as a midwife (*maia*) and as a physician (*iatros*).

50. Hippocrates *Fleshes* 19 (Loeb VIII, 165).

51. Hippocrates *Diseases of Women I* 68.

52. Hippocrates *Nature of the Child* 13.

53. See pages 274ff.

54. Hippocrates *Diseases of Women I* 20 (belonging to the old part).

55. Ibid., 21 (layer C).

56. See ibid., 40 (layer C); cf. also *Sterile Women*, 213 (layer C), twice.

57. See Hippocrates *Epidemics I* 9.

58. See Hippocrates *Epidemics IV* 13.

59. See Hippocrates *Precepts* 6 (passage cited earlier in connection with the poor).

60. As attested by an inscription of the third century B.C., the existence of which has been known since the beginning of the century thanks to Herzog, but which was published only recently by J. Benedum, *ZPE* 25, no. 1 (1977): 265–270, and L. Robert, *Revue de philologie* 52 (1978): 242–251.

61. Hippocrates *Epidemics V* 35 (Loeb VII, 183).

62. Hesiod *Works and Days* 102–104; see the translation by David Tandy and Walter Neale (henceforth "Tandy-Neale"), 65–67.

63. For the Greek text see Page *PMG* 813.

64. See Aeschylus *Prometheus Bound* 478–483.

65. See Plato *Republic* 1.346a–d; Aristotle *Politics* 3.6.1278b40–1279a1.

66. Hippocrates *Epidemics I* 11 (Loeb I, 165).

67. Hippocrates *Breaths* 1 (Loeb II, 227).

68. C. V. Daremberg, *La médicine: Histoire et doctrines* (Paris, 1865; reprinted New York: Arno Press, 1967), 347.

69. Hippocrates *In the Surgery* 6 (Loeb III, 63).

70. Hippocrates *Physician* 5 (Loeb VIII, 307).

71. This is a manuscript in the collections of the Vatican, *Urbinas* 64; for the text, see I. L. Heiberg, *Hippocratis opera* [= *CMG* 1.1] (Leipzig/Berlin, 1927), 5.

72. See Antiphon *On the Chorus Boy* 17.

73. See Plato *Laws* 11.933d.

74. Euripides *Ion* 1015 (Grene-Lattimore IV, 53). On the possibility that a physician might be paid by enemies of the patient to kill him, see Plato *Statesman* 298a–b and Aristotle *Politics* 3.16.1287a39ff.

75. See Aristophanes *Clouds* 766; frag. 28.

76. See Theophrastus *Historia plantarum* 9.16.8.

77. See pages 122ff.

78. See page 90.

79. Hippocrates *On Joints* 70 (Loeb III, 367). The quotation that follows is found here as well.

80. Herodotus 3.130; see Grene's translation, *The History* (Chicago, 1987), 266, and page 21.

81. Hippocrates *On Joints* 62 (Loeb III, 351).

82. Hippocrates *Superfoetation* 8.

83. Hippocrates *On Joints* 47 (Loeb III, 301).

84. See ibid.

85. Hippocrates *Epidemics VI* 4.7 (Loeb VII, 249–251).

86. Hippocrates *Aphorisms* 2.38 (Loeb IV, 117–119).

87. Hippocrates *Epidemics VI* 5.7 (Loeb VII, 257).

88. See pages 79ff.

89. Plato *Gorgias* 456b; see the Hackett translation by D. J. Zeyl (Indianapolis, 1997), 801.

90. See Hippocrates *Prognostic* 2, 7, 16.

91. Rufus of Ephesus *Quaestiones medicinales* 13; see the Teubner edition by H. Gärtner (Leipzig, 1970), 16.

92. Hippocrates *Epidemics VI* 2.24 (Loeb VII, 235); the bracketed interpolation is mine.

93. Hippocrates *On Fractures* 5 (Loeb III, 107).

94. Hippocrates *Epidemics I* 11 (Loeb I, 165).

95. Hippocrates *Aphorisms* 1.1 (Loeb IV, 99).

96. Hippocrates *In the Surgery* 3 (Loeb III, 61–63).

97. Hippocrates *On Joints* 30 (Loeb III, 255–257).

98. See Hippocrates *Haemorrhoids* 2.

99. Hippocrates *On Fractures* 9 (Loeb III, 121).

100. Hippocrates *On Joints* 14 (Loeb III, 235–237).

101. See ibid., 37.

102. Hippocrates *Decorum* 14 (Loeb II, 297).

103. See Hippocrates *Prorrhetic II* 3–4.

104. Ibid., 4 (Loeb VIII, 229).

105. Hippocrates *Decorum* 14 (Loeb II, 297).

106. Hippocrates *Art* 7 (Loeb II, 201–203).

107. Diels-Kranz 68B234; see J. Barnes, *Early Greek Philosophy* (Harmondsworth, 1987), 274.

108. Hippocrates *On Joints* 14 (Loeb III, 235–237).

Seven. The Physician and the Disease

1. Hippocrates *Art* 11 (Loeb II, 211).

2. Hippocrates *Nature of Man* 9 (Loeb IV, 25).

3. Hippocrates *Breaths* 1 (Loeb II, 229); cf. *Aphorisms* 2.22.

4. Homer *Iliad* 2.721–723 (Lattimore, 95).

5. Aeschylus *Philoctetes* frag. 253 Radt (= Aristotle *Poetics* 1458b23).

6. Compare with this the name of another disease attested earlier in the Hippocratic corpus, "podagra," which literally means "the action of capturing the foot." The foot was the prey seized by the disease, which in turn was compared to a wild beast. The same archaic conception is at the root of these two names of diseases.

7. See in particular Hippocrates *Ulcers* 10.

8. Jean Hamburger, ed., *Dictionnaire de médecine* (Paris, 1975), 569.

9. The author of *Diseases I* ranks leprosy alongside another skin affliction, lichen, among diseases that were not fatal; see the third chapter of this treatise.

10. This comment is taken from M. Grmek, "La réalité nosologique au temps d'Hippocrate," in L. Bourgey and J. Jouanna, eds., *La Collection hippocratique et son rôle dans l'histoire de la médecine* (Leyden, 1975), 237–255. (This volume contains the proceedings of the 1972 Strasbourg Colloquium on Hippocrates; see the bibliography for further details.)

11. The only thing that is certain is that it was not plague in the modern sense of the term; that is to say, the infectious disease originating in certain rodents due to *Yersinia pestis* and transmitted to human beings via fleas. The particular species of rat affected by *Yersinia pestis* in the great medieval plagues of Europe—namely, the black rat—was unknown in classical Greece.

12. The principal account of epilepsy in the Hippocratic Collection is the treatise *The Sacred Disease*.

13. Hippocrates *Internal Affections* 10–12 (three consumptions); 52–54 (three tetanuses); 35–38 (four jaundices); 14–17 (four diseases of the kidney).

14. See Galen *Commentary on Hippocrates' Regimen in Acute Diseases* 1.7.

15. Pindar *Pythian Odes* 3.47–50; see F. J. Nisetich, *Pindar's Victory Songs* (Baltimore, 1980), 171.

16. Hippocrates *Diseases I* 2 (Loeb V, 101–103).

17. Hippocrates *Aphorisms* 3.20–23 (Loeb IV, 129–131).

18. Hippocrates *Nature of Man* 8 (Loeb IV, 23–25).

19. See Hippocrates *Airs, Waters, Places* 3.

20. See ibid., 4.

21. Cities facing east, by contrast, are the healthiest; see ibid., 5–6.

22. See ibid., 3–4.

23. Hippocrates *Aphorisms* 3.24–31 (Loeb IV, 131–135).

24. Hippocrates *Breaths* 2 (Loeb II, 229).

25. Ibid., 15 (Loeb II, 253).

26. See Hippocrates *Ancient Medicine* 1.

27. Jones follows the manuscripts here in putting "of the disease" (*nousou*), which is absurd in the context. The phrase is better interpreted as "of the year" (*eniautou*); cf., for example, *Aphorisms* 3.15.

28. Hippocrates *Humours* 12 (Loeb IV, 83–85).

29. See Hippocrates *Nature of Man* 15.

30. Ibid., 9 (Loeb IV, 25–27).

31. Hippocrates *Breaths* 6 (Loeb II, 233). The translation has been modified since Jones, anachronistically, contrasts "endemic" (i.e., pestilential) fevers with "epidemic" fevers; this distinction was first made by Galen (see note 38 below).

32. See Hippocrates *Regimen in Acute Diseases* 1.

33. See Thucydides 2.47–54.

34. These two passages are found in *Breaths* 6 and *Regimen in Acute Diseases* 2.

35. See Hippocrates *Speech of the Envoy* (Littré IX, 409).

36. See Hippocrates *Letters* 1 (Littré IX, 313); *Letters* 2 (Littré IX, 313); *Letters* 11 (Littré, IX, 328).

37. See Hippocrates *Speech of the Envoy* (Littré IX, 419); *Decree of the Athenians* (Littré IX, 400). Regarding this pestilence see also pages 31ff.

38. Galen, in the preamble to the first book of his *Commentary on Epidemics I of Hippocrates*, explicitly notes the dual sense given by the author of *Airs, Waters, Places* to the concept of "general disease," for the first time using the terms "endemic disease" and "epidemic disease" to distinguish its two aspects.

39. This probably was not the original title, because the term "epidemic" is not employed in the Hippocratic corpus; but it does not contradict the vocabulary of these books, where one meets in connection with diseases the Greek verb *epidemein* once (in *Epidemics I*) and once the Greek form for the adjective "epidemic" (in *Epidemics VII*).

40. See Hippocrates *Prognostic* 2, 3, 5, 6, 8, 24.

41. Hippocrates *Airs, Waters, Places* 3, 4 (Loeb I, 75, 77).

42. See *Prognostic* 2 (Loeb II, 9): "In acute diseases the physician must conduct his inquiries in the following way."

43. Hippocrates *Regimen in Acute Diseases* 5 (Loeb II, 67).

44. The third chapter of *Diseases I* (Loeb V, 105) opposes diseases of long duration to ones that are rapidly decided: "The following diseases are inevitably long [*macra*]: consumption, dysentery, gout, swellings at the joints . . . , white phlegm, sciatica, strangury. . . . But ardent fever, phrenitis, pneumonia, angina, staphylitis, and pleurisy reach their crises quickly." Among the latter group of diseases that are quickly decided one notes "acute diseases." But diseases of long duration were not yet called "chronic" (*chronia*).

45. Pindar *Pythian Odes* 3.47–53; see note 15 above.

46. See chapter 8.

47. See Hippocrates *Sacred Disease* 1.

48. Sophocles *Ajax* 582–583 (Grene-Lattimore II, 241).

49. See Aeschylus *Agamemnon* 848–850.

50. Plato *Gorgias* 480c; see the Hackett translation by D. J. Zeyl (Indianapolis, 1997), 825.

51. See Galen *Commentary on the Aphorisms of Hippocrates* 7.44.

52. Heraclitus frag. 58 Diels-Kranz; see J. Barnes, *Early Greek Philosophy* (Harmondsworth, 1987), 103.

53. Plato *Gorgias* 456b; see the Hackett translation by Zeyl, 801.

54. On this triad see, for example, *Airs, Waters, Places* 11 (Loeb I, 105): "[O]ne should neither purge, nor apply cautery or knife to the bowels, before at least ten days are past."

55. Hippocrates *Aphorisms* 7.87 (Loeb IV, 217).

56. Hippocrates *Nature of Man* 20 [= *Regimen in Health* 5 (Loeb IV, 51)].

57. Ibid., 5 (Loeb IV, 15).

58. See Hippocrates *Internal Affections* 6.

59. Hippocrates *Regimen in Acute Diseases* 23 (Loeb II, 81–83).

60. This report was cited at page 49 in connection with schools of medicine.

61. See Xenophon *Anabasis* 6.4.11.

62. See *Nature of Man* 6; *Aphorisms* 5.4; *Prenotions of Cos* 554.

63. Hippocrates *Epidemics V* 15 (Loeb VII, 165–167); translation slightly modified to indicate that the drug was administered in stronger form (*ischuron*) the second time.

64. Hippocrates *Affections* 33 (Loeb V, 57).

65. See ibid., 28 (Loeb V, 51), where for treating strangury the author recommends "the diuretic medications recorded in the *Medication Book* as stopping pain"; cf. ibid., 20 (Loeb V, 37): "Also, give the diuretic medications said to soften the spleen."

66. Hippocrates *Diseases of Women I* 85; cf. ibid., 89.

67. Hippocrates *Epidemics V* 17 (Loeb VII, 169).

68. Antyllus (later than first century A.D.), cited by Oribasius 8.13.

69. See Hippocrates *Diseases II* 22; also chapter 19 of the same book, which recommends celery juice as well as flower of copper and myrrh.

70. See Hippocrates *Epidemics VI* 6.13; cf. *Epidemics IV* 40.

71. See pages 92ff.

72. Hippocrates *Nature of Man* 11 (Loeb IV, 33).

73. The sublingual region was bled especially in cases of angina: see *Regimen in Acute Diseases (Appendix)* 6. On incisions made to the head, see *Diseases II* 18.

74. Hippocrates *Diseases of Women I* 77.

75. Hippocrates *Regimen in Acute Diseases (Appendix)* 3 (Loeb VI, 265).

76. Hippocrates *Epidemics V* 6 (Loeb VII, 157).

77. Hippocrates *Art* 2 (Loeb II, 205).

78. Hippocrates *Diseases II* 12 (Loeb V, 211).

79. Hippocrates *Internal Affections* 18 (Loeb VI, 133).

80. Hippocrates *Epidemics V* 7 (Loeb VII, 157–159).

81. See Hippocrates *Regimen in Acute Diseases* 1.

82. See Plato *Republic* 3.405cff.

83. See Hippocrates *Regimen in Acute Diseases* 1.

84. Hippocrates *Regimen* 39 (Loeb IV, 307).

85. See ibid., 39–56.

86. See Hippocrates *Affections* 39–61.

87. Hippocrates *Regimen* 40 (Loeb IV, 307–311).

88. See Hippocrates *Nature of Man* 9; *Regimen in Acute Diseases* 10.

89. Hippocrates *Regimen in Acute Diseases* 10 (Loeb II, 71).

90. See Hippocrates *Ancient Medicine* 5.

91. Ibid.

92. See Hippocrates *Regimen* 52; *Affections* 40, 48.

93. See Hippocrates *Regimen in Acute Diseases* 17.

94. See ibid., 10.

95. Hippocrates *Aphorisms* 2.21 (Loeb IV, 113).

96. Hippocrates *Affections* 61 (Loeb V, 91).

97. See Homer *Odyssey* 10.519.

98. See Hippocrates *Regimen in Acute Diseases* 15.

99. See ibid., 16.

100. See Plato *Phaedrus* 227d.

101. Hippocrates *Epidemics VI* 3.18 (Loeb VII, 243).

102. Hippocrates *Regimen* 2 (Loeb IV, 229).

103. Hippocrates *Regimen* 61 (Loeb IV, 349–351).

104. See, for example, *Diseases of Women II* 117.

105. See Hippocrates *Regimen* 35.

106. Hippocrates *Regimen in Acute Diseases* 65 (Loeb II, 121).

107. See Hippocrates *Regimen* 57; cf. *Epidemics VII* 78.

108. See Hippocrates *Nature of Man* 18, 19 (= *Regimen in Health* 3, 4).

109. See Hippocrates *Regimen* 57.

110. Hippocrates *Affections* 53 (Loeb V, 83).

111. See, for example, *Regimen* 89; many other such passages could be cited.

112. See, for example, *Diseases II* 61; also *Nature of Women*, 3.

113. Hippocrates *Art* 5.

114. Hippocrates *Prognostic* 10 (Loeb II, 23).

115. Hippocrates *Aphorisms* 2.3 (Loeb IV, 109); cf. 7.72.

116. Hippocrates *Regimen* 60 (Loeb IV, 347).

117. See Hippocrates *Nature of Man* 22 (= *Regimen in Health* 7).

118. See Hippocrates *Affections* 36.

119. Hippocrates *Regimen* 58 (Loeb IV, 345).

120. Hippocrates *Epidemics VI* 5.15 (Loeb VII, 259).

121. See Hippocrates *On Joints* 50.

122. See Hippocrates *Superfoetation* 13.

123. Hippocrates *Diseases of Girls* 1.

124. See pages 121ff.

125. See Hippocrates *Aphorisms* 5.29–62. The treatise *Coan Prenotions* also has a section on women (503–544).

126. See Euripides *Ion* 304.

127. See Aristophanes *Thesmophoriazusai* 502–515.

128. Hippocrates *Aphorisms* 5.59 (Loeb IV, 175); cf. *Nature of Women* 96.

129. See Aristotle *De generatione animalium* 2.7.747a7–9.

130. Hippocrates *Nature of Women* 99.

131. Hippocrates *Sterile Women* 214.

132. Plato *Theaetetus* 149d; see the Hackett translation by M. J. Levett, rev. Myles F. Burnyeat (Indianapolis, 1997), 166.

133. Hippocrates *Diseases of Women I* 17.

134. See Hippocrates *Sterile Women* 220.

135. Ibid., 218.

136. Ibid., 220.

137. Hippocrates *Aphorisms* 5.41 (Loeb IV, 169).

138. Hippocrates *Sterile Women* 216.

139. Ibid., 215.

140. Ibid., 216; cf. *Aphorisms* 5.42.

141. Hippocrates *Aphorisms* 5.48 (Loeb IV, 171).

142. See ibid., 5.29, 5.31.

143. See ibid., 5.30.

144. Ibid., 5.37–38 (Loeb IV, 167).

145. On midwives, see pages 122ff. Among the postpartum affections, one may mention the absence of lochial purgation (*Nature of Women* 9), prolapse of the womb

(*Nature of Women* 4 and 5), inflammation of the womb (*Nature of Women* 27 and 29), scirrhosity of the womb (*Nature of Women* 37).

146. Hippocratic physicians thought that an incision made to a vein behind the ear could cut off the pathway followed by the sperm in its descent from the head: see *Airs, Waters, Places* 22; *Generation* 2; cf. also *Places in Man*, 3. For further detail, see pages 271–272.

147. See Hippocrates *Aphorisms* 5.63.

148. Aristotle *De generatione animalium* 2.7.747a3–6; see the Loeb translation by A. L. Peck (Cambridge, Mass., 1953), 247.

149. Hippocrates *Places in Man* 47 (Loeb VIII, 95).

150. See Hippocrates *Aphorisms* 5.62.

151. See Hippocrates *Sterile Women* 217.

152. See Hippocrates *Diseases of Women II* 144; *Sterile Women* 248; *Nature of Women* 5.

153. See Soranus *Diseases of Women* 4.36.

154. See, for example, *Nature of Women* 9.

155. See, for example, ibid., 36.

156. See Hippocrates *Sterile Women* 230.

157. For example, Thasos (wine, nuts) and Miletus (wool).

158. See Homer *Odyssey* 4.230–232. Among distant lands, Egypt was the most frequently cited in the Hippocratic Collection, and it was from Egypt that the most varied products came: Egyptian crocus, Egyptian thorny fruit, Egyptian fava bean, Egyptian acorn, Egyptian oil, Egyptian white oil, Egyptian myrrh, Egyptian white myrrh; also mentioned, in addition to plants and their derivatives, were Egyptian salt, Egyptian alum, Egyptian saltpeter, Egyptian soil.

159. From Ethiopia came primarily cumin, but also a variety of daucus and a root called "Ethiopian root." The medicine called "Mead" or "Indian" was pepper.

Eight. Hippocratic Rationalism and the Divine

1. Hippocrates *Diseases of Women II* 151.

2. See Herodotus 3.33. Even after Hippocrates, the technical name of the affection was to remain the "sacred disease," at least among certain authors. Aristotle's disciple Theophrastus (*Historia plantarum* 9.11.3) mentions the plant called Heracles, whose root is good against the "sacred disease." The fact that Theophrastus says nothing more specific about the disease is proof that this name was still usual in the fourth century.

3. The expression appears in six different Hippocratic treatises of various origins, two coming from the school of Cos (*Airs, Waters, Places* and the treatise devoted to this very topic, *The Sacred Disease*), one reputed to belong to the school of Cnidus (*Diseases of Women II*), and the other three being of disputed provenance (*Breaths, Prorrhetic II,* and *Diseases of Girls*).

4. On disturbance of the motions of the blood, see Hippocrates *Breaths* 14; and on disturbance of the motions of the air, see *The Sacred Disease* 7. For a discussion of the part of the body affected, see ibid., 17.

5. See, for example, Hippocrates *Breaths* 14.

6. Hippocrates *Diseases of Girls* 1.

7. Hippocrates *Regimen in Acute Diseases* 8 (Loeb II, 69). He adds that this kind of contradiction is also found in connection with the inspection of entrails.

8. See Cicero *De divinatione* 2.39.

9. Hippocrates *Sacred Disease* 2 (Loeb II, 141).

10. Diels-Kranz 88B25.12ff.

11. See Sophocles *Oedipus Tyrannus* 387–388.

12. Hippocrates *Sacred Disease* 4 (Loeb II, 147).

13. Ibid., 2 (Loeb II, 141).

14. On the recruitment of public physicians, see pages 76ff.

15. Hippocrates *Sacred Disease* 2 (Loeb II, 141–143).

16. Ibid., 4 (Loeb II, 147–149).

17. See pages 68 and 145.

18. Euripides *Hippolytus* 141–147 (Grene-Lattimore III, 173).

19. See Plato *Republic* 2.364b–c; *Laws* 10.909b (cf. 10.908d and 11.933).

20. Hippocrates *Sacred Disease* 21 (Loeb II, 183).

21. Hippocrates *Airs, Waters, Places* 22 (Loeb I, 129).

22. See Herodotus 1.105 and 4.67.

23. Hippocrates *Airs, Waters, Places* 22 (Loeb I, 127).

24. Ibid. (Loeb I, 127).

25. Hippocrates *Sacred Disease* 21 (Loeb II, 183).

26. Ibid. (Loeb II, 183).

27. See Thucydides 2.47.4. It is true that in the same passage the historian calls attention to the impotence of medicine.

28. See ibid., 5.104–105.

29. Hippocrates *Sacred Disease* 3 (Loeb II, 145).

30. Ibid., 4 (Loeb II, 149).

31. Heraclitus frag. 5 (Diels-Kranz 22B5); see J. Barnes, *Early Greek Philosophy* (Harmondsworth, 1987), 118. The quote that follows is from the same source.

32. Hippocrates *Sacred Disease* 4 (Loeb II, 149–151).

33. Hippocrates *Prognostic* 1 (Loeb II, 7–9); the bracketed words translate a phrase found in the manuscripts that Jones considered an interpolation. The same ambiguity with regard to the meaning of the word "divine" is found at the beginning of *Nature of Women*: "Here is what I say about the nature of women and their diseases: the divine is the principal cause in human beings; then come the constitutions of women and their colors." This reference to the divine occurs, however, in an introduction that is more recent than the body of the work.

34. Euripides (frag. 292 Nauck) actually distinguishes between two sorts of diseases: diseases caused by the gods and spontaneous diseases.

35. See Hippocrates *Regimen* 87.

36. Ibid., 89 (Loeb IV, 437).

37. See Hippocrates *Prognostic* 25; also Galen *Commentary on the Prognostic of Hippocrates* 1.4.

38. On Hippocrates' Asclepiad origins, see pages 10ff.

39. See especially Pindar *Pythian Odes* 3, composed around 475 B.C.

40. It was the geographer Strabo (9.5.17) who declared that the sanctuary at Tricca was the oldest.

41. See Herodas *Mimiambi* 2.95–97: "Now you will show to what extent Kos and Merops are strong . . . and how Asklepios came here from Trikka"; and 4.1–2: "Greetings, Lord Paeeon, who rulest Trikka and hast settled sweet Kos and Epidauros" (see the Loeb translation by J. Rusten, I. C. Cunningham, and A. D. Knox [Cambridge, Mass., 1993], 239, 255).

42. See the earlier allusion in Aristophanes' *Wasps* of 422 (l.123).

43. Aristophanes *Plutus* 411 and 621.

44. Ibid., 727–741.

45. Pausanias *Periegesis* 2.27.3; see the Loeb translation by W. H. S. Jones (Cambridge, Mass., 1964), 1:393.

46. R. Herzog, "Die Wunderheilungen von Epidauros," *Philologus*, Suppl. 22, 3 (1931): no. 4.

47. See Aristophanes *Plutus* 716ff.

48. Herzog, "Die Wunderheilungen," no. 22.

49. Ibid., 20.

50. Ibid., 17. The modern medical term is "spasmodic ulcer."

51. Ibid., 43.

52. Ibid., 21.

53. On the blind, see ibid., nos. 4, 9, 11, 18, 20, 22, 32, 40, 55, 65, 69; the paralyzed and lame: 3, 15, 16, 35, 36, 37, 38, 57, 64, 70; the mute: 5, 44, 51; women who are barren or who cannot give birth: 1, 2, 31, 34, 39, 42; abscesses, ulcers, empyemas: 17, 30, 45, 48, 66; intestinal worms: 23, 25, 41; headache: 29; dropsy: 21, 49; consumption: 33; epilepsy: 62; lithiasis: 8, 14; gout: 43.

54. On visitors from Epidaurus, see ibid., nos. 8, 35, 49, 66; Argos: 37, 62; Troezen: 23, 34, 48; Hermione: 20; Halieis: 18, 33; Pellene: 2; Caphyae: 41; Messene: 42; Sparta: 21; Athens: 4; Thebes: 28; Kirrha: 38; Epirus: 31; Thessaly: 6; Pherae: 25; Heraclea: 30; Torone: 13; Lampsacus: 15; Aegina: 26; Ceos: 39; Mytilene: 19; Chios: 63; Thasos: 22; Cnidus: 32.

55. Ibid., 3.

56. Ibid., 36.

57. Aeschines *Against Ctesiphon* 107ff.; the text is preserved in *Anthologia Graeca* 6.330 (see the Loeb translation by W. R. Paton [Cambridge, Mass., 1960], 1:475). It comes from a votive inscription in the sanctuary at Epidaurus; cf. *IG* IV² 255 (= Herzog 75).

58. Herzog 23.

59. Aelian *On the Nature of Animals* 9.33; see the Loeb translation by A. F. Scholfield (Cambridge, Mass., 1959), 2:253.

60. Herzog 23.

61. Ibid., 62.

62. In the *Plutus* of Aristophanes (883ff.), a righteous man who buys a magic ring from a famous seller of medicines, Eudemos, believes himself to be protected against snake bites—and demogogues.

63. Hippocrates *Epidemics V* 23 (Loeb VII, 175).

64. Ibid., 46 (Loeb VII, 187).

65. See Herzog 12.

66. See pages 18ff.

67. Hippocrates *Sacred Disease* 4 (Loeb II, 149).

68. See note 42 above.

69. Hygieia and Panacea, who are also invoked in *The Oath*, are present in the sanctuary of Asclepius at Cos; see Herodas *Mimiambi* 4.5ff.

70. See Theocritus *Epigrams* 8 (= *Anthologia Graeca* 6.337).

71. See pages 33ff.

72. On the pestilence as a general disease, as opposed to particular diseases, see the discussion at pages 150ff.

73. See Aeschylus *Persians* 715; *Suppliants* 659.

74. Sophocles *Oedipus Tyrannus* 22–30 (Grene-Lattimore II, 11–12).

75. Ibid., 168ff. (Grene-Lattimore II, 18).

76. See Homer *Iliad* 1.50–52.

77. See Hesiod *Works and Days* 238ff.

78. See Hippocrates *Breaths* 6.

79. See Sophocles *Oedipus Tyrannus* 97.

80. Hippocrates *Breaths* 6 (Loeb II, 235).

81. Homer *Iliad* 1.62–63 (Lattimore, 60–61).

82. Diogenes Laertius *Vitae philosophorum* 1.110; see the Loeb translation by R. D. Hicks (Cambridge, Mass., 1959), 1:115–117.

83. See Thucydides 2.47.4.

84. Hippocrates *Nature of Man* 9 (Loeb IV, 27–29).

85. From an Agence France-Presse dispatch reported in the 29 July 1989 edition of *Le Monde*.

86. The probable date of *Oedipus Tyrannus* is around 425 B.C. Certain critics have seen in the pestilence described by Sophocles an echo not of the great "plague" of 429 but of its recurrence in 427–426.

87. See Thucydides 2.47–54.

88. See page 33 and note 35 on page 427.

89. Thucydides 2.48.3; see the translation by R. Crawley (1876), rev. R. C. Feetham (1903), *The History of the Peloponnesian War* (New York, 1970), 99.

90. Hippocrates *Breaths* 1 (Loeb II, 229). The bracketed phrase is found in the

manuscripts; it was omitted by Jones, who considered it a gloss. See my edition of the *Breaths* (Budé V, 1 [1988]), 404 and note 1.

91. Thucydides 2.47.4; see the Crawley-Feetham translation cited above (note 89), 98, slightly modified.

92. See ibid., 2.51.4.

Nine. *Hippocrates and the Birth of the Human Sciences*

1. Sophocles *Ajax* 125–126, 131–133 (Grene-Lattimore, II, 225).

2. Hippocrates *Sacred Disease* 21 (Loeb II, 183).

3. Hippocrates *Airs, Waters, Places* 21 (Loeb I, 127).

4. Hippocrates *Nature of Man* 7 (Loeb IV, 21–23).

5. See G. Sarton, *A History of Science: Ancient Science through the Golden Age of Greece* (Cambridge, Mass., 1952), 368.

6. Hippocrates *Airs, Waters, Places* 1–2 (Loeb I, 71–73).

7. To each type of city corresponds also a typology of diseases: see pages 147ff.

8. Hippocrates *Airs, Waters, Places* 5 (Loeb I, 81).

9. Ibid., 6 (Loeb I, 83).

10. Ibid., 4 (Loeb I, 79).

11. Ibid., 5 (Loeb I, 81).

12. Ibid.

13. See Hesiod *Works and Days* 225–247.

14. Ibid., 235 (Tandy-Neale, 77); Hippocrates *Airs, Waters, Places* 5 (Loeb I, 81).

15. See Hesiod *Works and Days* 243; Hippocrates, *Airs, Waters, Places* 6.

16. See ibid., 10–11.

17. Ibid., 10 (Loeb I, 99).

18. See ibid., 5.

19. Ibid., 6 (Loeb I, 83).

20. Ibid., 11 (Loeb I, 105).

21. Ibid., 2 (Loeb I, 73).

22. Ibid., 11 (Loeb I, 105).

23. Ibid., 2 (Loeb I, 73).

24. Note the roughly contemporaneous use of the term in Aristophanes *Clouds* 201.

25. Homer *Iliad* 22.31 (Lattimore, 436).

26. See Plato *Protagoras* 315c; cf. 318e.

27. See Aristophanes *Clouds* 194–201.

28. See Plato *Protagoras* 318e.

29. Plato *Laws* 5.747d; see the Hackett translation by T. J. Saunders (Indianapolis, 1997), 1427.

30. Vitruvius *On Architecture* 1.1.10; see the Loeb translation by F. Granger (Cambridge, Mass., 1962), 1:15.

31. See Hippocrates *Airs, Waters, Places* 12–24.

32. The other account is Herodotus 5.16 (concerning the lacustrian villages of Lake Prasias in northern Greece).

33. Hippocrates *Airs, Waters, Places* 15 (Loeb I, 113–115).

34. Ibid., 12 (Loeb I, 105–107).

35. Ibid. (Loeb I, 107).

36. Ibid., 16 (Loeb I, 115).

37. Ibid. (Loeb I, 115–117).

38. Ibid., 23 (Loeb I, 133).

39. Ibid., 20 (Loeb I, 125).

40. Ibid., 17 (Loeb I, 117–119).

41. The term "macrocephalic" has since acquired another meaning, denoting now a disproportionately large head. The modern term corresponding to the ancient sense of "macrocephalic" is "turricephalic."

42. Ibid., 14 (Loeb I, 111); translation slightly modified. See Plato (*Alcibiades* 1.121c–d) for a comparable custom at the court of the Persian king: "When the eldest son and heir to the throne is born, . . . the boy is brought up . . . by the most highly respected eunuchs in the royal household. They attend to all the needs of the infant child, and are especially concerned to make him as handsome as possible, shaping and straightening his infant limbs" (from the Hackett translation by D. S. Hutchinson [Indianapolis, 1997], 578–579).

43. Pindar's phrase is preserved in Plato *Gorgias* 484b; it was cited earlier by Herodotus (3.38), though without the words "mortal and immortal" (see the note by Grene in his translation *The History* [Chicago, 1987], 228).

44. See Hippocrates *Airs, Waters, Places* 17; Herodotus 4.102.

45. See Hippocrates *Airs, Waters, Places* 17; Herodotus 4.117.

46. See Herodotus 4.1–82.

47. See Hippocrates *Airs, Waters, Places* 18–22.

48. Ibid., 18 (Loeb I, 119–121).

49. Herodotus 4.46; see Grene, trans., *The History*, 298.

50. Herodotus 4.29; see Grene, trans., *The History*, 290.

51. See Hippocrates *Airs, Waters, Places* 18.

52. See Herodotus 4.46.

53. Ibid., 2.77; see Grene, trans., *The History*, 163.

54. Hippocrates *Aphorisms* 3.1 (Loeb IV, 123).

55. Herodotus 9.122; see Grene, trans., *The History*, 664.

56. Hippocrates *Airs, Waters, Places* 24 (Loeb I, 137).

57. Ibid. (Loeb I, 137).

58. Herodotus 5.78; see Grene, trans., *The History*, 389.

59. See pages 188ff.

60. See Aeschylus *Persians* 345ff. With this tragedy, staged only eight years after the battle of Salamis, Aeschylus had the distinction of being the first Greek author to

pose the question clearly and the first one to give it an answer. Although he did not neglect human factors such as courage, Aeschylus explained the Greek victory mainly by the intervention of a god.

61. With regard to Themistocles, see Herodotus 8.109; with regard to Demaratus, 7.101–104.

62. Aristotle *Politics* 7.7.1327b24–34; see the Loeb translation by H. Rackham (Cambridge, Mass., 1959), 565–567.

63. The expression is due to L. Edelstein (see *The Idea of Progress in Classical Antiquity* [Baltimore, 1967], 35; for his analysis of the quarrel between ancients and moderns within the Hippocratic Collection, see 37–40).

64. On the polemic against a new philosophical medicine, see pages 282ff.

65. Aeschylus *Prometheus Bound* 479–480 (Grene-Lattimore I, 329).

66. Sophocles *Antigone* 398–399 (Grene-Lattimore II, 174–175).

67. Hippocrates *Ancient Medicine* 3 (Loeb I, 17–21); translation slightly modified.

68. Ibid., 5 (Loeb I, 21–23).

69. See Euripides *Suppliant Women* 202.

70. See Aeschylus *Prometheus Bound* 478–481.

71. See ibid., 442ff.; Euripides *Suppliant Women* 201ff.

72. Aeschylus *Prometheus Bound* 474–480 (Grene-Lattimore I, 328–329).

73. Compare ibid., 482 (*kraseis*), and *Ancient Medicine* 5 (*kresesi*).

74. Sophocles *Antigone* 389 (Grene-Lattimore II, 174).

75. Hippocrates *Ancient Medicine* 14 (Loeb I, 37).

76. Euripides *Telephus* frag. 715 Nauck. Probably the notion was already widespread among thinkers in the fifth century. But we have only indirect evidence of this: the *Anonymus Iamblichi*, which may date back to the fifth century (see Diels-Kranz 89.6.1), and, much more problematically, the passage in Diodorus of Sicily on the first men (1.8.9 = Diels-Kranz 68B5), the source of which has been put by some scholars as far back as the fifth century.

77. Aeschylus *Prometheus Bound* 480 (Grene-Lattimore I, 329).

78. See Hippocrates *Ancient Medicine* 12.

79. Hippocrates *Places in Man* 46 (Loeb VIII, 93).

80. See Hippocrates *Art* 8.

81. Hippocrates *Ancient Medicine* 2 (Loeb I, 15).

82. Compare the use of the expression "it is probable" (*eikos*) in Thucydides 1.4; 10.3 (bis); 10.4; and in Hippocrates *Ancient Medicine* 3 (bis).

83. See Thucydides 1.5–6.

84. See Hippocrates *Ancient Medicine* 5.

85. See Plato *Protagoras* 320cff.

86. Regarding the references to the food of animals, see *Protagoras* 321b: "Then [Epimetheus] provided them with various forms of nourishment, plants for some, fruit from trees for others, roots for still others. And there were some to whom he gave the consumption of other animals as their sustenance." The allusion to medicine is

found at 322c: "[O]ne person practicing the art of medicine suffices for many ordinary people." See the Hackett translation by S. Lombardo and K. Bell (Indianapolis, 1997), 757, 758.

87. Diodorus of Sicily 1.8; see the Loeb translation by C. H. Oldfather (Cambridge, Mass., 1960), 1:29–31.

88. Diels-Kranz 68B144 (= Philodemus *De musica* 4.31).

89. See Diels-Kranz 60A4 (= Hippolytus *Refutation of All Heresies* 1.9.5): the first living creatures (including men) had "the same way of life inasmuch as they were [all] nourished by the mud. They were short-lived. . . . Men were [later] separated from the other animals and established leaders and laws and [arts] and cities and the rest" (adapted from J. Barnes, *Early Greek Philosophy* [Harmondsworth, 1987], 241).

90. See Diels-Kranz 60A4 (= Hippolytus *Refutation* 1.9.5): "On the subject of animals, he says that, as the earth grew warm, it was first in the lower part, where the hot and cold were mixing, that many animals including men appeared" (from J. Barnes, *Early Greek Philosophy*, 241).

Ten. Challenges to Medicine and the Birth of Epistemology

1. See pages 119–120.

2. See Hippocrates *Art* 1 and 8.

3. See Plato *Sophist* 232d–e.

4. Hippocrates *Art* 4 (Loeb II, 195).

5. Cicero *De natura deorum* 2.12; the passage is referenced as II.IV.12 in the Loeb translation by H. Rackham (Cambridge, Mass., 1956), 134.

6. Hippocrates *Art* 5 (Loeb II, 197).

7. See ibid., 8.

8. See pages 108ff.

9. Hippocrates *Art* 2 (Loeb II, 191–193); the Jones translation has been slightly modified, following my edition of *The Art* (Budé V, 1 [1988]), 226 and note 2.

10. On the Sophists, see *Dissoi logoi* (Diels-Kranz 90.6); on the adversaries of the Sophists, see Plato *Protagoras* 319c–e; *Meno* 93d–94b; *Laches* 185b–187b; also Xenophon *Memorabilia* 3.5.21 and 4.2.2.

11. See Hippocrates *Art* 8 (Loeb II, 205): "Those experienced in this craft [medicine] have no need either of such foolish blame or of such foolish praise; they need praise only from those who have considered where the operations of craftsmen reach their end and are complete, and likewise where they fall short."

12. Hippocrates *Art* 2 (Loeb II, 193); Jones translation again slightly modified (see note 9 above).

13. These positions are clearly presented by Plato in the *Cratylus*.

14. Hippocrates *Art* 11 (Loeb II, 211).

15. Diels-Kranz 68B11; adapted from J. Barnes, *Early Greek Philosophy* (Harmondsworth, 1987), 253–254.

16. Hippocrates *Art* 11 (Loeb II, 211).

17. Ibid. (Loeb II, 211).

18. See ibid., 12.

19. Euripides *Alcestis* 785–786: thus a standard French rendering; cf. Grene-Lattimore III, 42 ("Fortune is dark; she moves, but we cannot see the way, nor can we pin her down by science and study her"). See also Agathon, frag. 6 and 8 (Snell).

20. Hippocrates *Ancient Medicine* 1 (Loeb I, 13).

21. Ibid., 12 (Loeb I, 33).

22. Hippocrates *Art* 4 (Loeb II, 195).

23. Hippocrates *Places in Man* 46 (Loeb VIII, 93).

24. There did exist a goddess *Tuchè* in Hesiod's time, sometimes said to be the daughter of Oceanus (Hesiod), sometimes the daughter of Zeus (Pindar); but she was unimportant and, as the ancient sense of the word suggests, a goddess of success. By contrast, from the fourth century and especially during the Hellenistic era, another goddess *Tuchè* emerged who was the personification of the notion of *tuchè* in the modern sense, with its positive and negative sides; and, although a personification, she was an object of worship.

25. Galen *Exhortation to the Study of the Arts* 2–5 (excerpts).

26. Hippocrates *Art* 5 (Loeb II, 199).

27. Ibid. (Loeb II, 199).

28. Hippocrates *Ancient Medicine* 1 (Loeb I, 13).

29. Ibid., 3–4 (Loeb I, 19–21).

30. Hippocrates *Breaths* 1 (Loeb II, 227).

31. Hippocrates *Ancient Medicine* 11 (Loeb I, 27–29).

32. Homer *Iliad* 11.514 (Lattimore, 248).

33. Plato *Protagoras* 322b–d; see the Hackett translation by S. Lombardo and K. Bell (Indianapolis, 1997), 758.

34. Hippocrates *Art* 6 (Loeb II, 199–201).

35. Diels-Kranz 67B2; see J. Barnes, *Early Greek Philosophy*, 243.

36. See Aristotle *Metaphysics* 1.1.981a28–30: "For the experienced know the fact, but not the wherefore; but the artists know the wherefore [*dioti*] and the cause" (from the Loeb translation by Hugh Tredennick [Cambridge, Mass., 1961], 7).

37. Hippocrates *Art* 11 (Loeb II, 211).

38. Hippocrates *Breaths* 1 (Loeb II, 229); translation slightly modified.

39. Hippocrates *Ancient Medicine* 20 (Loeb I, 55); the bracketed interpolation is mine.

40. See Cicero *Brutus* 46; also Quintilian *Institutio Oratoria* 3.1.8.

41. Plato *Gorgias* 465a; see the Hackett translation by D. J. Zeyl (Indianapolis, 1997), 808–809 (emphasis added).

42. Ibid., 500e–501a; see the Zeyl translation, 845. Again, the emphasis is mine.

43. See page 6.

44. Plato *Phaedrus* 271b; see the Hackett translation by A. Nehamas and P. Woodruff (Indianapolis, 1997), 548. The emphasis is mine once more.

45. Compare Hippocrates *Art* 5 and Plato *Phaedrus* 274b3.

46. See ibid., 270b.

47. To these two types of knowledge correspond two types of physicians, distinguished by Plato in a celebrated passage of the *Laws* (4.720a–d; see also 9.857c–d).

Eleven. Medicine in Crisis and the Reaction against Philosophy

1. Heraclitus *On the Universe* 16 (Loeb IV, 475 [= Diels-Kranz 22B40]).

2. Diels-Kranz 12A27 [= Aëtius 3.16.1 (D.381); reconstructed from Plutarch *Epitom.* 3.16].

3. Diels-Kranz 21A46 [= Aëtius 3.4.4 (D.371); reconstructed from Stobaeus *Ecl.* 1.31].

4. See Diels-Kranz 64A17 (= Alexander of Aphrodisius *Commentary on the Meteorologica of Aristotle* 353a32): "Diogenes says that the cause of the salty character of the sea is as follows: as the sun attracts upwards the fresh part [of the sea], the result of this is that the remaining and subsistent part is salty."

5. Hippocrates *Airs, Waters, Places* 8 (Loeb I, 91–93).

6. See what was said earlier about Democedes of Croton at page 25.

7. See Diels-Kranz 24A1 (= Diogenes Laertius *Vitae philosophorum* 8.83; Diels-Kranz 24A3 (= Aristotle *Metaphysics* 1.5.986a). Note that Alcmaeon's *On Nature* was dedicated to the Pythagoreans (see Diels-Kranz 24B1).

8. See Diels-Kranz 24A3 (= Aristotle *Metaphysics* 1.5.986a).

9. See ibid.

10. See Diels-Kranz 24A1 (= Diogenes Laertius *Vitae philosophorum* 8.83).

11. See Diels-Kranz 24B4 (= Plutarch *Epitom.* 5.30; and Stobaeus *Ecl.* 4.35–36).

12. See Diels-Kranz 31A3 (= Galen *On the Therapeutic Method* 1.1); cf. also Diels-Kranz 31A1 (= Diogenes Laertius *Vitae philosophorum* 8.58).

13. According to some, this took the form of a poem (see Diels-Kranz 31A1 [= Diogenes Laertius 8.77]; according to others, it was a work of prose (Diels-Kranz 31A2 [= *Suda* s.v. Empedocles]).

14. See Diels-Kranz 31A1 (= Diogenes Laertius *Vitae philosophorum* 8.69).

15. See Diels-Kranz 31A1 (= Diogenes Laertius *Vitae philosophorum* 8.70).

16. See Diels-Kranz 31A14 (= Plutarch *Curiosity* 515c, *Adversus Coloten* 1126b; and other authors).

17. See Diels-Kranz 31A2 (= *Suda* s.v. Empedocles).

18. See Diels-Kranz 31A1 (= Diogenes Laertius *Vitae philosophorum* 8.61).

19. Diels-Kranz 31B111; see J. Barnes, *Early Greek Philosophy* (Harmondsworth, 1987), 162.

20. Hippocrates *Sacred Disease* 4 (Loeb II, 147).

21. See Diels-Kranz 31B100.

22. See Diels-Kranz 59A43 (= Aristotle *Metaphysics* 1.3.984a11–13).

23. Diels-Kranz 59A43 (= Aristotle *De caelo* 3.3.302a28); see G. S. Kirk, J. E. Raven, and M. Schofield, *The Presocratic Philosophers: A Critical History with a Selection of Texts* (Cambridge, 2nd ed., 1983), 373.

24. In addition to Diels-Kranz 59A43, cited in the preceding note, see Diels-Kranz 59A44 (= Lucretius 835–838).

25. Diels-Kranz 59B10 (= scholium to Gregory of Nazianzus *Patrologia Graeca* 36.911 Migne); see J. Barnes, *Early Greek Philosophy* (Harmondsworth, 1987), 234.

26. See Diels-Kranz 59A43 (= Aristotle *De caelo* 3.3.302a28ff.).

27. Several versions were given of this trial; see in particular Diels-Kranz 59A1 (= Diogenes Laertius 2.12–14).

28. See Diels-Kranz 59A16 (= Plutarch *Life of Pericles* 6).

29. Hippocrates *Sacred Disease* 14 (Loeb II, 169).

30. See page 263.

31. See Diels-Kranz 64A1 (= Diogenes Laertius 9.57).

32. See Diels-Kranz 64A4 (= Simplicius *Phys.* 151.20).

33. See Diels-Kranz 64B6 (= Aristotle *Historia animalium* 2.2.511b30ff.).

34. See Diels-Kranz 64A19 (= Theophrastus *On the Senses* 43).

35. See Diels-Kranz 64A29a (= [Galen] *De humoribus* 19.495 Kühn).

36. This papyrus was referred to earlier in connection with the Hippocratic question; see page 59ff.

37. On Samos, see Diels-Kranz 38A1 (= Aristoxenus and Iamblichus); on Rhegium, 38A1 and 38A5 (= Sextus Empiricus); on Croton, 38A11 (= *Anonymus Londinensis* 11.22); on Metapontum, 38A1 and 38A16 (= Censorinus).

38. See Diels-Kranz 38A2 (= scholium to Aristophanes *Clouds* 94ff.).

39. See, in particular, Diels-Kranz 38A16 (= Censorinus 7.2).

40. See Diels-Kranz 38A7.

41. See, in particular, Diels-Kranz 44A4a (= Plutarch *Socrates' Daimonion* 583a); Diels-Kranz 44A1a (= Plato *Phaedo* 61d–e).

42. See Diels-Kranz 44A27 (= *Anonym. Lond.* 18.8ff.).

43. See Diels-Kranz 44A27 (= *Anonym. Lond.* 18.30ff.).

44. See Diels-Kranz 44A16 (= Stobaeus *Ecl.* 1.15.6) and 44A17 (= Plutarch *Epit.* 3.11); Diels-Kranz 44A17 (= Stobaeus *Ecl.* 1.21).

45. See, in particular, Diels-Kranz 44B1 (= Diogenes Laertius 8.85).

46. See Diels-Kranz 68A33 (= Diogenes Laertius 9.45–49). Regarding Democritus's nickname, see *Suda* 447 (s.v. Democritus).

47. See Diels-Kranz 68A10 (= *Suda* s.v. Hippocrates). On the relations between Democritus and Hippocrates according to the *Letters*, see page 20.

48. See Diels-Kranz 68A2 (= *Suda* s.v. Democritus).

49. See Diels-Kranz 68A10 (= *Suda* s.v. Hippocrates).

50. Hippocrates was born in 460 and Democritus in 470–469 or between 460 and 457 (cf. Diels-Kranz 68A1 [= Diogenes Laertius 9.41]).

51. Diels-Kranz 31A75 [= Aëtius 5.18.1 (D.427); reconstructed from Plutarch *Epitom.* 5.18].

52. Hippocrates *Eight Months' Child* 12.

53. See Hippocrates *Generation / Nature of the Child* 7; cf. *Regimen* 27.

54. See Aeschylus *Eumenides* 658–661.

55. See Hippocrates *Airs, Waters, Places* 14; and *Sacred Disease* 2.

56. Hippocrates *Generation / Nature of the Child* 2.

57. See pages 188ff.

58. Hippocrates *Airs, Waters, Places* 22 (Loeb I, 127–129).

59. Hippocrates *Fleshes* 6 (Loeb VIII, 143).

60. See Aristotle *Historia animalium* 7.3.583b23–25; *De generatione animalium* 4.6.775a11–12.

61. Compare Hippocrates *Regimen* 27 and *Superfoetation* 14.

62. This was in any case the opinion of Theophrastus during the Hellenistic period (see Diels *Dox.* 422 [= Plutarch *Epit.* 5.10]); cf. the opinion of Democritus cited in the following note.

63. See Diels-Kranz 68A141 (= Plutarch *Epit.* 5.3). Other similarities have been mentioned. The one that is considered closest concerns their respective opinions about twins (see Hippocrates *Generation / Nature of the Child* 31 and Diels-Kranz 68A151 [= Aelian *On the Nature of Animals* 12.16]). But these two texts diverge with regard to the main point: whereas the Hippocratic physician wishes to show that even pigs and dogs can have two or more offspring from a single act of coitus, Democritus (according to Aelian) says that a single act does not suffice, that there must be two or three. It is surprising that Diels, in his edition of the pre-Socratics, should have inserted this Hippocratic text in the doxography of Democritus alongside Aelian's text. It really does not belong here.

64. See Aristotle *De generatione animalium* 1.17.721b11–12: "There are some who assert that the semen is drawn from the whole of the body" (from the Loeb translation by A. L. Peck [Cambridge, Mass., 1953], 51).

65. Hippocrates *Nature of the Child* 13. Part of this passage was cited earlier at page 123.

66. Galen *On the Seed* 4 (Kühn IV, 525); *On the Formation of the Foetus* (Kühn IV, 653).

67. Hippocrates *Nature of the Child* 29.

68. Hippocrates *Regimen* 10 (Loeb IV, 247–249).

69. This is the first clear formulation in an entirely preserved Greek text of the micro/macrocosmic theory. Within the Hippocratic Collection, compare it with the more recent treatise *Sevens* (chapters 6 and 15), where it is the universe that is made in the image of man.

70. Plato *Phaedo* 96a–c; see the Hackett translation by G. M. A. Grube (Indianapolis, 1997), 135.

71. See page 268.

72. See Hippocrates *Fleshes* 1.

73. Ibid. (Loeb VIII, 133).

74. Ibid., 3 (Loeb VIII, 135).

75. Ibid., 14 (Loeb VIII, 153).

76. Ibid., 2 (Loeb VIII, 133).

77. See Hippocrates *Breaths* 14; cf. also *Diseases I* 30.

78. See Hippocrates *Sacred Disease* 14 and 17.

79. See Hippocrates *Fleshes* 15–18.

80. Compare Hippocrates *Regimen* 23.

81. Hippocrates *Fleshes* 15 (Loeb VIII, 153–155).

82. Ibid., 1 (Loeb VIII, 133).

83. Ibid., 18 (Loeb VIII, 157–159).

84. See ibid., 19.

85. Isocrates *Antidosis* 268; see the Loeb translation by G. Norlin (Cambridge, Mass., 1968), 2:333–335.

86. See Hippocrates *Sevens* 10.

87. See pages 232ff.

88. See Hippocrates *Ancient Medicine* 1.

89. Hippocrates *Ancient Medicine* 20 (Loeb I, 53).

90. See pages 277ff.

91. Hippocrates *Regimen* 2 (Loeb IV, 227).

92. Hippocrates *Ancient Medicine* 20 (Loeb I, 53–55). The end of this passage was cited earlier in connection with the discussion of causality (see page 255).

93. Hippocrates *Nature of Man* 1 (Loeb IV, 3).

94. See Isocrates *Antidosis* 268 (cited at page 282).

95. See Aristotle *De sensu* 436a19–b1.

96. Galen drew the opposite lesson from Hippocrates' teaching, however. He considered that a physician must also be a philosopher, and to make his point he gave Hippocrates as an example in his slender volume of this name, *Quod optimus medicus sit quoque philosophus.*

97. Celsus *De medicina* prooem. 7–8; see the Loeb translation by W. G. Spencer (Cambridge, Mass., 1960), 1:5.

Twelve. *From Observation of the Visible to Reconstruction of the Invisible*

1. On the physical conditions under which the physician encountered the patient, whether at the patient's bedside or in his office, see pages 85ff.

2. Hippocrates *In the Surgery* 1 (Loeb III, 59).

3. Hippocrates *Epidemics IV* 43 (Loeb VII, 137–139); the Smith translation has been slightly modified.

4. Hippocrates *Epidemics VI* 8.17 (Loeb VII, 285).

5. See pages 106ff.

6. Hippocrates *Prognostic* 2 (Loeb II, 9–11). The description is found in summary and dissociated form in section 209 of the compilation *Coan Prenotions*; cf. also 214.

7. Hippocrates *Prognostic* 4 (Loeb II, 15); Jones translation slightly modified, emphasis added. This is the only Hippocratic treatise where carphology is attested in the narrow sense of the term ("to pick up whisps of straw or twigs on the bed"). The

verb *karphologein* is not found elsewhere in the collection. By contrast, other treatises note the gesture of the hand snatching or picking up bits of wool from the blankets (cf. *Regimen in Acute Diseases [Appendix]* 8; *Epidemics VII* 25; *Internal Affections* 48; *Critical Days* 3) or plucking sticks of straw from the walls (cf. *Epidemics VII* 25).

8. Jean Hamburger, ed., *Dictionnaire de médecine*, "Carphologie" (Paris, 1975).

9. Ibid., "Hippocratisme digital."

10. Hippocrates *Prognostic* 17 (Loeb II, 35). Another version of this description is found in *Coan Prenotions* 396.

11. See Hippocrates *Places in Man* 14.

12. See Hippocrates *Coan Prenotions* 396; *Diseases II* 47, 48, 50, 61; *Internal Affections* 10, 23.

13. Aretaeus *On the Causes and Symptoms of Chronic Diseases* 1.8; see Francis Adams, ed. and trans., *The Extant Works of Aretaeus, the Cappadocian* (London, 1856), 311. Aretaeus also indicates the incurving of the nails in peripneumonia (*Causes and Symptoms of Acute Diseases* 2.1). Galen, a century later, was to explain the incurving of the nails by the melting of the skin of the finger that served to support it; see his (erroneous) commentary on chapter 17 of Hippocrates' *Prognostic* (2.60).

14. See Hippocrates *Coan Prenotions* 396; *Diseases II* 2.47, 2.48, 2.61; *Internal Affections* 10, 23.

15. P. Marie, "De l'ostéo-arthropathie hypertrophiante pneumique," *Revue de médecine* 10 (1890): 1–36.

16. Hippocrates *Prognostic* 7 (Loeb II, 17). The emphasis is mine.

17. Numerous examples are to be found in *Nature of Women* and *Diseases of Women*.

18. Hippocrates *On Fractures* 27 (Loeb III, 159).

19. Hippocrates *Internal Affections* 44 (Loeb VI, 221).

20. See Hippocrates *Diseases III* 15.

21. See Hippocrates *Diseases II* 49.

22. See Hippocrates *Coan Prenotions* 223.

23. Hippocrates *Diseases II* 61 (Loeb V, 307): dropsy of the lung.

24. Ibid., 59: collapse of a lung against the side.

25. Hippocrates *Diseases II* 47 (Loeb V, 273); see also *Coan Prenotions* 424.

26. This is the Greek verb *kludazomai* (or its composite form *enkludazomai*): see Hippocrates *Diseases III* 16b; *Internal Affections* 23; *Diseases I* 15; *Places in Man* 14.

27. See R. T. H. Laënnec, *De l'auscultation médiate* (1st ed., Paris, 1819), II, 120.

28. Ibid., II, 161, n. (a): the text is in Latin in the original.

29. Laënnec, *De l'auscultation médiate* (2nd rev. ed., Paris, 1826), II, 315.

30. From Laënnec's "Réponse à l'Examen de Broussais," cited in A. Rouxeau, *Laënnec après 1806* (Paris, 1920), 326.

31. Hippocrates *Coan Prenotions* 621.

32. Hippocrates *Internal Affections* 47, 49.

33. Hippocrates *Diseases of Women II* 115.

34. Hippocrates *Diseases II* 49.

35. See, for example, Hippocrates *Prognostic* 11.

36. Ibid., 13.

37. Hippocrates *Diseases II* 57 (Loeb V, 301).

38. See Hippocrates *Epidemics VI* 8.8: "Tears, voluntary, involuntary, many, few, hot, cold; thickness, *taste*" (my emphasis). And just prior to this: "Excretions: . . . hot, *salty, sweet*, thin, thick, uniformly or not" (my emphasis again).

39. Aristophanes *Plutus* 696–706.

40. Hippocrates *Prognostic* 15 (Loeb II, 33). The emphasis is mine, as again in note 42 below.

41. Ibid., 22 (Loeb II, 45–47).

42. Ibid., 25 (Loeb II, 55).

43. Hippocrates *Epidemics I* 23 (Loeb I, 181); the Jones translation has been slightly modified.

44. See pages 28ff.

45. See Galen *Critical Days* 2.4. In *Epidemics V*, such as it has come down to us, there are actually many more; but many of the cases are repeated in *Epidemics VII* and Galen may not have taken these cases into account.

46. Hippocrates *Epidemics V* 62 (Loeb VII, 197).

47. The *bregma* is the front part of the skull at the top of the head where the bone is thinnest and where the brain sustains lesions with the greatest intensity (cf. Hippocrates *On Wounds in the Head* 2).

48. A cyathus is a vase and a unit of measure (equal to 0.045 liters).

49. Hippocrates *Epidemics V* 50 (Loeb VII, 191).

50. Hippocrates *Epidemics VII* 25 (Loeb VII, 327–331); the Smith translation has been slightly modified.

51. Indications of the hour such as "that of the filling of the marketplace" (i.e., from 10 A.M. to 1 P.M.) or "before the marketplace was empty" are common in Greek; but they are not found in the Hippocratic Collection apart from books V and VII of the *Epidemics*.

52. See Hippocrates *Prognostic* 3.

53. See ibid., 9.

54. See ibid., 2 (cited at page 293).

55. Ibid., 6 (Loeb II, 15).

56. See ibid., 4 (cited at page 294).

57. Hippocrates *Art* 11 (Loeb II, 209–211). The immediately preceding extract reproduces the opening sentences of this chapter.

58. The sole use of the term "anatomy" (*anatomè*) to denote the internal structure of the human body is in the title of a brief one-page treatise (Littré VIII, 538–541), the recent character of which—Hellenistic or Roman period—cannot be doubted.

59. The fact that embalming was not practiced in Greece does not mean that the Greeks were unaware of it; Herodotus describes the practice of embalming in detail in his section on Egypt (*Historiae* 2.86).

60. Aristotle *Historia animalium* 1.16.494b22–24; see the Loeb translation by A. L. Peck (Cambridge, Mass., 1965), 57.

61. The same false idea was already to be found in the Hippocratic Collection at *Diseases IV* 40.

62. Aristotle *De partibus animalium* 3.4.667b2–6; see the Loeb translation by A. L. Peck (Cambridge, Mass., 1961), 247.

63. See page 265.

64. See Aristotle *De partibus animalium* 3.4.667b11–12; cf. also 4.2.677a9.

65. See Hippocrates *Nature of Man* 11.

66. See Hippocrates *Sacred Disease* 3.

67. Galen *Anatomical Procedures* 2.1; see Charles Singer, trans., *Galen: On Anatomical Procedures* (Oxford, 1956), 31.

68. See Hippocrates *Sacred Disease* 11 (cited at page 265).

69. Hippocrates *Internal Affections* 23 (Loeb VI, 149).

70. See also Hippocrates *Epidemics VI* 4.6 (comparison of the intestine in man and dog). An instance of animal dissection occurs also in the treatise *The Heart*; but this treatise is much more recent, dating from the Hellenistic period. In itself the intervention is interesting, for the author uses, apparently for the first time in the history of medicine, an artificial coloring in order to follow the course of liquids within the body. Thus, for example, this passage from chapter 2: "If, after having colored some water with cyan [a dark-blue substance] or minium, one gives it to an animal that is completely parched to drink, particularly to a pig—a beast that is neither fussy nor clean—and then, while it is still drinking, one opens its mouth, one will note that the trachea is colored by the drink; but the intervention is not done on just any animal." Nonetheless, the demonstrative value of the procedure is disappointing, because the author wants to prove that, while the greater part of the liquid swallowed goes into the stomach, a small part passes into the trachea; it is impossible, however, for even a small amount of a liquid to pass into the trachea.

71. The absence of such a distinction is obvious in the oldest treatises. Nonetheless, certain treatises distinguish arteries from veins. The distinction is mentioned in the surgical treatises (see, for example, *On Joints* 45) and in *Epidemics V* 46; however, we do not know what it actually involved in these two passages: the author of *On Joints* says there that he will speak of the communications between veins and arteries in another work, unfortunately lost. By contrast, in chapter 31 of the post-Hippocratic treatise *Nutriment*, there is a clear distinction between the veins, which carry blood, and the arteries, which carry air.

72. Used in the plural, the Greek word for arteries corresponded to what we call the bronchial tubes.

73. This pulse is known from chapter 31 of the *Nutriment*; but, as indicated

previously, this treatise is from a period following the Hippocratic age, showing signs especially of Stoic influence.

74. For one example among others, see Hippocrates *Coan Prenotions* 125.

75. The chief descriptions are to be found in Hippocrates *Epidemics II* 4.1 (= *Nature of Bones* 10); *Nature of Man* 11 (= *Nature of Bones* 9); *Sacred Disease* 3; *Fleshes* 5.

76. See Hippocrates *Places in Man* 47 (Loeb VIII, 95): "Diseases of women, as they are called. The uterus is the cause of all these diseases."

77. See Hippocrates *Nature of Women* 3 (liver); 8 (hip); 14 (loins); 38 (ribs); 48 (head); 49 (legs and feet); 62 (heart).

78. See Hippocrates *Diseases of Women I* 7.

79. See Hippocrates *Diseases of Women II* 145.

80. See Hippocrates *On Joints* 45; cf. *Mochlicon* 1.

81. Hippocrates *On Joints* 46 (Loeb III, 293).

82. See, for example, Hippocrates *Prognostic* 5.

83. Hippocrates *Breaths* 4 (Loeb II, 231–233).

84. See ibid., 2–5.

85. See pages 184ff.

86. See Hippocrates *Sacred Disease* 7.

87. See the recent treatise entitled *Anatomy*. It was only with Aristotle that the distinction was clearly made (*De partibus animalium* 3.3.664a–b). Otherwise the term "esophagus" (literally, "carrying food"), found in Aristotle, is attested in only two treatises of the Hippocratic Collection, *Anatomy* and *Places in Man*.

88. See Hippocrates *Sacred Disease* 4.

89. See, for example, Hippocrates *Diseases I* 34.

90. See, for example, Hippocrates *Fleshes* 3 (Loeb VIII, 135) where the sequence "pharynx, oesophagus, stomach [*gaster*] and intestines" makes its specialized meaning explicit.

91. See, for example, Hippocrates *Ancient Medicine* 11.

92. Significant in this connection is the treatise *Fleshes*, which explains the original formation of man. The author dedicates a chapter to each of the important internal organs: brain (4); heart (5); lungs (7); liver (8); spleen and kidney (9). This is not true of the stomach, which is mentioned only in passing in chapter 3.

93. These three models of explanation are unified in Hippocrates *Ancient Medicine* 11.

94. See Aristotle *Meteorologica* 4.3.381b7.

95. Hippocrates *Ancient Medicine* 18 (Loeb I, 47).

96. See ibid., 22.

97. See, for example, Hippocrates *Nature of Man* 7.

98. This does not prevent the word from being used in certain passages of the Hippocratic Collection to denote "inflammation." This double sense was indeed remarked by Galen in his *Hippocratic Glossary*.

99. Another four-humor theory (blood, bile, water, phlegm) is attested in *Generation / Nature of the Child* 3 and *Diseases IV* 32.

100. Phlegm, cold and wet, predominates in winter, a cold and wet season; blood, wet and hot, predominates in spring, also wet and hot; yellow bile, hot and dry, predominates in summer, a hot and dry season; black bile, dry and cold, predominates in fall, likewise a dry and cold season. This schematism was to be pushed still further after Hippocrates by putting the four humors into systematic relation with four ages and, especially, four temperaments.

101. Hippocrates *Haemorrhoids* 1 (Loeb VIII, 381).

102. Hippocrates *Ancient Medicine* 22 (Loeb I, 57–59); the emphasis is mine. The same comparison between the head and a cupping glass is found in *Diseases IV* 35.

103. Diels-Kranz 59B21a.

104. See page 264.

105. Herodotus 2.33; see the Grene translation *The History*, 144.

106. He was also the author of *Diseases IV* and of the C layer of the gynecological treatises.

107. Hippocrates *Generation / Nature of the Child* 4.

108. Homer *Iliad* 22.220, 237, 250.

109. See Hippocrates *Generation / Nature of the Child* 18; repeated in *Diseases of Women I* 6 (layer C) and 72 (layer C). For the reference to sacrificial practice, see also *Fleshes* 8.

110. The term "carotids" (literally, "causing a heavy sleep") appeared later in the medical vocabulary of the Greeks (first attestation in Aretaeus, first century B.C.). The impropriety of the term was denounced very shortly thereafter; see Rufus of Ephesus in the first century A.D.: "The name carotids ("causing a heavy sleep") was formerly applied to the hollow vessels that pass through the neck, because their compression produces a heavy sleep and aphonia; but it is known today that this state results not from the arteries, but from the sensitive nerves located nearby; so that if one wished to change the name it would not be an error" (*De corporis humani appellationibus* 210). The term survived, however.

111. See page 314.

112. See Hippocrates *Breaths* 8.

113. See Hippocrates *Diseases IV* 52.

114. Ibid., 51.

115. See Aristotle *De generatione animalium* 2.4.740b13ff.

116. Hippocrates *Nature of the Child* 17.

117. Hippocrates *Art* 13 (Loeb II, 215).

118. C. V. Daremberg, *Hippocrate* (Paris, 1843), 9.

Thirteen. Health, Sickness, and Nature

1. Etymology reveals that the word denoting health in Greek (*hygieia*) is in fact a compound whose second element (-*gi*-) stems from the Indo-European root signifying "life," like the initial element (*bi*-) of "biology" (literally, "science of life"), and

whose first element (*hy-*, from the Indo-European *su-*) means "well." Thus, the Greek term that we translate by "health" literally means "the state of one who is well in life." This positive sense has passed into French (and English) terms derived from the Greek. To quote the fine definition found in Jean Hamburger's dictionary of medicine, the term "hygiene" strictly refers to "the branch of medicine that studies the means of maintaining human beings in good health by protecting them against disease." From this definition, in which one notes the expression "good health," it is clear that the word "hygiene" shares a positive sense with the Greek word *hygieia*, even if the latter has a broader meaning than the modern word derived from it— *hygieia* referring to good health in general and "hygiene" to the art of keeping healthy people in good health.

2. The adjective *hygiès*, meaning "healthy," is often used in the nosological treatises to refer to a patient who is cured of his disease in the expression *hygiès ginesthai* (literally, "to become healthy"), and to refer to a physician who cures a patient in the expression *hygiea poiein* (literally, "to make the patient healthy"). An equivalent use can be found in our own speech today when we talk of a patient who "recovers his health." But aside from the fact that the notion of a return to a previous state of health is not expressed in the Greek, the use of the concept of health to express the idea of curing or healing is much less common in English than in Greek.

3. Plato *Gorgias* 451e: thus the Hackett translation by D. J. Zeyl (Indianapolis, 1997), 797. Plato omits the end: "[F]ourth is to be in the prime of life in the company of one's friends." The complete text is given in the scholium *ad. loc.*; see E. Diehl, ed., *Anthologia Lyrica Graeca* (Leipzig, 1925), 2^2.6.16.

4. For the end of the fifth century and the beginning of the fourth, see the hymn to Health of Ariphron of Sicyon cited at page 125, and that of his contemporary Licymnius of Chios (Page *PMG* 769).

5. See Herodas *Women Making a Dedication and Sacrifice to Asclepius* 3ff. and 20ff.

6. Plato *Gorgias* 452a; see the Hackett translation by Zeyl, 797.

7. Hippocrates *Regimen* 69 (Loeb IV, 383).

8. Hippocrates *Affections* 1 (Loeb V, 7).

9. The Latin title by which it is commonly known is *De sanitate tuenda*; the original Greek title is *Hygieinon*.

10. The small treatise entitled in Littré's edition *Régime Salutaire* (VI, 70–87)— called *Regimen in Health* in English—is only the last part of *Nature of Man*. The initial list of one manuscript, however, bears the title of a lost Hippocratic treatise named *On Health*.

11. Hippocrates *Nature of Man* 17 (= *Regimen in Health* 2 [Loeb IV, 49]).

12. See Hippocrates *Regimen* 68.

13. Quoted in Oribasius 3.168ff. (= Frag. 141 Wellmann).

14. See pages 331ff.

15. See page 238.

16. See Hippocrates *Nature of Man* 22 (= *Regimen in Health* 7).

17. Hippocrates *Art* 3 (Loeb II, 193).

18. Epictetus 2.17.8; see the Loeb translation by W. A. Oldfather (Cambridge, Mass., 1961), 1:339.

19. Hippocrates *Ancient Medicine* 14 (Loeb I, 39).

20. D. Diderot, *Lettre sur les sourds et muets à l'usage de ceux qui entendent et qui parlent* (Paris, 1751).

21. Hippocrates *Nature of Man* 4 (Loeb IV, 11–13).

22. Hippocrates *Regimen* 69 (Loeb IV, 383).

23. Diels-Kranz 24B4 [= Aëtius 5.30.1 (D.442)]. For more on Alcmaeon see page 262.

24. Of course, Alcmaeon's definition of health is not identical to that of the Hippocratic physician. While for Alcmaeon health seems to be defined by reference to political equality in an isonomic regime, there is apparently no particular political connotation in the definition of health given by the physician. Attempts to locate political models of biological thought in the Hippocratic Collection have produced rather disappointing results. But it remains the case that Alcmaeon's fundamental perspective, according to which biological processes are expressed in terms of struggle between forces that dominate (or are dominated) when they are not in balance with each other, is the same as the one regularly encountered among the Hippocratic physicians.

25. Galen *On Preserving Health* 1.4 (Kühn VI, 11–12).

26. Chrysippus *De affectibus*, quoted in Galen *De placitis Hippocratis et Platonis* 5.2; also fragment 471 in *Stoicorum veterum fragmenta*, ed. J. von Arnim, vol. 3 (Leipzig, 1903), 121.

27. See pages 146ff. on the various principles of classification for diseases, some of which take causes into account.

28. Hippocrates *Airs, Waters, Places* 11 (Loeb I, 105). On the notion of change in this treatise see page 215; compare *Humours* 15 and *Aphorisms* 3.1.

29. Hippocrates *Regimen in Acute Diseases* 35 (Loeb II, 91).

30. For Herodotus, see the comparison at page 228 between his account and that of *Airs, Waters, Places*.

31. See Thucydides 7.87.

32. Hippocrates *Regimen in Acute Diseases* 28, 30 (Loeb II, 85–89); a comparable account is to be found in chapters 10 and 11 of *Ancient Medicine*.

33. See Hippocrates *Regimen in Acute Diseases* 9 (= 28 in Jones's numbering, as above); cf. also *Aphorisms* 2.50.

34. See Hippocrates *Epidemics I* 10 (= 23 in Jones's numbering, as cited at page 303).

35. Erasistratus *On Paralysis* 2, cited by Galen in the first chapter of his treatise *On Habits*; see Arthur J. Brock, trans., *Greek Medicine: Being Extracts Illustrative of Medical Writers from Hippocrates to Galen* (London, 1929), 185. In some versions the final sentence of this passage is followed by another: "So it is clear that habit is powerful in all our physical and mental behaviors."

36. See in particular Plato *Republic* 8.556e.
37. See, for example, Hippocrates *Breaths* 8 and *Ancient Medicine* 16.
38. See Philostratus *On Athletic Training* 43.
39. Hippocrates *Aphorisms* 1.3 (Loeb IV, 99–101).
40. Hippocrates *Nature of Man* 22 (= *Regimen in Health* 7 [Loeb IV, 55]).
41. Aeschylus *Agamemnon* 1001–1003 (Grene-Lattimore I, 66).
42. See Hippocrates *Nutriment* 34.
43. Hippocrates *Regimen* 69 (Loeb IV, 383).
44. Ibid., 2 (Loeb IV, 231).
45. Ibid., 70 (Loeb IV, 383–385). The emphasis is mine.
46. See Hippocrates *On Joints* 56.
47. Hippocrates *Aphorisms* 6.2 (Loeb IV, 181).
48. Hippocrates *Ancient Medicine* 10, 12 (Loeb I, 29–33).
49. Compare chapters 10 and 12 with chapter 14.
50. Hippocrates *Art* 11 (Loeb II, 211); cited earlier at page 141.
51. On the approach of disease, see *prospelazein* in Hippocrates *Regimen* 67. On the attack, see *ephodos*: this term, which denotes the attack of heroes in a religious conception of disease (see *Sacred Disease* 4) is also used in a rational perspective to designate the attack of fever (*Prognostic* 20); see also *prospiptein*, "to rush at" (*Generation* 11). Verbs signifying "to seize": *lambanein* and its compounds very frequently occur. Verbs signifying "to hold": *echein, katechein* are likewise very common.
52. Verb signifying "to dominate" in connection with disease: *epikratein* (see Hippocrates *Regimen in Acute Diseases [Appendix]* 3, 11; *Diseases IV* 53). Verb signifying "to resist" in connection with disease: *antechein* (see *Ancient Medicine* 3; *Regimen in Acute Diseases [Appendix]* 3); also *exarkein* (see *Aphorisms* 1.9, 10).
53. Hippocrates *Regimen in Acute Diseases (Appendix)* 5 (Loeb VI, 267).
54. Hippocrates *Ancient Medicine* 6 (Loeb I, 23).
55. On the nourishment of fever, see for example Hippocrates *Diseases IV* 46, 49, 51.
56. Ibid., 51.
57. Certain terms designating the recurrence of disease are quite colorful. The disease can once again become angry at the patient, for example (*palinkotos, palinkoteo, palinkotaino, palinkotesis, palinkotie*).
58. See for example Hippocrates *Breaths* 14, where an epileptic fit is described as a tempest (*cheimon*); see also *Prognostic* 24, where patients are caught in the storm of the disease (*cheimazesthai*).
59. Verb signifying "to begin": *archesthai* (see Hippocrates *Internal Affections* 50); "to go": *erchomai* (see *Places in Man* 4); "to turn": *trepesthai* (see *Aphorisms* 7.49); "to settle": *pegnusthai* (see *Places in Man* 1), *aposterizesthai* (see *Prorrhetic II* 2); "to move again": *metallassein* (see *Places in Man* 1).
60. Hippocrates *Nature of Man* 4 (Loeb IV, 13).
61. Hippocrates *Places in Man* 1 (Loeb VIII, 19–21).

62. See Hippocrates *Glands* 11 (Loeb VIII, 117–119): "Fluxes from the head are sometimes secreted through the natural passages of the ears, eyes, or nose: these are three possibilities; others flow through the palate into the throat or into the oesophagus, others through the vessels into the spinal marrow, or to the hips: seven possibilities in all."

63. Verb signifying "to reach one's height": *akmazein* (see Hippocrates *Aphorisms* 1.8).

64. See Hippocrates *Nature of Man* 8 (cited at page 147).

65. Hippocrates *Affections* 8 (Loeb V, 17).

66. Hippocrates *Epidemics I* 11 (Loeb I, 163–165).

67. The most complete description of these various fevers is found in Hippocrates *Epidemics I* 11 (= 24–25 in Jones's numbering [Loeb I, 181–183]).

68. Hippocrates *Fleshes* 19 (Loeb VIII, 163). The line immediately following about the fundamental period of human life is found at the beginning of this chapter.

69. The leading specialist in septenary theory in the Hippocratic Collection is the author of the treatise *Sevens*. For him, all things in both the universe and in man are explained by the number seven.

70. Outside the Hippocratic Collection, on the importance of the number seven in the development of the embryo and of man, see Alcmaeon (Diels-Kranz 24A15 = Aristotle *Historia animalium* 7.1.581a), Empedocles (Diels-Kranz 31B153a = Theon of Smyrna) and especially Hippon (Diels-Kranz 38A16 = Censorinus *De die natali* 7.2).

71. Hippocrates *Prognostic* 20 (Loeb II, 43).

72. It goes without saying that the mode of calculation does not by itself explain the series of critical days. Another partisan of reckoning by hebdomads, the author of *Sevens*, gives (in chapter 26) a series that begins with 7 (first hebdomad) and continues 9, 11, 14 (second hebdomad), 21 (third hebdomad), and so on.

73. To understand the detail of the calculation in the *Prognostic*, it is necessary to know that the units of measure (in this case tetrads) may be counted either as "linked" (e.g., 1, 2, 3, 4 / 4, 5, 6, 7) or as "disjoint" (e.g., 1, 2, 3, 4 / 5, 6, 7, 8). The calculation of the author of the *Prognostic* is as follows: first tetrad (1, 2, 3, 4); second linked tetrad (4, 5, 6, 7); third disjoint tetrad (8, 9, 10, 11); fourth linked tetrad (11, 12, 13, 14); fifth linked tetrad (14, 15, 16, 17). As the periods (hebdomads or triads) may be counted by linking or by disjunction, an identical series of critical days can be interpreted by taking either the hebdomad or the tetrad—or both—as a base. Thus, the series of critical days indicated in the *Prognostic* (1, 4, 7, 11, 17) is also adopted in *Aphorisms* 2.24, but it is justified through a calculation mixing hebdomads with tetrads: "the seventeenth is to be watched, being the fourth from the fourteenth [i.e., it forms a continuous tetrad counting from 14, the last element of the second hebdomad] and the seventh from the eleventh [i.e., counting from 11 to 17 yields a hebdomad]."

74. Hippocrates *Regimen in Acute Diseases (Appendix)* 21 (Loeb VI, 285).

75. See Hippocrates *Epidemics I* 12.

76. See Hippocrates *Prognostic* 20.

77. On the analogy between these latter two domains for the purposes of counting up critical days, see for example Hippocrates *Eight Months' Child* (= *Seven Months' Child* 9): "For women, the conception of the embryo, abortion, and childbirth are reckoned in the same periods as diseases, healing, and death for all people"; see also *Prognostic* 20.

78. Hesiod *Works and Days* 824 (Tandy-Neale, 135).

79. See also Hippocrates *Critical Days* 11.

80. Hippocrates *Eight Months' Child* (= *Seven Months' Child* 9).

81. The days 14, 28, and 42 constitute the end of the second, fourth, and sixth hebdomads respectively.

82. On the importance of the decade among the Pythagoreans, see Aristotle *Metaphysics* 1.5.986a8ff. The sole Hippocratic treatise where the decade figures in the calculation of critical days is the *Fleshes*; but even here (chapter 19) it is a question of decades of hebdomads.

83. Compare Hippocrates *Ancient Medicine* 19, where both crises and the *number* of periods are said to be of great importance in such diseases, and *Ancient Medicine* 9, where it is said to be necessary to aim at some measure; but in the latter case there is no measure—either by *number* or weight—to which one can refer in order to know what is exact, apart from bodily sensation.

84. See Hippocrates *Regimen* 2.

85. Hippocrates *On Joints* 78 (Loeb III, 383).

86. Ibid., 14 (Loeb III, 235).

87. See, for example, Hippocrates *Diseases of Women I* 65: "In following this treatment the woman recovers, but she no longer gives birth."

88. Hippocrates *Art* 3 (Loeb II, 193).

89. This theme was sketched earlier at pages 135–136.

90. Hippocrates *Epidemics I* 11 (Loeb I, 165); this passage was cited earlier in connection with the relation between the physician and the patient (at page 136). The emphasis here, as in the passages that follow, is of course mine.

91. Hippocrates *Nature of Man* 9 (Loeb IV, 25).

92. Hippocrates *Breaths* 1 (Loeb II, 229). Note that the bracketed phrase does not appear in the Loeb translation by Jones, who considers it a gloss; he notes, however, its presence in most surviving manuscripts. Compare *Aphorisms* 2.22 (Loeb IV, 113): "Diseases caused by repletion are cured by depletion; those caused by depletion are cured by repletion, and in general contraries are cured by contraries."

93. See Hippocrates *Places in Man* 42 (Loeb VIII, 85): "Another principle is the following: a disease arises because of similars, and, by being treated with similars, patients recover from such diseases." It should be noted, however, that this author does not regard homeopathy and allopathy as mutually exclusive. The nature of the treatment depends on the nature of the cause of the disease. Certain diseases are caused by contraries, others by similars. Therapy by similars was already sufficiently

known in the fifth century B.C. to have found expression in the theater with Sophocles: physicians "evacuate bitter bile with a bitter clyster" (Frag. 854 Radt = Plutarch *Tranquillity of Mind* 7.468b).

94. See Hippocrates *Prognostic* 1.

95. See for example Hippocrates *Breaths* 6 (Loeb II, 235): "[W]henever the air has been infected with such pollutions as are hostile [*polemia*] to the human race, then men fall sick."

96. Hippocrates *Sacred Disease* 21 (Loeb II, 183).

97. Ibid.

98. Hippocrates *Places in Man* 45 (Loeb VIII, 91).

99. See pages 328–331.

100. Ibid.

101. Hippocrates *Regimen in Acute Diseases* 26, 27 (Loeb II, 83–85).

102. Hippocrates *Regimen in Acute Diseases* 28 (Loeb II, 85).

103. Hippocrates *Ancient Medicine* 10 (Loeb I, 29).

104. See for example Hippocrates *On Fractures* 2, 3.

105. Hippocrates *Places in Man* 2 (Loeb VIII, 21–23).

106. Galen *Med. Phil.* 1.

107. Hippocrates *On Fractures* 7 (Loeb III, 113); compare 35 (Loeb III, 181): "There are great differences between . . . one bodily constitution and another as to power of endurance"; and *On Joints* 8 (Loeb III, 213): "One should bear in mind that there are great natural diversities as to the easy reduction of dislocations."

108. Hippocrates *Humours* 16 (Loeb IV, 89).

109. Hippocrates *Epidemics I* 23 (Loeb I, 181); the whole passage was cited earlier at page 303.

110. Hippocrates *Epidemics VI* 5.1 (Loeb VII, 255). The author of *Epidemics VI* was not the first to emphasize the innate wisdom of nature; see earlier the comic poet Epicharmus (Diels-Kranz 23B4, 6ff.): "Nature alone knows about this wisdom; for it has taught itself."

111. Aristotle *De partibus animalium* 2.13.657a36–b2; see the Loeb translation by A. L. Peck (Cambridge, Mass., 1961), 183.

112. Hippocrates *Nutriment* 15, 39.

113. In chapter 10 of the treatise *The Heart*, the physician admires the way in which the sigmoid valves are adapted to their purpose; but this is a recent treatise, contemporary with Aristotle or later. In a treatise dating from the ancient period, *On Joints*, it is said in chapter 52 (Loeb III, 319), in connection with an unreduced inward dislocation of the thigh, that "the body finds out for itself the easiest posture." While the author adds that this is not a premeditated attitude, he does not share the view of the author of *Nutriment* that nature has no need of a teacher. Nature does in fact have a teacher: injury. "[T]he lesion itself teaches [the patient] to choose the easiest [attitude] available" (Loeb III, 317).

114. Aristotle *De partibus animalium* 1.1.639b19–21; see the Loeb translation by A. L. Peck (Cambridge, Mass., 1961), 57.

115. With regard to the expression "necessities of nature," see for example Hippocrates *Fleshes* 19.

116. Hippocrates *Breaths* 1 (Loeb II, 229). On art in general as an imitation of nature, see *Regimen* 11ff.

117. Hippocrates *Art* 13 (Loeb II, 215).

118. F. Bacon, *De dignitate et augmentis scientiarum* (London, 1623), II, 2.

119. Hippocrates *Epidemics I* 11 (Loeb I, 165).

Fourteen. The Legacy of Hippocratism in Antiquity

1. See pages 5–7. On the other accounts prior to the Hellenistic period, see chapter 4.

2. The two most important glossators of the third century B.C. were the Herophilean Bacchius of Tanagra (see page 63) and the dissident Herophilean Philinus of Cos, founder of the empiricist sect. But the first to have composed a glossary of Hippocrates was a grammarian, also of Cos, named Xenocrites (per the information given by Erotian in the preface to his *Glossary*). No doubt it was not accidental that two native Coan scholars should have devoted works to Hippocrates of Cos. Herophileans continued to produce scholarly works on Hippocrates after the time of Bacchius, among them Callimachus (third to second century B.C.), Zeno (second century B.C.), and Heraclides of Eritrea (first century B.C.).

3. Thus Cicero *Ad Atticum* 16.15.5: "[B]ut even Hippocrates forbids medical treatment in hopeless cases" (see D. R. Shackleton Bailey, ed., *Cicero's Letters to Atticus* [Cambridge, 1967], 6:209); *De natura deorum* 3.38.91: "[A]nd the bestowal of health upon many sick persons I ascribe to Hippocrates rather than to Aesculapius" (see the Loeb translation by H. Rackham [Cambridge, Mass., 1956], 377); and *De oratore* 3.33.132: "Do you really suppose that in the time of the great Hippocrates of Cos there were some physicians who specialized in medicine and others in surgery and others in ophthalmic cases?" (see the Loeb translation by H. Rackham [Cambridge, Mass., 1960], 2:103).

4. On this glossary, see pages 63ff.

5. The two most important references by Galen to these editions are found in his *Commentaries on Hippocrates' Nature of Man* (1.2) and on *Epidemics VI* (Arabic part). Many other allusions are sprinkled throughout his work. Some have seen the edition of Artemidorus as the source of our medieval manuscripts, but this hypothesis has been challenged.

6. Celsus *De medicina* prooem. 2–3, 5–8; see the Loeb translation by W. G. Spencer (Cambridge, Mass., 1960), 1:3–7.

7. Ibid., 66.

8. See also Seneca *Epistulae* 95.20 ("the greatest of physicians, the founder of medicine") and later Theodorus Priscianus 2.25 ("the guarantor of our profession").

9. Pliny *Natural History* 29.1–2; see the Loeb translation by W. H. S. Jones (Cambridge, Mass., 1963), 8:183–185.

10. Our source for this is Galen, who affirms it in a rather large number of passages in his work. These physicians devoted themselves particularly to the exegesis of Hippocratic texts.

11. In addition to Apollonius of Citium, whom we have already mentioned, one should note the following scholars of this school whose works of Hippocratic exegesis were used by Erotian: Glaucias (second century B.C.), Zeuxis (second century B.C.), Heraclides of Tarentum (first century B.C.).

12. Soranus has in mind several passages of Hippocrates here: *Aphorisms* 5.42, *Sterile Women* 216, *Superfoetation* 19. On these tests see pages 173ff.

13. Soranus *Diseases of Women* 1.15.

14. It was of particular interest to philosophers. In connection with Stoicism, see Epictetus 2.17.8 (cited at page 325; cf. 1.8.11: "See with what art Hippocrates expresses himself"); with Epicurianism, see Demetrius of Laconia, who cites the *Prognostic (PHerc.* 831), *Prorrhetic I*, and *Epidemics VI (PHerc.* 1012).

15. Plutarch *Life of Cato the Elder* 23.4 (cited at page 23).

16. The passages (with their Hippocratic equivalents) are as follows: 1. Plutarch 82d (= *Epidemics V* 27); 2. Plutarch 90c (= *Epidemics VI* 3.19); 3. Plutarch 127d10 (= *Aphorisms* 2.5); 4. Plutarch 291c (= *Breaths* 1); 5. Plutarch 455e (= *Prognostic* 2); 6. Plutarch 515a (= *Epidemics·VI* 3.19); 7. Plutarch 682e (= *Aphorisms* 1.3); 8. Plutarch 699c; 9. Plutarch 1047d; 10. Plutarch 1091c (= *Aphorisms* 1.3); 11. Plutarch 1099d (= *Aphorisms* 2.46).

17. Plutarch refers to this in his *Aitia romana* (291c).

18. See Plutarch *How to Profit from Your Enemies* 90c (a passage wrongly set aside in the Budé edition) and *Talkativeness* 515a.

19. Hippocrates *Epidemics VI* 3.19 (Loeb VII, 243).

20. Plutarch *The Control of Anger* 455e6ff.; see Robin Waterfield, trans., *Plutarch: Essays* (Harmondsworth, 1992), 182.

21. Montaigne, *Essais* (Paris, 1588), II, 31; see M. A. Screech, ed. and trans., *The Essays of Michel de Montaigne* (London, 1991), 810.

22. Plutarch *Progress in Virtue* 82d; see Waterfield, *Plutarch: Essays*, 138 (translation slightly modified).

23. Hippocrates *Epidemics V* 27 (Loeb VII, 179).

24. Quintilian *Institutio Oratoria* 3.6.64 (see the Loeb translation by H. E. Butler [Cambridge, Mass., 1963], 1:443); cf. Celsus 8.4.3–4.

25. W. Peek *Griechische Versinschriften* 1632.

26. During the same period, the Latin poet Aulus Gellius, in his *Noctes Atticae* (19.2.8), spoke of the "divine science" of Hippocrates and cited a passage that is not preserved in the Hippocratic Collection: "Coitus is a small epilepsy" (same passage found later in Macrobius *Saturnalia* 2.8.16). A half-century later, the Greek encyclopedist Athenaeus, a native of Naucratis in Egypt, described Hippocrates as "very holy" (9.399b), which did not, however, prevent him from making specific references to his work.

27. Peek *Griechische Versinschriften* 2040.

28. C. V. Daremberg, *Oeuvres anatomiques, physiologiques et médicales de Galien*, 2 vols. (Paris, 1854–1856), 1:1.

29. Galen *Med. Phil.* 1.

30. These four treatises, among others, are referred to: *Airs, Waters, Places, Places in Man, Prognostic*, and *Regimen in Acute Diseases*.

31. Galen *On My Own Books* 1.

32. Ibid., 6.

33. Galen *On the Order of My Own Books* 3.

34. See page 135 on his judgment of Hippocrates at the end of his treatise *Medical Questions*.

35. Palladius *Commentary on Epidemics VI of Hippocrates* 6.3.

36. Saint Jerome *Against John of Jerusalem* 38.

37. Ibid., 39.

38. Dante, *The Divine Comedy*, Purgatory XXIX, 136ff. ("*sommo Ippocrate*").

39. See Oribasius *Collectiones medicae* 1 (preface): "Galen prevails over all those who have treated the same subject because he avails himself of the most exact methods and definitions, given that he follows Hippocratic principles and opinions."

40. See Aëtius 5.83.

41. Ibid., 5.1.

42. This passage from *Epidemics VI* was cited and commented on earlier in the previous chapter at pages 346–347.

43. We should mention at this juncture a contemporary of Aëtius, the physician Alexander of Tralles, who cites Hippocrates sixteen times in his *Therapeutica* (in twelve books) and in two other treatises, one entitled *De febribus* ("On Fevers") and the other *De oculis* ("On the Eyes"). Hippocrates remained an authority for Alexander, who referred to him as "divine" or the "very divine Hippocrates." For him Galen and Hippocrates were the two greatest physicians, whose works rendered superfluous those of other physicians, such as Erasistratus and Asclepiades (see *On Fevers* 1 in Puschmann, ed., *Alexander von Tralles* (1878–1879), I, 291, 5–7).

44. *Anthologia Graeca* 11.382; see the Loeb translation by W. R. Paton (Cambridge, Mass., 1960), 4:253–255.

45. The *Aphorisms* were also commented on by the Byzantine Theophilus Protospatharius (ninth century?), who described Hippocrates as the "Prometheus of medicine" (*De corp. hum. fabr.* 5.20).

46. This information is given by Stephanus in the preface to his *Commentary on the Prognosticon of Hippocrates*. One began with the *Aphorisms*, which deals with all parts of medicine. Next came the works that treat of the normal condition of human beings: *Nature of Man, Nature of the Child, Humours, Nutriment*. One went on then to the works that treat of the pathological, a distinction being made between those concerning sporadic diseases (*Prognostic, Regimen in Acute Diseases, On Joints, On Fractures*) and those concerning general diseases, which in turn were subdivided into endemic

diseases (*Airs, Waters, Places*) and epidemic diseases (*Epidemics*). One finished with *Diseases of Women*.

47. In Paul of Aegina, there are forty-four citations of Hippocrates as against sixty-eight of Galen; in Aëtius, thirty-six citations of Hippocrates as against one hundred ninety-four of Galen.

48. On this procedure see page 137.

49. Paul of Aegina 6.112; see Francis Adams, *The Seven Books of Paulus Aegineta* (London, 1846), 2:479–480.

50. Cited by M.-H. Marganne, "De la réduction des luxations de la mâchoire: precédents antiques à la 'manoeuvre de Nélaton,' " *Revue médicale de Liège* 40 (1985): 105–108.

51. See chapter 1 of Ali ibn Ridwan, *Sur le chemin vers le bonheur par la profession médicale*, ed. A. Dietrich (Göttingen, 1982), 14–18.

52. Seven treatises were translated: *Airs, Waters, Places, Aphorisms, Diseases of Women, Nature of Man, Prognostic, Regimen, Sevens.*

53. See Cassiodorus *De institutione divinarum litterarum* 1.31: "Post haec, legite Hippocratem atque Galenum latina lingua conversos."

54. This was the treatise *Superfoetation*.

55. The Arabic translation thus preserved Galen's *Commentaries* on Hippocrates that are lost in Greek (on *Epidemics II, Airs, Waters, Places,* and fragments of a commentary on *The Oath*, whose authenticity is disputed).

56. This manuscript is *Parisinus graecus* 2141.

57. The first edition that appeared in Lyons in 1532 (*Hippocratis ac Galeni libri aliquot ex recognitione Fr. Rabelaesi*) went through six editions in the course of the sixteenth century, not only at Lyons but also at Venice, Salamanca, and Frankfurt. It consisted of the Latin translation (taken from earlier editions) of four great Hippocratic treatises (*Aphorisms, Prognostic, Regimen in Acute Diseases, Nature of Man*) as well as the Greek text of the *Aphorisms*. The Bibliothèque Nationale de Paris possesses a copy of the *princeps* edition of Hippocrates annotated by Rabelais himself.

58. See F. Robert, "Littré et Hippocrate," *Hist. Sc. Med.* 15 (1981): 221–226; J. Jouanna, "Littré, éditeur et traducteur de Hippocrate," *Revue de synthèse* (1982): 285–301; see also Jean Hamburger's chapter on Hippocrates in *Monsieur Littré* (Paris, 1988), 49–65.

59. See J. Pigeaud, "L'hippocratisme de Cardan: Étude sur le Commentaire d'*Airs, eaux, lieux* par Cardan," *Res Publica Litterarum* (University of Kansas) 8 (1985): 219–229.

60. See the ninth *mémoire* in volume II of the 1824 edition (132–232).

61. See Jean Brethe de la Gressaye, ed., *Oeuvres complètes du Montesquieu: L'Esprit des lois*, 4 vols. (Paris, 1950–1961), II, 173.

62. [Adamantios] Coray, *Traité d'Hippocrate Des airs, des eaux, des lieux, traduction nouvelle avec le texte grec*, vol. 1 (Paris, Year IX [1800]), III.

63. See M. Grmek, *La première révolution biologique* (Paris, 1990), particularly the

chapter "Hippocrate en France au XVIIe siècle" (285–299). For a specific example of the corruption of the Hippocratic text to suit a particular point of view, see J. Roger, *Les sciences de la vie dans la pensée française du XVIIIe siècle* (Paris, 1963), 27, n. 81.

64. What Sydenham valued in Hippocrates was that he had "clearly stated the symptoms of each disease without the help of any hypothesis or any system, as one sees in his books of the *Diseases, Affections*, etc." (see the preface to his first edition of the Hippocratic works [Amsterdam, 1683]). But his reading of Hippocrates is sometimes rather peculiar. For example, chapter 20 of *Ancient Medicine*, where the Hippocratic author denounces philosophically inclined medicine, he interprets as a criticism of those who "give more credit to a curious study of anatomy than to practical observations" (*Treatise on Dropsy*). Obviously, human anatomical knowledge is not at all at issue in this section.

65. Sydenham, *Methodus curandi febres: Variolae anomalae An[ni] 1674[–]75* [1st ed., Amsterdam, 1666], V, 4.

66. "Formerly Hippocrates was of Cos, now he is of Montpellier." Under the inscription is a bronze bust of Hippocrates placed on a marble column. This is an ancient bust, found in digs at Velletri (in Roman times the town of Velitrae, in Latium), and offered to the medical faculty at Montpellier by the local government under the First Empire. The inaugural address was delivered by Barthez ("Discours sur la génie d'Hippocrate prononcé le 4 messidor de l'an IX, dans l'école de médecine de Montpellier," in P. J. Barthez, *Nouveaux éléments de la science de l'homme* (Paris, 3rd enlarged ed., 1858), II, 233–281.

67. See L. Dulieu, *La médecine à Montpellier* (Avignon, 1983), III, 1, 230: Galen disappeared from the course list after 1684, whereas Hippocrates lasted until 1771.

68. On Laënnec and direct auscultation in Hippocrates, see page 300. On Laënnec and Hippocrates more generally, see J. Pigeaud, "L'Hippocratisme de Laennec," *Bull. Ass. Guillaume Budé* (1975): 357–363. It will be recalled that Laënnec did his medical thesis on *La doctrine d'Hippocrate* (1804).

69. It suffices to read M.-S. Houdart's work on Hippocrates (*Études historiques et critiques sur la vie et la doctrine d'Hippocrate*, 2nd ed. [Paris, 1840]) to appreciate the intensity of these struggles. Houdart, an admirer of Broussais, considered that it had fallen to the "illustrious founder of the physiological school" to "utterly shatter the scepter of Hippocratism" (303).

BIBLIOGRAPHY

I. GENERAL BIBLIOGRAPHY

A. A number of general works on Hippocrates or on medicine in antiquity deserve to be mentioned:

Amundsen, D. W. *Medicine, Society and Faith in the Ancient and Medieval Worlds.* Baltimore, 1995.

Ayache, L. *Hippocrate.* Paris, 1992.

Baissette, G. *Hippocrate.* Paris, 1931. (A fine novel about Hippocrates.)

Bourgey, L. *Observation et expérience chez les médecins de la Collection hippocratique.* Paris, 1953.

Brock, N. van. *Recherches sur le vocabulaire médical du grec ancien: soins et guérison.* Paris, 1961.

Cohn-Haft, L. *The Public Physicians of Ancient Greece.* Northampton, Mass., 1956.

Cordes, P. IATROS: *Das Bild des Arztes in der griechischen Literatur von Homer bis Aristoteles.* Stuttgart, 1994.

Corvisier, J.-N. *Santé et société en Grèce ancienne.* Paris, 1985.

Deichgräber, K. *Die Epidemien und das Corpus Hippocraticum.* Berlin, 1933; 2nd edition (with "Nachwort und Nachträge," 173–187), 1971.

———. *Ausgewählte Kleine Schriften.* Hildesheim, 1984.

Di Benedetto, V. *Il medico et la malattia: La scienze di Ippocrate.* Turin, 1986.

Diller, H. *Kleine Schriften zur antiken Medizin.* Berlin, 1973.

Ducatillon, J. *Polémiques dans la Collection hippocratique.* Lille/Paris, 1977.

Dumenil, M.-P. *Le sang, les vaisseaux, le coeur dans la Collection hippocratique: Anatomie et physiologie.* Paris, 1983.

Edelstein, L. *Peri Aeron und die Sammlung der hippokratischen Schriften.* Berlin, 1931.

———. "Nachträge (Hippokrates)." In *Real-Encyclopedie der classischen Altertumwissenschaft,* Suppl. 6 (1953): 1290–1345.

———. *Ancient Medicine* (collected papers). Baltimore, 1967.

Flashar, H. *Melancholie und Melancholiker in den medizinischen Theorien der Antike.* Berlin, 1966.

———, ed. *Antike Medizin.* Darmstadt, 1971. (An important collection of specialized papers.)

Foucault, M. *Histoire de la sexualité.* Paris, 1976.

Gossen, H. "Hippokrates." In *Real-Encyclopedie der classischen Altertumwissenschaft,* VIII (1913): 1801–1852.

Gourevitch, D. *Le triangle hippocratique dans le monde gréco-romain: Le malade, sa maladie et son médecin. BÉFAR* (École française de Rome) 251. Rome, 1984.

——, ed. *Maladie et maladies: Histoire et conceptualisation (Mélanges en l'honneur de M. Grmek)*. Geneva, 1992.

Grensemann, H. *Knidische Medizin*. 2 vols. Berlin, 1975; Stuttgart, 1987.

Grmek, M. D. *Les maladies à l'aube de la civilization orientale*. Paris, 1983.

——, ed. *Storia del pensiero medico occidentale*. Vol. I: *Antichità e Medioevo*. Bari, 1993.

Harris, C. R. S. *The Heart and the Vascular System in Ancient Greek Medicine*. Oxford, 1973.

Heidel, W. A. *Hippocratic Medicine: Its Spirit and Method*. New York, 1941.

Joly, R. *Le niveau de la science hippocratique*. Paris, 1966.

——. "Hippocrates of Cos." In C. C. Gillispie, ed., *Dictionary of Scientific Biography*. Volume VI. New York, 1972.

Jouanna, J. *Hippocrate: Pour une archéologie de l'école de Cnide*. Paris, 1974.

——. "Hippocrate." In *Encyclopaedia Universalis*. 2nd edition. Paris, 1989.

Koelbing, H. M. *Arzt und Patient in der antiken Welt*. Zurich, 1977.

Krug, A. *Heilkunst und Heilkult: Medizin in der Antike*. Munich, 1984.

Kudlien, F. *Der Beginn des medizinischen Denkens bei den Griechen*. Zurich/Stuttgart, 1967.

Lain Entralgo, P. *La Medicina hipocrática*. Madrid, 1970.

Langholf, V. *Medical Theories in Hippocrates: Early Texts and the "Epidemics."* Berlin, 1990.

Lichtenthaeler, C. *Der Eid des Hippokrates: Ursprung und Bedeutung*. Cologne, 1984. (Lichtenthaeler also published a series of fourteen Hippocratic studies in French and German [Geneva, 1948–1991].)

Lloyd, G. E. R. *Early Greek Science: Thales to Aristotle*. London, 1970.

——. *Magic, Reason, and Experience: Studies in the Origin and Development of Greek Science*. Cambridge, 1979.

——. *Science, Folklore, and Ideology: Studies in the Life Sciences of Ancient Greece*. Cambridge, 1983.

——. *Demystifying Mentalities*. Cambridge, 1990.

——. *Methods and Problems in Greek Science: Selected Papers*. Cambridge, 1991.

Majno, G. *The Healing Hand: Man and Wound in the Ancient World*. Cambridge, Mass., 1975.

Manuli, P., and M. Vegetti. *Cuore, sangue e cervello: Biologia e antropologia nel pensiero antico*. Milan, 1977.

Martiny, M. *Hippocrate et la médecine*. Paris, 1964.

Müri, W. *Der Arzt im Altertum*. 3rd edition. Munich, 1962.

Phillips, E. D. *Aspects of Greek Medicine*. Philadelphia, 1973; reprinted, 1987.

Pigeaud, J. *La maladie de l'âme*. Paris, 1981.

——. *Folie et cures de la folie chez les médecins de l'Antiquité gréco-romaine: La manie*. Paris, 1987.

Pinault, J. R. *Hippocratic Lives and Legends.* Leiden, 1992.

Pohlenz, M. *Hippokrates und die Begründung der wissenschaftlichen Medizin.* Berlin, 1938.

Potter, P. *Short Handbook of Hippocratic Medicine.* Québec, 1988.

Roselli, A. *La chirurgia ippocratica.* Florence, 1975.

Sarton, G. *A History of Science: Ancient Science through the Golden Age of Greece.* Cambridge, 1952.

Sendrail, M. *Histoire culturelle de la maladie.* Toulouse, 1980.

Skoda, F. *Médecine ancienne et métaphore: Le vocabulaire de l'anatomie et de la pathologie en grec ancien.* Paris, 1988.

Smith, W. D. *The Hippocratic Tradition.* Ithaca, 1979.

Staden, H. von. *Herophilus: The Art of Medicine in Early Alexandria.* Cambridge, 1989.

Thivel, A. *Cnide et Cos? Essai sur les doctrines médicales dans la Collection hippocratique.* Paris, 1981.

Vintro, E. *Hipocrates y la nosologia hipocrática.* Barcelona, 1972.

Vitrac, B. *Médecine et philosophie au temps d'Hippocrate.* Paris, 1989.

B. The best introduction to the modern study of Hippocrates is the series of conference proceedings volumes of the international Hippocratic Colloquia that have taken place every three years since 1972:

Bourgey, L., and J. Jouanna, eds. *La Collection hippocratique et son rôle dans l'histoire de la médecine: Colloque de Strasbourg (23–27 octobre 1972).* Leiden, 1975.

Joly, R., ed. *Corpus Hippocraticum: Actes du Colloque hippocratique de Mons (22–26 septembre 1975).* Mons, 1977.

Grmek, M. D., and F. Robert, eds. *Hippocratica: Actes du Colloque hippocratique de Paris (4–9 septembre 1978).* Paris, 1980.

Lasserre, F., and P. Mudry, eds. *Formes de pensée dans la Collection hippocratique: Actes du IVe Colloque international hippocratique (Lausanne, 21–26 septembre 1981).* Geneva, 1983.

Baader, G., and R. Winau, eds. *Die hippokratischen Epidemien: Theorie-Praxis-Tradition . . . : Ve Colloque international hippocratique (Berlin, 10–15 September 1984).* Stuttgart, 1988. (= *Sudhoffs Archiv,* Special Issue 27.)

Potter, P., G. Maloney, and J. Desautels, eds. *La maladie et les maladies dans la Collection hippocratique: Actes du VIe Colloque international hippocratique (Québec, 28 septembre–3 octobre 1987).* Québec, 1990.

López Férez, J. A., ed. *Tratadós Hipocrático (Estudios acerca de su contenido, forma e influencia): Actas del VIIe colloque international hippocratique (Madrid, 24–29 de Septiembre de 1990).* Madrid, 1992.

Wittern, R., and P. Pellegrin, eds. *Hippokratische Medizin und antike Philosophie: Verhandlungen des VIII. Internationalen Hippokrates-Kolloquiums in Kloster Banz / Staffelstein vom 23. bis 28. September 1993.* Vol. I of *Medizin der Antike,* ed. G. Preiser. Hildesheim, 1996.

See also in this connection:

Imbert-Valassopoulos, C., ed. *Hippocrate et son héritage*. Franco-Hellenic Colloquium in the History of Medicine, Fondation Marcel Mérieux (Lyons, 9–12 October 1985). Lyons, n.d.

Demont, P., ed. *Médecine antique*. Five studies by J. Jouanna, A. Debreu, P. Demont, and M. Perrin. Amiens, 1991.

Eijk, P. van der, H. F. J. Hortmanshoff, and P. H. Schrijvers, eds. *Ancient Medicine in Its Socio-cultural Context*. Papers read at the congress held at the University of Leiden, 13–15 April 1992. 2 vols. Amsterdam, 1995.

Ginouvès, R., A.-M. Guimier-Sorbets, J. Jouanna, and L. Villard. *L'eau, la santé et la maladie dans le monde grec*. BCH (École française d'Athènes), Suppl. 28 (1994).

C. The basic edition of Hippocrates is the Greek-French edition of Émile Littré, *Oeuvres complètes d'Hippocrate*, 10 vols. (Paris, 1839–1861). The French translation has been separately published as *Hippocrate: Oeuvres complètes*, edited with commentary by P. Theil and T. Vetter, 4 vols. (Paris: 1979–1989). Littré's edition has not been entirely superseded, though many of the treatises have been reedited on a sounder manuscript basis in a number of collections: Teubner (Greek text only), *CMG* (initially, Greek text only; later, Greek with translation into a modern language), Loeb (Greek-English), and Budé (Greek-French). For editions of specific treatises, see the list in appendix 3.

A selection of treatises in English translation may be found in the Pelican Classics volume *Hippocratic Writings*, edited with an introduction by G. E. R. Lloyd and translated by J. Chadwick, W. N. Mann, I. M. Lonie, and E. T. Withington. London, 1978; reprinted 1983.

There exist a complete concordance and a complete index of Greek words:

Kühn, J. H., and U. Fleischer, *Index Hippocraticus; cui elaborando interfuerunt sodales* THESAURI LINGUAE GRAECAE *Hamburgensis: Curas postremas adhibuerunt K. Alpers A. Anastassiou D. Irmer V. Schmidt*. 4 vols. Göttingen, 1986–1989.

Maloney, G., and W. Frohn. *Concordance des oeuvres hippocratiques*. 6 vols. Hildesheim, 1989.

The most complete bibliography concerning Hippocrates is to be found in:

Maloney, G., and R. Savoie, eds. *Cinq cent ans de bibliographie hippocratique*. Québec, 1982. (To be completed for recent years in collaboration with the *Newsletter* of the Society for Ancient Medicine at the University of Pennsylvania, now published at the University of Michigan as the *Society for Ancient Medicine Review*.)

Bruni Celli, B. *Bibliografia Hipocrática*. Caracas, 1984.

Leitner, H. *Bibliography to the Ancient Medical Authors.* Bern/Stuttgart/Vienna, 1973 (for the editions).

II. SUPPLEMENTARY BIBLIOGRAPHY BY CHAPTER

Neither the general works nor the conference proceedings volumes already cited are mentioned in what follows.

One. Hippocrates of Cos

Dugand, J.-E. *Essai sur la vie d'Hippocrate.* Doctoral thesis. Nice, 1987.

Gamberale, M. "Ricerche sul *genos* degli Asclepiadi." *Rend. Accad. Lincei* 33 (1978): 83–95.

———. "La genealogia di Ippocrate di Cos e gli Asclepiadi di Rodi." *Rend. Accad. Lincei* 35 (1980): 109–116.

Huet, G. "La légende de la fille d'Hippocrate à Cos." *Bibl. de l'École des chartes* (Paris) 79 (1919): 45–59.

Jouanna, J. "Collaboration ou résistance au barbare: Artémise d'Halicarnasse et Cadmos de Cos chez Hérodote et Hippocrate." *Ktema* 9 (1984): 15–26.

Kudlien, F. "Hippokrateszitate in der altgriechischen Komödie?" *Episteme* 4 (1971): 279–284.

Petersen, C. "Zeit und Lebensverhältnisse des Hippokrates." *Philologus* (1849): 209–265.

Pugliese Carratelli, G. "Gli Asclepiadi e il Sinecismo di Cos." *La parola del Passato* 12 (1957): 333–342.

———. "Il damos Coo di Isthmos." *Ann. Scuola Arch. di Atene,* n.s., 25–26 (1963–1964): 147–202.

———. "La norma etica degli Asklapiadai di Cos." *La parola del Passato* 46 (1991): 81–94.

———. "ΑΠΟΓΟΝΟΙ ΑΣΚΛΗΠΙΟΥ ΚΑΙ ΗΡΑΚΛΕΟΥΣ." In U. Albini et al., eds., *Storia, poesia e pensiero nel mondo antico: Studi in onore di Marcello Gigante,* 543–547. Naples, 1994.

Robert, F. "Hippocrate et le clergé d'Asclépios à Cos." *CR Acad. Inscr.* (1939): 91–99.

Schöne, H. I. "Bruchstücke einer neuen Hippokratesvita." *Rheinisches Museum* 58 (1903): 55–66.

Sherwin-White, S. M. *Ancient Cos.* Göttingen, 1978.

Sudhoff, K. "Eine mittelalterliche Hippokrates-Vita." *Archiv für Geschichte der Medizin* 8 (1915): 404–413.

———. *Kos und Knidos.* Munich, 1927.

Two. Hippocrates the Thessalian

Bousquet, J. "Inscriptions de Delphes." *BCH* 80 (1956): 579–591. (See, in particular, no. 7, "Delphes et les Asclépiades.")

Brunn, W. von. "Das Grabmal des Hippokrates." *Münchener Medizinische Wochenschrift* 88 (1947): 474–475.

Cavaignac, E. "Le Presbeutikos et la Biographie d'Hippocrate." *Le Courrier d'Épidaure* (Paris) 16, no. 3–4 (1949): 16–25.

Chamoux, F. "Perdiccas." In M. Renard, ed., *Hommages à Albert Grenier*, 386–396. Brussels, 1962.

Fronimopoulos, J., and J. Stefanellis. "Four Legends about Hippocrates, Collected by Mr. Zarakas of the Village Pili—Cos." *Documenta Ophthalmologica* 68 (1988): 3–8.

Herzog, R. "Die Grabschrift des Thessalos von Kos." *Quellen und Studien zur Geschichte der Naturwissenschaften und der Medizin* 3, no. 4 (1933): 54–58 [= 262–266].

Hillert, A. "Antike Ärztedarstellungen." *Marburger Schriften zur Medizingeschichte* 25 (1990): 24–40. (On the most recent developments in the representation of Hippocrates, with bibliography.)

Mesk, J. "Aegritudo Perdicae." *Wiener Studien* 57 (1939): 166–172.

Meyer-Steineg, T. "Hippokrates-Erzählungen." *Archiv für Geschichte der Medizin* 6 (1912): 1–11. (Tales of an islander recorded on Cos in 1910.)

Pomtow, H. "Hippokrates und die Asklepiaden in Delphi." *Klio* 15 (1918): 303ff.

Rubin Pinault, J. "How Hippocrates Cured the Plague?" *Journal of the History of Medicine and Allied Sciences* 41 (1986): 52–75.

Wickersheimer, E. "Légendes hippocratiques du Moyen Âge." *Archiv für Geschichte der Medizin* 45 (1961): 164–175.

Three. Hippocrates and the School of Cos

Fraser, P. M. *Ptolemaic Alexandria*. Vol. I, 343–346. Oxford, 1952. (On the school of Cos after Hippocrates.)

Grensemann, H. "Polybos." In Pauly-Wissowa, Suppl. 14 (1974): 428–436.

———. "Die sogenannten 'Sentenzen der Knidier', oder Knidische Medizin im Corpus Hippocraticum: Eine Replik." *Würzburger medizinhistorische Mitteilungen* 10 (1992): 137–160. (Reply to the article by Kollesch cited below.)

Joly, R. "Hippocrates and the School of Cos: Between Myth and Skepticism." In *Nature Animated II*, ed. M. Ruse, 29–47. Dordrecht, 1983.

Jouanna, J. "Le problème des écoles médicales en Grèce classique: réinterpretation de témoignages épigraphiques et littéraires." *Actes du Xᵉ Congrès de l'Association Guillaume Budé* (Toulouse, 8–12 avril 1978), 312–314. Paris, 1980.

Kollesch, J. "Knidos als Zentrum der frühen wissenschaftlichen Medizin im antiken Griechenland." *Gesnerus* 46 (1989): 11–28.

Kudlien, F. *Der griechische Arzt im Zeitalter des Hellenismus*. Wiesbaden, 1979.

Lonie, I. M. "Cos versus Cnidus and the historians." *History of Science* 16 (1978): 42–75 and 77–92.

Mansfeld, J. "The historical Hippocrates and the origin of scientific medicine." In *Nature Animated II*, ed. M. Ruse, 49–76. Dordrecht, 1983.

Rosenthal, F. "An ancient commentary on the Hippocratic Oath." *Bulletin of the History of Medicine* 30 (1956): 52–87.

Smith, W. D. "Galen on Coans versus Cnidians." *Bulletin of the History of Medicine* 47 (1973): 569–578.

Wellmann, M. "Hippokrates, des Thessalos Sohn." *Hermes* 61 (1926): 329–334.

Four. *Writings in Search of an Author*

Blass, F. "Die pseudohippokratische Schrift *Peri physon* und der Anonymus Londinensis." *Hermes* 36 (1901): 405–410.

Capelle, W. "Zur hippokratischen Frage." *Hermes* 57 (1922): 247–265.

Diels, H. "Über die Excerpte von Menons *Iatrika* in dem Londoner Papyrus 137." *Hermes* 28 (1893): 406–434.

———. "Über einen neuen Versuch, die Echtheit einiger hippokratischen Schriften nachzuweisen." *Königl. Preuss. Akad. Wiss.* (Berlin) (1910): 1140–1155.

Gomperz, T. "Die hippokratische Frage und der Ausgangspunkt ihrer Lösung." *Philologus* 70 (1911): 213–241.

Herter, H. "The problematic mention of Hippocrates in Plato's *Phaedrus*." *Illinois Classicial Studies* 1 (1976): 22–42.

Joly, R. "La question hippocratique et le témoignage du *Phèdre*." *Revue des études grecques* 74 (1961): 69–92.

Jouanna, J. "La *Collection hippocratique* et Platon." *Revue des études grecques* 90 (1977): 15–28.

———. "Remarques sur les réclames dans la tradition hippocratique: Analyse archéologique du texte des manuscrits." *Ktema* 2 (1977): 381–396.

Langholf, V. "Kallimachos, Komödie und hippokratische Frage." *Med.-hist. Journal* 21 (1986): 3–30.

Lloyd, G. E. R. "The Hippocratic Question." *Classical Quarterly*, n.s., 25 (1975): 171–192.

Schöne, H. "Echte Hippokratesschriften." *Deutsche Medizinische Wochenschrift* 36 (1910): 418–466.

Steckerl, F. "Plato, Hippocrates and the Menon Papyrus." *Classical Philology* 40 (1945): 166–180.

Five. *The Physician and the Public*

Bucheim, L. "Das Verdikt der 'nicht behandelbaren Krankheit' in der altägyptischen Medizin." *Sudhoffs Archiv* 49 (1965): 170–184.

Jouanna, J. "Rhétorique et médecine dans la *Collection hippocratique*: Contribution à l'histoire de la rhétorique au Ve siècle." *Revue des études grecques* 97 (1984): 26–44.

Lanza, D. *Lingua e discorso nell'Atene delle professioni.* Naples, 1979.

Thivel, A. "Diagnostic et pronostic à l'époque d'Hippocrate et à la nôtre." *Gesnerus* 42 (1985): 479–497.

Wittern, R. "Die Unterlassung ärztlicher Hilfeleistung in der griechischen Medizin der klassischen Zeit." *Münch. med. Wochenschrift* 121 (1979): 731–734.

Six. The Physician and the Patient

Deichgräber, K. "Medicus gratiosus: Untersuchungen zu einem griechischen Arztbild." *Akademie der Wissenschaften und der Literatur: Abhandlungen der Geistes- und sozialwissenschaftlichen* (Mainz), no. 3 (1970): 1–119.

——. "Die Patienten des Hippokrates: Historisch-prosopographische Beiträge zu den *Epidemien* des *Corpus Hippocraticum*." *Abhandl. der Akad. der Wiss. und der Lit.* (Mainz), no. 9 (1982): 1–42.

Ducatillon, J. "Du *régime*, livre III: Les deux publics." *Revue des études grecques* 82 (1969): 33–42.

Joly, R. "Esclaves et médecins dans la Grèce antique." *Sudhoffs Archiv* 53 (1969): 1–14.

Kudlien, F. *Die Sklaven in der griechischen Medizin der klassischen und hellenistischen Zeit.* Wiesbaden, 1968.

——. "Medical ethics and popular ethics in Greece and Rome." *Clio Medica* 5 (1970): 91–121.

Mueri, W. *Arzt und Patient bei Hippokrates.* Bern, 1936.

Seven. The Physician and the Disease

Artelt, W. *Studien zur Geschichte der Begriffe "Heilmittel" und "Gift."* Leipzig, 1937.

Byl, S. "Rheumatism and gout in the *Corpus Hippocraticum*." *Antiquité classique* 57 (1988): 89–102.

Byl, S., and W. Szafran. "La Phrénitis dans le Corpus hippocratique: Étude philologique et médicale." *Vesalius* 2, no. 2 (1996): 98–105.

Craik, E. "Hippocratic Diaita." In J. Wilkins, D. Harvey, and M. Dobson, ed., *Food in Antiquity*, 343–350. Exeter, 1995.

Demand, N. *Birth, Death and Motherhood in Classical Greece.* Baltimore, 1994.

Dierbach, J. H. *Die Arzneimittel des Hippokrates.* Heidelberg, 1824.

Goltz, D. "Studien zur altorientalischen und griechischen Heilkunde, Therapie, Arzneibereitung, Rezeptstruktur." *Sudhoffs Archiv*, Special Issue 16 (1974).

Grmek, M. D. "Les ruses de guerre biologiques dans l'Antiquité." *Revue des études grecques* 92 (1979): 141–163.

——. "Les cas de tétanos dans le livre V des *Epidémies* hippocratiques." In *Histoire de la médecine: Leçons méthodologiques*, ed. D. Gourevitch. Paris, 1995.

Grmek, M. D., and R. Wittern. "Die Nierenkrankheit des attischen Strategen Nikias und die Nierenleiden im *Corpus Hippocraticum*." *Arch. Intern. Hist. Sci.* 26 (1977): 3–22.

Hanson, A. E. "Continuity and change: three case studies in Hippocratic gynecological therapy and theory." In *Women's History and Ancient History*, ed. S. B. Pomeroy, 73–110. Chapel Hill, 1991.

——. "Obstetrics in the *Hippocratic Corpus* and Soranos." *Forum* 4, no. 1 (1994): 93–110.

Jouanna, J. "La maladie sauvage dans la *Collection hippocratique* et la tragédie grecque." *Métis* 3 (1988): 343–360.

King, H. "Food and Blood in Hippocratic Gynaecology." In *Food in Antiquity*, ed. J. Wilkins, D. Harvey, and M. Dobson, 351–358. Exeter, 1995.

Lloyd, G. E. R. The female sex: medical treatment and biological theories in the fifth and fourth centuries B.C. Part II of *Science, Folklore and Ideology*. Cambridge, 1983.

Lorenz, G. *Antike Krankenbehandlung in historisch-vergleichender Sicht: Studien zum Konkret-anschaulichen Denken.* Heidelberg, 1990.

Preiser, G. *Allgemeine Krankheitsbezeichnungen im Corpus Hippocraticum.* Berlin, 1976.

Riddle, J. M. *Contraception and Abortion from the Ancient World to the Renaissance.* Cambridge, Mass., 1992.

Staden, Heinrich von. "Matière et signification: Rituel, sexe et pharmacologie dans le *Corpus hippocratique*." *L'Antiquité classique* 60 (1991): 42–61.

Stannard, J. "Hippocratic Pharmocology." *Bull. Hist. Med.* 35 (1961): 497–518.

Temkin, O. *The Falling Sickness: A History of Epilepsy from the Greeks to the Beginnings of Modern Neurology.* Baltimore, 1945; 2nd revised edition, 1971.

Eight. Hippocratic Rationalism and the Divine

Dodds, E. R. *The Greeks and the Irrational.* Berkeley and Los Angeles, 1951.

Edelstein, E. J., and L. *Asclepius: A Collection and Interpretation of the Testimonies.* Baltimore, 1945.

Eijk, P. J. van der. "The 'Theology' of the Hippocratic Treatise *On the Sacred Disease*." *Apeiron* 23 (1990): 87–119.

Grmek, M. D. "Les vicissitudes des notions d'infection, de contagion et de germe dans la médecine antique." In *Mémoires V du Centre Jean-Palerne: Textes médicaux latins antiques,* 53–70. Saint-Étienne, 1984.

Herzog, R. *Die Wunderheilungen von Epidauros* [= *Philologus*, Suppl. 22, no. 3 (1931): 1–164]. Leipzig, 1931.

Jouanna, J. "Hippocrate de Cos et le sacré." *Journal des savants* (January–June 1989): 3–22.

——. "Médecine hippocratique et tragédie grecque." In *Anthropologie et théâtre antique* (Actes du Colloque international de Montpellier, 6–8 March 1986). *Cahiers du Gita* 3 (1987): 109–131.

Kudlien, F. "Das Göttliche und die Natur im hippokratischen *Prognostikon*." *Hermes* 105 (1977): 268–274.

Lanata, G. *Medicina magica e religione popolare in Grecia fino all'età di Ippocratica.* Rome, 1967.

Lichtenthaeler, C. *Thucydide et Hippocrate vus par un historien-médecin.* Geneva, 1965.

Martin, R., and H. Metzger. L'évolution du culte d'Asclépios en Grèce. Chapter II of *La religion grecque.* Paris, 1976.

Nestle, W. "Hippocratica." *Hermes* 73 (1938): 1–38.

Parker, R. *Miasma, Pollution and Purification in Early Greek Religion.* Oxford, 1983.

Rechenauer, G. *Thukydides und die hippokratische Medizin.* Hildesheim, 1991.

Temkin, O. *The Falling Sickness: A History of Epilepsy from the Greeks to the Beginnings of Modern Neurology.* Baltimore, 1945; 2nd revised edition, 1971.

Weidauer, K. *Thukydides und die hippokratischen Schriften: Der Einfluss der Medizin auf Zielsetzung und Darstellungsweise des Geschichtswerks.* Heidelberg, 1954.

Nine. Hippocrates and the Birth of the Human Sciences

Desautels, J. *L'image du monde selon Hippocrate.* Québec, 1982.

Edelstein, L. *The Idea of Progress in Classical Antiquity.* Baltimore, 1967.

Guthrie, W. K. C. *In the Beginning: Some Greek Views on the Origins of Life and the Early State of Man.* London, 1957.

Herter, H. "Die kulturhistorische Theorie der hippokratischen Schrift von der *Alten Medizin.*" *Maia* 15 (1963): 464–483.

Jouanna, J. "Les causes de la défaite des Barbares chez Eschyle, Hérodote et Hippocrate." *Ktema* 6 (1981): 3–15.

Romilly, J. de. "Thucydide et l'idée de progrès." *Annali della scuola normale superiore di Pisa (Lettere, storia e filosofia)* 35 (1966): 143–191.

——. "La vue d'en haut: découverte des sciences de l'homme." Chapter III of *La construction de la vérité chez Thucydide.* Paris, 1990.

Sassi, M. M. *La scienza dell'uomo nella Grecia antica.* Turin, 1988.

Ten. Challenges to Medicine and the Birth of Epistemology

Demont, P. "Die *Epideixis* über die *Techne* im V. und IV. JR." In *Vermittlung und Tradierung von Wissen in der griechischen Kultur,* ed. W. Kullmann and J. Althoff, 181–209. Tübingen, 1993.

Heinimann, F. "Eine vorplatonische Theorie der τέχνη." *Museum Helveticum* 18 (1961): 105–130.

Herter, H. "Die Treffkunst des Arztes in hippokratischer und platonischer Sicht." *Sudhoffs Archiv Gesch. Med.* 47 (1963): 247–290.

Jori, A. *Medicina e medici nell'Antica Grecia: Saggio sul Perì Téchnes ippocratico.* Istituto Italiano per gli Studi Storici. Naples, 1996.

Jouanna, J. "Le médecin modèle du législateur dans les *Lois* de Platon." *Ktema* 3 (1978): 77–91.

Pigeaud, J. "Le style d'Hippocrate ou l'écriture fondatrice de la médecine." In *Les savoirs de l'écriture en Grèce ancienne,* ed. M. Detienne, 305–329. Lille, 1988.

Romilly, J. de. "La médecine comme modèle intellectuel dans la Grèce antique." In *Rencontres avec la Grèce antique,* 201–216. Paris, 1995.

Eleven. Medicine in Crisis and the Reaction against Philosophy

Joly, R. *Recherches sur le traité pseudo-hippocratique du Régime.* Volume 156 of *Bibliothèque de la faculté de philosophie et lettres de l'université de Liège.* Paris, 1960.

Jones, W. H. S. *Philosophy and Medicine in Ancient Greece.* Baltimore, 1946.

Kühn, J. H. *Systeme- und Methodenprobleme im Corpus Hippocraticum* [= *Hermes*, Einzelschriften XI]. Wiesbaden, 1956.

Lesky, E. *Die Zeugungs- und Vererbungslehren der Antike und ihr Nachwirken.* Wiesbaden, 1950. [= *Abhandl. der Akad. der Wiss. und der Lit.* (Mainz), no. 19 (1950): 1227 (1)–1425 (201)].

Lloyd, G. E. R. "Aspects of the interrelations of medicine, magic and philosophy in ancient Greece." *Apeiron* 9 (1975): 1–16.

Longrigg, J. "Philosophy and medicine." *Harvard Studies in Classical Philology* 67 (1963): 147–175.

———. *Greek Rational Medicine: Philosophy and Medicine from Alcmaeon to the Alexandrians.* London, 1993.

Mansfeld, J. *The Pseudo-Hippocratic Tract ΠΕΡΙ ΕΒΔΟΜΑΔΩΝ ch. 1–11 and Greek Philosophy.* Assen, 1971.

Stückelberger, A. *Vestigia Democritea: Die Rezeption der Lehre von den Atomen in der antiken Naturwissenschaft und Medizin.* Basel, 1984.

Twelve. From Observation of the Visible to Reconstruction of the Invisible

Coury, C. *L'hippocratisme digital.* Paris, 1960.

———. "Le signe du doigt hippocratique." *Pagine Stor. Med.* 12 (1968): 3–12.

Grmek, M. D. "L'expérimentation biologique quantitative dans l'Antiquité." In *La première révolution biologique*, 17–43. Paris, 1990.

———. *Le chaudron de Médée: L'expérimentation sur le vivant dans l'Antiquité.* Paris, 1997.

Kudlien, F. "Antike Anatomie und menschlicher Leichnam." *Hermes* 97 (1969): 78–94.

Regenbogen, O. "Eine Forschungsmethode antiker Naturwissenschaft." *Quellen und Studien zur Geschichte der Mathematik.* Abt. B, I, 2 (1930): 131–182.

Senn, G. "Uber Herkunft und Stil der Beschreibungen von Experimenten im *Corpus Hippocraticum*." *Arch. Gesch. Med.* 22 (1929): 217–289.

Thirteen. Health, Sickness, and Nature

Jouanna, J. "Hippocrate et la santé." In *La santé*, ed. L. Braun, 17–47. Centre de documentation en histoire de la philosophie (Cahiers du Séminaire de philosophie, vol. 8). Strasbourg, 1988.

Kudlien, F. "The old Greek concept of relative health." *Journal of the History of Behavioral Sciences* 9, no. 1 (1973): 53–59.

———. "Die Beudeutung des Ungeraden in der hippokratischen Krisenarithmetik." *Hermes* 108 (1980): 200–205.

Sobel, H. *Hygieia: Der Göttin der Gesundheit.* Darmstadt, 1990.

Wöhrle, G. *Studien zur Theorie der antiken Gesundheitslehre* [= *Hermes*, Einzelschriften LVI]. Stuttgart, 1990.

Fourteen. The Legacy of Hippocratism in Antiquity

Byl, S. *Recherches sur les grands traités biologiques d'Aristote: sources écrites et préjugés.* Brussels, 1980.

Deichgräber, K. *Die grieche Empirikerschule.* 2nd edition. Berlin/Zurich, 1965.

Flashar, H. "Beiträge zur spätantiken Hippokratesdeutung." *Hermes* 110 (1962): 402–418.

Ilberg, J. "Die Hippokratesausgaben des Artemidoros Kapiton und Dioskurides." *Rheinisches Museum für Philologie,* n.f., 45 (1890): 111–137.

Irigoin, J. "Hippocrate et la *Collection hippocratique.*" *Annuaire du Collège de France* (1987–1988): 629–647.

——. "Hippocrate, Galien, et quelques autres médecins grecs." *Annuaire du Collège de France* (1988–1989): 585–603.

Iskandar, A. Z. "An attempted reconstruction of the late Alexandrian medical curriculum." *Medical History* 20 (1976): 235–258.

Jacquart, D., and F. Micheau. *Le médecine arabe et l'occident médiéval.* Paris, 1996.

Jouanna, J. "Médicine et politique dans la *Politique* d'Aristote." *Ktema* 5 (1980): 257–266.

——. "Remarques sur la valeur relative des traductions latines pour l'édition des textes hippocratiques." In *Le latin médical,* ed. G. Sabbah, 11–26. Saint-Étienne, 1991.

Kibre, P. *Hippocrates latinus: A repertorium of Hippocratic writings in the Latin Middle Ages.* New York, 1985; rev. edition, 1995.

Manetti, D., and A. Roselli. "Galeno commentatore di Ippocrate." *ANRW,* II, 37, 2 (1994): 1528–1635.

Marganne, M.-H. "De la réduction des luxations de la mâchoire: précédents antiques à la 'manoeuvre de Nélaton'." *Rev. Méd. Liège* 40 (1985): 105–108.

Nutton, V. "What's in an oath?" *Journal of the Royal College of Physicians of London* 29 (1995): 518–524.

Sezgin, F. *Medizin-Pharmazie Zoologie-Tierheilkunde.* Vol. III of *Geschichte des arabischen Schrifttums,* 27–39. Leiden, 1970.

Strohmaier, G. "La tradition hippocratique en latin et en arabe." In *Le latin médical,* ed. G. Sabbah, 27–39. Saint-Étienne, 1991.

Temkin, O. "Geschichte des Hippokratismus im ausgehenden Altertum." *Kylos* 4 (1932): 1–80.

——. "Hippokrates." *Reallexicon für Antike und Christentum* 15 (1991): cols. 466–481.

——. *Hippocrates in a World of Pagans and Christians.* Baltimore, 1991.

Ullmann, M. "Die Periode der Übersetzungen." Chapter 2 of *Die Medizin im Islam,* especially 25–35. Leiden, 1970.

Wolska-Conus, W. "Les commentaires de Stéphanos d'Athènes au *Prognostikon* et aux *Aphorismes* d'Hippocrate." *Revue des Études Byzantines* 50 (1992): 5–86.

——. "Stéphanos d'Athènes (d'Alexandrie) et Théophile le Prôtospathaire: Commentateurs des *Aphorismes* d'Hippocrate sont-ils indépendants l'un de l'autre?" *Revue des Études Byzantines* 52 (1994): 5–68.

———. "Sources des commentaires de Stéphanos d'Athènes et de Théophile le Prô-tospathaire aux *Aphorismes* d'Hippocrate." *Revue des Études Byzantines* 54 (1996): 5–66.

Aelian
On the Nature of Animals: 9.33, 200; *12.16*
(= DK 68A151), 462 n. 63
Varia Historia: 4.20, 20 (n. 61)
Aelius Aristides
Asclepiads: 11ff., 11 (n. 24), 12
To the Rhodians on Concord: 45, 421 n. 28
Aeschines
Against Ctesiphon: 107ff. (= Anthologia
Graeca *6.330*), 13 (n. 31), 200
Aeschylus
Agamemnon: 848–850, 155; *1001–1003*,
332; *1623*, 102 (n. 104)
Eumenides: 62, 102 (n. 104); *658–661*, 271
Persians: 354ff., 231; *715*, 204
Philoctetes (frag. 253 Radt), 142
Prometheus Bound: 442ff., 232 (n. 71);
473–475, 92; *474–480*, 236 (n. 72);
478–481, 236 (n. 70); *478–483*, 126;
479–480, 233; *480*, 238; *482*, 237
(n. 73)
Suppliants: 263, 102 (n. 104); *659*, 204
Aëtius of Amida
3.4.4 (D.371), 260 (n. 3); *3.16.1 (D.381)*,
260 (n. 2); *5.1*, 358–9; *5.18.1 (D.427)*,
270 (n. 51); *5.30.1 (D.442)*, 327 (n. 23);
5.83, 358; *5.95*, 33 (n. 35)
Agathias
(Anthologia Graeca *11.382*), 359
Agathon
Frag. 6 and 8 Snell, 250 (n. 19)
Alcmaeon
DK 24A1 (= *Diogenes Laertius 8.83*), 262
(nn. 7, 10); DK 24A3 (= *Aristotle*
Metaphysics *1.5.986a*), 262 (nn. 7–9);
DK 24A15 (= *Aristotle* Historia Ani-
malium *7.1.581a*), 339 (n. 70); DK
24B1, 460 n. 7; DK 24B4 (= *Aëtius*
5.30.1 [D.442]), 327; DK 24B4
(= *Plutarch* Epitom. *5.30* and Stobaeus
Ecl. *4.35–36*), 262 (n. 11)

Alexander of Aphrodisius
Commentary on the Meteorologica *of Aris-
totle: 353a32*, 460 n. 4
Alexander of Tralles
On Fevers: 1, 477 n. 43
Anaxagoras
DK 59A1 (= *Diogenes Laertius 2.12–14*),
263–4 (n. 27); DK 59A16 (= *Plutarch*
Life of Pericles 6), 264 (n. 28); DK
59A43 (= *Aristotle* De caelo
3.3.302a28ff.), 264 (nn. 23–24, 26);
DK 59A43 (= *Aristotle* Metaphysics
1.3.984a11–13), 264 (n. 22); DK 59A44
(= *Lucretius 835–838*), 264 (n. 24); DK
59B10 (= schol. Gregory of Nazianzus
36.911 Migne), 264 (n. 25); DK
59B21a, 318
Anaximander
DK 12A27 (= *Aëtius 3.16.1 [D.371]*),
260
Andreas
Genealogy of Physicians, 26 (n. 5)
Anonymus Iamblichi
DK 89.6.1, 457 n. 76
Anonymus Londinensis
4.31–40 and 4.40–5.34, 432 n. 35; *5.35–
6.18 and 6.31–43*, 59–60; *6.43–45 and
7.1ff.*, 435 n. 13; *11.22*, 266 (n. 37);
12.8–36, 48 (n. 30); *18.8ff.*, 267
(n. 42); *18.30ff.*, 267 (n. 43); *19.1–18*,
400; *19.2ff.*, 62
Anthologia Graeca
6.136 and 6.142, 118 (n. 30); *6.330*, 200
(n. 57); *6.337* (= *Theocritus* Epigrams
8), 203 (n. 70); *7.135*, 37 (n. 54); *7.508*,
419 n. 17; *11.382*, 359 (n. 44)
Antiphon
On the Chorus Boy: 17, 129 (n. 72)
Antyllus
(*Oribasius* Collectiones medicae *8.13*),
159 (n. 68)

wrote any of the dozens of treatises attributed to him.

Jacques Jouanna contends that a great deal can be concluded about the life and works of Hippocrates. Published to both critical and popular acclaim in France in 1992, *Hippocrates* reveals a man who was not only the greatest of the ancient physicians but also a philosopher of unrecognized ability and consequence who influenced both Plato and Aristotle; a historian who was the equal of Herodotus and Thucydides as a writer and superior to them in his powers of observation and analysis; and a master of tragical narrative who bears comparison with Aeschylus, Sophocles, and Euripides, the great playwrights of the classical period. Now that Hippocrates has at last emerged from the hagiographic mists of Byzantium and medieval Europe, the justice of his reputation as one of the greatest figures of antiquity can be more fully appreciated.

JACQUES JOUANNA is a professor of Greek literature and civilization at the Sorbonne (University of Paris–IV). He is also the director of the Research Group in Greek Medicine at the Centre National de la Recherche Scientifique and a member of the Institut de France (Académie des Inscriptions et Belles-Lettres).

Medicine and Culture